METHODS IN MOLECULAR BIOLOGY

Series Editor
John M. Walker
School of Life and Medical Sciences
University of Hertfordshire
Hatfield, Hertfordshire, AL10 9AB, UK

For further volumes:
http://www.springer.com/series/7651

Metagenomics

Methods and Protocols

Second Edition

Edited by

Wolfgang R. Streit

Mikrobiologie & Biotechnologie, Biocenter Klein Flottbek, University of Hamburg, Hamburg, Germany

Rolf Daniel

Göttingen Genomics Laboratory, Department of Genomic and Applied Microbiology, Institut für Mikrobiologie und Genetik, Georg-August-Universität Göttingen, Göttingen, Germany

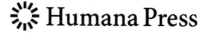 Humana Press

Editors
Wolfgang R. Streit
Mikrobiologie & Biotechnologie
Biocenter Klein Flottbek
University of Hamburg
Hamburg, Germany

Rolf Daniel
Göttingen Genomics Laboratory
Department of Genomic and Applied
  Microbiology
Institut für Mikrobiologie und Genetik
Georg-August-Universität Göttingen
Göttingen, Germany

ISSN 1064-3745   ISSN 1940-6029   (electronic)
Methods in Molecular Biology
ISBN 978-1-4939-8274-5   ISBN 978-1-4939-6691-2   (eBook)
DOI 10.1007/978-1-4939-6691-2

Preface

Metagenomics is a key technology to the DNA-based exploration of the genomic potential from not-yet-cultivated microbes for ecology and biotechnology. Since the term "metagenome" was coined almost two decades ago, metagenomics has dramatically changed our view on many research areas such as microbial ecology, community biology, and microbiome research, and it has resulted in the rapid identification of many novel biomolecules with potential value to bio-based industrial processes. Function-driven metagenomics has been the focus of many laboratories around the world to quickly encounter novel functional genes encoding enzymes with new and/or improved traits. In this way, the diversity of biocatalysts and other valuable biomolecules useful for downstream applications increased significantly. Industries demand enzymes that can be directly applied in biotechnological processes and catalyze a wide variety of different reactions. Ideally, these biocatalysts/bioactive molecules should be highly active with a broad range of substrates under harsh reaction conditions and, at the same time, should possess a predictable substrate specificity and enantioselectivity. Today, only a limited number of truly well-suited enzymes fulfill these requirements. To identify novel biomolecules different strategies are employed: While the sequence-based detection of novel enzymes and other biomolecules certainly provides rapid access to novel genes and enzymes, it suffers from the fact that only sequences with putative function and similarities to already known genes are recovered. Function-based screens overcome this bottleneck but are limited by low hit rate due to the often poor capabilities of the employed host to express foreign genes and to produce active recombinant proteins. Thus, function-driven detection of novel biocatalysts or other valuable biomolecules is still a very time-consuming process that slows down development times for novel products. However, it has the huge advantage that functional biocatalysts and bioactive compounds are recovered.

In recent years, various novel technologies have been developed to access the metagenomes of microbial communities using high-throughput technologies often in combination with next-generation sequencing approaches. Within the second edition of this book, we provide up-to-date technologies on various function-based technologies currently used in metagenomics. Our goal is that this book serves as a manual for researchers who are interested in establishing metagenomics in their laboratories. All working steps involved are presented in the chapters: Starting from the DNA isolation from soils and marine samples followed by the construction and screening of the libraries for diverse enzymes and biomolecules. The book provides a comprehensive overview of current methods used to isolate DNA and construct large-insert and small-insert libraries from terrestrial and marine habitats, including plant and fungal microbiomes. It further summarizes methods for establishing metagenome libraries in non-*E. coli* hosts such as *Streptomyces*, and it highlights novel molecular tools ready to use for function-driven mining of metagenomic DNA. Lastly, several chapters provide detailed insights into screening protocols for a wide array of different genes encoding enzymes with relevance to biotechnology and ecology. Protocols are offered for the screening of lipases/esterases, cellulases, hydrogenases, ligninolytic enzymes, glycosyl transferases, and quorum-quenching enzymes involved in the destruction of N-acyl homoserine lactone-based cell–cell communication signals. Furthermore, the book provides detailed screening protocols for phosphatases, poly-hydroxyalkanoate metabolism-related enzymes, stereoselective hydrolases, and microbial signals for the discovery of secondary metabolites. Finally, detailed insights into the pipeline necessary for the reconstruction of metabolic pathways are given.

In our view, this book provides a comprehensive collection of up-to-date protocols for metagenomics and tools for the recovery of many major types of biocatalysts and allows an easy setup of these screens in any microbiology laboratory.

Hamburg, Germany   *Wolfgang R. Streit*
Göttingen, Germany   *Rolf Daniel*

Contents

Contributors

NICOLE ADAM • *Molecular Biology of Microbial Consortia, Biocenter Klein Flottbek, University of Hamburg, Hamburg, Germany*

JOZEF ANNÉ • *Lab. Molecular Bacteriology, Department Microbiology and Immunology, Rega Institute, KU Leuven (University of Leuven), Leuven, Belgium*

RAFAEL BARGIELA • *Institute of Catalysis, Consejo Superior de Investigaciones Científicas (CSIC), Madrid, Spain*

KRISTEL BERNAERTS • *Department of Chemical Engineering, KU Leuven (University of Leuven), Leuven, Belgium*

UWE T. BORNSCHEUER • *Department of Biotechnology and Enzyme Catalysis, Institute of Biochemistry, Greifswald University, Greifswald, Germany*

DOMINIQUE BÖTTCHER • *Department of Biotechnology and Enzyme Catalysis, Institute of Biochemistry, Greifswald University, Greifswald, Germany*

TREVOR C. CHARLES • *Department of Biology, University of Waterloo, Waterloo, ON, Canada*

YIN CHEN • *School of Life Sciences, University of Warwick, Coventry, UK*

JIUJUN CHENG • *Department of Biology, University of Waterloo, Waterloo, ON, Canada*

DON A. COWAN • *Institute for Microbial Biotechnology & Metagenomics, University of the Western Cape, South Africa; Centre for Bioprocess Engineering Research, University of Cape Town, South Africa*

SARA COYOTZI • *Department of Biology, University of Waterloo, Waterloo, ON, Canada*

ROLF DANIEL • *Göttingen Genomics Laboratory, Department of Genomic and Applied Microbiology, Institut für Mikrobiologie und Genetik, Georg-August-Universität Göttingen, Göttingen, Germany*

SANDRA DENMAN • *Centre for Ecosystems Society and Biosecurity, Forest Research, Surrey, UK*

JAMES DOONAN • *School of Biological Sciences, Bangor University, Bangor, Gwynedd, UK*

THOMAS DREPPER • *Institute of Molecular Enzyme Technology, Heinrich-Heine-University Düsseldorf, Jülich, Germany*

MARC G. DUMONT • *Centre for Biological Sciences, University of Southampton, Southampton, UK*

ÖZGE EYICE • *School of Biological and Chemical Sciences, Queen Mary University of London, London, UK*

MANUEL FERRER • *Institute of Catalysis, Consejo Superior de Investigaciones Científicas (CSIC), Madrid, Spain*

MIKKEL A. GLARING • *Department of Plant and Environmental Sciences, University of Copenhagen, Frederiksberg, Denmark*

PETER N. GOLYSHIN • *School of Biological Sciences, Bangor University, Bangor, Gwynedd, UK*

JOSE A. GUTIÉRREZ-BARRANQUERO • *BIOMERIT Research Centre, University College Cork–National University of Ireland, Cork, Ireland*

ROBERT J. HUDDY • *Institute for Microbial Biotechnology & Metagenomics, University of the Western Cape, South Africa; Centre for Bioprocess Engineering Research, University of Cape Town, South Africa*

NELE ILMBERGER • *Microbiology & Biotechnology, Biocenter Klein Flottbek, University of Hamburg, Hamburg, Germany*

KARL-ERICH JAEGER • *Institute of Molecular Enzyme Technology, Heinrich-Heine-University Düsseldorf, Jülich, Germany*

ELEANOR JAMESON • *School of Life Sciences, University of Warwick, Coventry, UK*

NADINE KATZKE • *Institute of Molecular Enzyme Technology, Heinrich-Heine-University Düsseldorf, Jülich, Germany*

ANDREAS KNAPP • *Institute of Molecular Enzyme Technology, Heinrich-Heine-University Düsseldorf, Jülich, Germany*

JAN KORMANEC • *Institute of Molecular Biology, Slovak Academy of Sciences, Bratislava, Slovak Republic*

DANIELA LANGFELDT • *Institut für Allgemeine Mikrobiologie, Christian-Albrechts-Universität zu Kiel, Kiel, Germany*

ANITA LOESCHCKE • *Institute of Molecular Enzyme Technology, Heinrich-Heine-University Düsseldorf, Jülich, Germany*

ANDRIY LUZHETSKYY • *Actinobacteria Metabolic Engineering Group, Helmholtz Institute for Pharmaceutical Research Saarland (HIPS), University of Saarland, Saarbrücken, Germany; Department of Pharmaceutical Biotechnology, University of Saarland, Saarbrücken, Germany*

JAMES E. MCDONALD • *School of Biological Sciences, Bangor University, Bangor, Gwynedd, UK*

J. COLIN MURRELL • *School of Environmental Sciences, University of East Anglia, Norwich, UK*

HEIKO NACKE • *Institut für Mikrobiologie und Genetik, Georg-August-Universität Göttingen, Göttingen, Germany*

JOSH D. NEUFELD • *Department of Biology, University of Waterloo, Waterloo, ON, Canada*

RICARDO NORDESTE • *Department of Biology, University of Waterloo, Waterloo, ON, Canada*

FERGAL O'GARA • *BIOMERIT Research Centre, University College Cork–National University of Ireland, Cork, Ireland; School of Biomedical Sciences, Curtin Health Innovation Research Institute, Curtin University, Perth, Australia*

PHIL M. OGER • *Univ Lyon, INSA-Lyon, UCBL, Villeurbanne Cedex, France; Univ Lyon, ENS-Lyon, Lyon, France*

MIRJAM PERNER • *Molecular Biology of Microbial Consortia, Biocenter Klein Flottbek, University of Hamburg, Hamburg, Germany*

BIRGIT PFEIFFER • *Institut für Mikrobiologie und Genetik, Georg-August-Universität Göttingen, Göttingen, Germany*

ULRICH RABAUSCH • *Microbiology and Biotechnology, Biocenter Klein Flottbek, University of Hamburg, Hamburg, Germany*

YURIY REBETS • *Helmholtz Institute for Pharmaceutical Research Saarland (HIPS), University of Saarland, Saarbrücken, Germany*

F. JERRY REEN • *BIOMERIT Research Centre, University College Cork–National University of Ireland, Cork, Ireland*

HENDRIK SCHÄFER • *School of Life Sciences, University of Warwick, Coventry, UK*

MARLEN SCHMIDT • *Department of Biotechnology and Enzyme Catalysis, Institute of Biochemistry, Greifswald University, Greifswald, Germany*

RUTH A. SCHMITZ • *Institut für Allgemeine Mikrobiologie, Christian-Albrechts-Universität zu Kiel, Kiel, Germany*

DOMINIK SCHNEIDER • *Institut für Mikrobiologie und Genetik, Georg-August-Universität Göttingen, Göttingen, Germany*

CAROLA SIMON • *Pohl-Boskamp GmbH, Hamburg, Germany*

MARIETTE SMART • *Institute for Microbial Biotechnology & Metagenomics, University of the Western Cape, South Africa; Centre for Bioprocess Engineering Research, University of Cape Town, South Africa*

PETER STOUGAARD • *Department of Plant and Environmental Sciences, University of Copenhagen, Frederiksberg, Denmark*

WOLFGANG R. STREIT • *Microbiology & Biotechnology, Biocenter Klein Flottbek, University of Hamburg, Hamburg, Germany*

MARTIN TAUBERT • *Institute of Ecology, Friedrich Schiller University Jena, Jena, Germany*

MARIA A. TRAINER • *Department of Biology, University of Waterloo, Waterloo, ON, Canada*

MARLA TRINDADE • *Institute for Microbial Biotechnology & Metagenomics, University of the Western Cape, South Africa; Centre for Bioprocess Engineering Research, University of Cape Town, South Africa*

STÉPHANE UROZ • *Interactions arbres microorganismes, INRA Université de Lorraine, Champenoux, France*

JAN K. VESTER • *Novozymes A/S, Bagsværd, Denmark*

GENIS A. CASTILLO VILLAMIZAR • *Institut für Mikrobiologie und Genetik, Georg-August-Universität Göttingen, Germany*

NANCY WEILAND-BRÄUER • *Institut für Allgemeine Mikrobiologie, Christian-Albrechts-Universität zu Kiel, Kiel, Germany*

BERND WEMHEUER • *Institut für Mikrobiologie und Genetik, Georg-August-Universität Göttingen, Göttingen, Germany*

FRANZISKA WEMHEUER • *Institut für Mikrobiologie und Genetik, Georg-August-Universität Göttingen, Göttingen, Germany*

PATRICK ZÄGEL • *Department of Biotechnology and Enzyme Catalysis, Institute of Biochemistry, Greifswald University, Greifswald, Germany*

Chapter 1

Construction of Small-Insert and Large-Insert Metagenomic Libraries

Carola Simon and Rolf Daniel

Abstract

The vast majority of the Earth's biological diversity is hidden in uncultured and yet uncharacterized microbial genomes. The construction of metagenomic libraries is a cultivation-independent molecular approach to assess this unexplored genetic reservoir. High numbers of novel biocatalysts have been identified by function-based or sequence-based screening of metagenomic libraries derived from various environments. Here, we describe detailed protocols for the construction of metagenomic small-insert and large-insert libraries in plasmids and fosmids, respectively, from environmental DNA.

Key words Metagenomic DNA, Small-insert library, Large-insert library, Plasmid, Fosmid, Whole genome amplification, WGA

1 Introduction

The construction and screening of metagenomic libraries that have been generated from DNA directly isolated from environmental samples has been proven to be a powerful tool for the recovery of novel biomolecules of biotechnological importance [1, 2]. In principle, metagenomic libraries provide access to the entire gene content of a habitat [3, 4]. The construction of metagenomic libraries involves the same steps as the cloning of genomic DNA derived from individual microorganisms. The required steps include fragmentation of environmental DNA by restriction digestion or shearing, insertion into an appropriate vector system, and transformation of the recombinant vectors into a suitable host, which is in most published studies on construction of metagenomic libraries *Escherichia coli* [4].

Although the generation of metagenomic libraries is conceptually simple, the community sizes of most metagenomes such as those derived from soil and sediment samples and, correspondingly, the large number of clones that are necessary for a significant coverage of the metagenome are great technological challenges [4, 5].

Wolfgang R. Streit and Rolf Daniel (eds.), *Metagenomics: Methods and Protocols*, Methods in Molecular Biology, vol. 1539, DOI 10.1007/978-1-4939-6691-2_1, © Springer Science+Business Media LLC 2017

Two types of libraries with respect to average insert size can be generated: small-insert libraries in plasmid vectors (less than 10 kb) and large-insert libraries in cosmid and fosmid vectors (up to 40 kb) or BAC vectors (more than 40 kb). The selection of a vector system for library construction depends on the quality of the isolated environmental DNA, the desired average insert size of the library, the copy number required, the host, and the screening strategy that will be used [3, 5]. Environmental DNA that is contaminated with humic or matrix substances after purification or DNA sheared during purification is only suitable for generation of small-insert libraries [3]. Small-insert metagenomic libraries are useful for the isolation of single genes or small operons encoding novel biomolecules. To identify complex pathways encoded by large gene clusters or large DNA fragments for the partial genomic characterization of uncultured microorganisms the generation of large-insert libraries is the appropriate method. Here, we describe one protocol for construction of small-insert libraries and one for large-insert fosmid libraries. Both methods have been proven to be suitable for cloning of DNA purified from various environmental samples, including soil, hydrothermal vents, ice, and human body [6–9].

2 Materials

2.1 Metagenomic DNA

The construction of metagenomic libraries derived from environmental samples and cloning of functional genes is dependent on the high quality of the extracted DNA, since the enzymatic modifications required during the construction of the libraries are sensitive to contamination by various biotic and abiotic components. High molecular environmental DNA is especially required for the construction of large-insert libraries. To start with library construction 5–10 μg of purified environmental DNA are required.

2.2 Generation of Small-Insert Metagenomic Libraries

1. Illustra GenomiPhi V2 DNA Amplification Kit (GE Healthcare, Munich, Germany).

2. Phi29 DNA polymerase (10 U/μL) and reaction buffer (10×) (Fermentas, St. Leon-Rot, Germany).

3. S1 nuclease (100 U/μL) and reaction buffer (5×) (Fermentas, St. Leon-Rot, Germany).

4. DNA polymerase I (10 U/μL) and reaction buffer (10×) (Fermentas, St. Leon-Rot, Germany).

5. Nebulizer (Invitrogen, Karlsruhe, Germany).

6. Shearing buffer: 10 mM Tris–HCl, pH 7.5, 1 mM EDTA, 10 % (w/v) glycerol. Store at room temperature.

7. Low melting point (LMP) Biozym Plaque *GeneticPure* Agarose (Biozym Scientific GmbH, Hess. Oldendorf, Germany).

8. Tris-acetate-ethylenediamine tetraacetic acid (TAE) buffer (50×): 242 g Tris-base, 57.1 mL acetic acid, 100 mL 0.5 M EDTA, pH 8. Add H_2O to 1 L. Store at room temperature.

9. GELase Agarose Gel-Digesting Preparation (EPICENTRE Biotechnologies, Madison, WI).

10. 3 M sodium acetate, pH 5.

11. 5 M NH_4OAc, pH 7.

12. T4 DNA polymerase (5 U/μL) (Fermentas, St. Leon-Rot, Germany).

13. 10 mM dNTP Mix (Fermentas, St. Leon-Rot, Germany).

14. Klenow Fragment (10 U/μL) (Fermentas, St. Leon-Rot, Germany).

15. Buffer O (10×) (Fermentas, St. Leon-Rot, Germany).

16. SureClean Plus (Bioline, Luckenwalde, Germany).

17. *Taq* DNA polymerase and reaction buffer with $(NH_4)_2SO_4$ (10×) (Fermentas, St. Leon-Rot, Germany).

18. 25 mM $MgCl_2$.

19. 100 mM dATP.

20. Antarctic phosphatase and buffer (10×) (New England Biolabs, Ipswich, MA).

21. Topo® XL PCR Cloning Kit (Invitrogen, Karlsruhe, Germany).

22. Bio-Rad Gene Pulser II (Bio-Rad, Munich, Germany).

23. Kanamycin stock solution: 25 mg/mL H_2O. Filter-sterilize and store at –20 °C.

24. Isopropyl-β-d-thiogalactopyranoside (IPTG) stock solution: 24 mg/mL in H_2O. Filter-sterilize, divide into 2 mL aliquots and store at –20 °C.

25. 5-Bromo-4-chloro-3-indolyl-β-d-galactoside (X-gal) stock solution: 20 mg/mL *N,N'*-dimethyl formamide. Filter-sterilize and store at –20 °C.

26. Lysogeny broth (LB) agar: 10 g NaCl, 10 g tryptone, 5 g yeast extract per liter, pH 7.2. Add 1.5 % agar. Sterilize by autoclaving.

27. LB agar supplemented with 50 μg/mL kanamycin, 48 μg/mL IPTG, and 40 μg/mL X-gal; add 1 mL of kanamycin, IPTG, and X-gal stock solution to 500 mL hot liquid LB agar after autoclaving.

2.3 Generation of Large-Insert Metagenomic Libraries

1. CopyControl™ Fosmid Library Production Kit (EPICENTRE Biotechnologies, Madison, WI). Store according to manufacturer's instructions.

2. Low melting point (LMP) Biozym Plaque *GeneticPure* Agarose (Biozym Scientific GmbH, Hess. Oldendorf, Germany).

3. Biometra Rotaphor (Biometra, Goettingen, Germany).

4. Tris-borate-EDTA (TBE) buffer (5×): 54 g Tris-base, 27.5 g boric acid, 20 mL 0.5 M EDTA, pH 8. Add H_2O to 1 L. Store at room temperature.

5. SureClean (Bioline, Luckenwalde, Germany).

6. LB broth supplemented with 10 mM $MgSO_4$.

7. Chloramphenicol stock solution: 6.25 mg/mL ethanol. Store at −20 °C.

8. LB agar supplemented with 12.5 μg/mL chloramphenicol; add 1 mL of chloramphenicol stock solution to 500 mL molten agar.

9. 3 M sodium acetate, pH 7. Store at room temperature.

10. Phage dilution buffer: 10 mM Tris–HCl, pH 8.3, 100 mM NaCl, 10 mM $MgCl_2$. Store at room temperature.

3   Methods

Library reconstruction comprises several separate steps. For successful cloning of environmental DNA it is recommended to avoid storage of the isolated DNA for longer periods between the individual steps. If this is not applicable, the purified DNA can be stored one to several days at 4 °C after each step. Before conducting the end-repair of insert DNA for construction of the plasmid library (*see* Subheading 3.1.5) or the size fractionation for fosmid library construction (*see* Subheading 3.2.2), the DNA can be stored at −20 °C. However, after end-repair or size fractionation the DNA should not be stored at −20 °C, as freezing and thawing will break the DNA strands. Similarly, unnecessary pipetting of the prepared DNA should be avoided. Where possible, the reagents should be added to the DNA rather than transferring the DNA. When DNA has to be transferred to a fresh microcentrifuge tube, use only large bore or cut off pipette tips to avoid further shearing of the DNA.

After completion of each step, the DNA concentration should be measured to ensure that a sufficiently high DNA concentration is recovered to conduct the remaining steps. Preferably, a large amount of DNA should be used to start as performing the separate procedures will result in loss of DNA. If less than 5 μg of environmental DNA are available, for reconstruction of small-insert libraries the amount of DNA can be increased by employing whole genome amplification (WGA). To improve cloning efficiency and to avoid abnormal insert size distribution, hyper-branched structures generated during WGA are resolved as described recently [10] with modifications.

In Subheadings 3.1.1–3.1.3 a protocol for WGA of the environmental DNA and resolving hyperbranched structures is given. However, if a sufficient amount of environmental DNA is available, metagenomic library construction starts with Subheading 3.1.4.

3.1 Generation of Small-Insert Metagenomic Libraries

3.1.1 Whole Genome Amplification of Environmental DNA

1. Conduct WGA of environmental DNA by using, e.g., the Illustra GenomiPhi V2 DNA Amplification Kit according to the manufacturer's instructions [11].

2. Purify the DNA with SureClean Plus according to the manufacturer's instructions [12]. Do not air-dry the pellet for longer than 5–10 min.

3. Resuspend the DNA pellet in 30 μL H$_2$O (*see* **Note 1**).

*3.1.2 Resolving Hyperbranched DNA Structures (See **Note 2**)*

1. Combine the following ingredients in a sterile microcentrifuge tube: the amplified and purified DNA from Subheading 3.1.1, **step 3**, 5 μL 10 mM dNTP Mix, 5 μL phi29 buffer (10×), and 1 μL phi29 DNA polymerase (10 U/μL). Add up to a final volume of 50 μL with H$_2$O. The reaction mix can be scaled up as needed.

2. Incubate at 30 °C for 2 h.

3. Inactivate the enzyme at 65 °C for 3 min.

4. Purify the DNA with SureClean (*see* Subheading 3.1.1, **steps 2** and **3**).

*3.1.3 S1 Nuclease Treatment (See **Note 2**)*

1. Set up the reaction mix as follows: the purified DNA from Subheading 3.1.2, **step 4**, 10 μL S1 nuclease buffer (5×), 2 μL S1 nuclease (100 U/μL). Add up to a final volume of 50 μL with H$_2$O.

2. Incubate at 37 °C for 30 min.

3. Purify the DNA with SureClean Plus (*see* Subheading 3.1.1, **steps 2** and **3**).

3.1.4 Shearing of Metagenomic DNA

1. Test the proportion of sheared DNA by running 1–2 μL of the DNA solution on a 0.8 % agarose gel. If more than 50 % of the DNA fragments display the desired insert size proceed with Subheading 3.1.5.

2. Assemble the nebulizer as indicated by the manufacturer.

3. Add 10–15 μg environmental DNA to 750 μL of shearing buffer and transfer into the bottom of the nebulizer (*see* **Note 3**).

4. Screw on cap of the nebulizer and place on ice to keep the DNA cold.

5. Connect the nebulizer to the compressed gas or air source and shear the DNA by applying 9–10 psi for approximately 10–15 s to obtain DNA fragments that are 3–8 kb in size. Check the

DNA on a 0.8 % agarose gel to ensure that the DNA is sheared sufficiently more than 50 % of the DNA fragments display the desired insert size. To vary the size of the DNA fragments either change the applied pressure or vary the time for shearing.

6. Transfer the DNA to two sterile microcentrifuge tubes.

7. Precipitate DNA by adding 1/10 volume of 3 M sodium acetate, pH 5, and 2.5 volumes of 96 % ethanol. Mix gently. Leave the DNA on ice for 20 min, then centrifuge in a microcentrifuge at top speed for 30 min at 4 °C.

8. Discard supernatant. Subsequently, wash the pellet twice with cold 70 % ethanol. After the second washing step carefully invert the tube and allow the pellet to air-dry for 5–10 min.

9. Gently resuspend the DNA in 36 µL H_2O.

3.1.5 End-Repair of Insert DNA

1. Add the following reagents to the resuspended DNA from Subheading 3.1.4, **step 9**: 5 µL Buffer O (10×), 1 µL 10 mM dNTP Mix, 1 µL T4 DNA polymerase (5 U/µL), and 1 µL DNA polymerase I (10 U/µL). Add H_2O to a final volume of 50 µL (*see* **Note 4**).

2. Incubate the reaction mix for 3 h at room temperature.

3. Inactivate the enzymes for 10 min at 75 °C.

3.1.6 Size Fractionation of the Insert DNA

1. Run the blunt-ended DNA on a 1 % LMP agarose gel prepared with 1× TAE buffer and a DNA size marker at each of the outside lanes of the gel. Do not include ethidium bromide in the gel.

2. Following electrophoresis, cut off the outer lanes of the gel containing the DNA ladder and stain with ethidium bromide. Visualize the DNA ladder with UV light and mark the position of the desired fragment sizes on both DNA ladders. After removing the gel slices from the UV light, reassemble the gel and cut out a gel slice containing DNA with the desired fragment size.

3. Weigh the gel slice in a tared tube.

4. Exchange the electrophoresis buffer in the gel slice with 1× GELase buffer by adding 3 µL of 1× GELase buffer per milligram of gel. Incubate at room temperature for 1 h and subsequently remove the buffer (*see* **Note 5**).

5. Melt the LMP gel by incubation at 70 °C for 3 min for each 200 mg of gel. If required, continue incubating at 70 °C for a few more minutes.

6. Transfer the molten agarose to 45 °C and equilibrate 2 min for each 200 mg of gel. Temperatures higher than 45 °C will inactivate the GELase enzyme.

7. Add 1 U of GELase enzyme for each 600 mg of gel. Keep the digested agarose solution at 45 °C and gently mix. Incubate for at least 1 h.

8. Transfer the reaction mix to 70 °C to inactivate the enzyme for 10 min.

9. Chill tube on ice for 5 min. Centrifuge in a microcentrifuge at top speed for 20 min to pellet any insoluble oligosaccharides. Carefully remove the supernatant and transfer to a new tube.

10. Precipitate the DNA by adding 1 volume of 5 M NH_4OAc, pH 7, to the molten agarose and 4 volumes of 96% ethanol (*see* **Note 6**). In the following, proceed as described in Subheading 3.1.4, **steps 7** and **8**.

11. Gently resuspend the DNA in 50 µL H_2O.

3.1.7 Addition of 3′
A-Overhangs to Blunt-
Ended,
Size-Fractionated DNA

1. Add the following reagents to the resuspended DNA from Subheading 3.1.6, **step 11**: 7 µL *Taq* DNA polymerase buffer (10×), 6 µL 25 mM $MgCl_2$, 1 µL 100 mM dATP, and 1 µL *Taq* DNA polymerase (5 U/µL). Add H_2O to a final volume of 70 µL.

2. Incubate at 72 °C for 30 min.

3. Purify DNA by using SureClean (*see* Subheading 3.1.1, **step 2**).

4. Resuspend DNA pellet in 30 µL H_2O (*see* **Note 7**).

3.1.8 Dephosphorylation
of Insert DNA

1. Prepare a reaction mix containing the following ingredients: 12.5 µL prepared insert DNA (approx. 500 ng), 1.5 µL Antarctic phosphatase buffer (10×), 1 µL Antarctic phosphatase (5 U/µL).

2. Incubate for 15 min at 37 °C.

3. Inactivate the enzyme at 65 °C for 5 min.

3.1.9 TOPO® Cloning

1. Set up the following cloning reaction in a sterile microcentrifuge tube: 4 µL dephosphorylated insert DNA and 1 µL pCR®-XL-TOPO® vector.

2. Mix gently without pipetting the solution and incubate for 5 min at room temperature.

3. Add 1 µL of the TOPO® Cloning Stop Solution (6×) and mix gently.

4. Briefly centrifuge the tube and place on ice. The ligation mix may be stored for 24 h at 4 °C.

5. Add 2 µL of the cloning reaction to one vial of Invitrogen's One Shot® electrocompetent *Escherichia coli* cells and mix gently. Do not pipet.

6. Transfer cells and DNA to a prechilled 0.1 cm electroporation cuvette.

7. Electroporate the cells. We use a Bio-Rad Gene Pulser II with the following settings: $200\,\Omega$, 25 µF, and 2.5 kV.

8. Immediately add 450 µL of room temperature S.O.C. medium (included in the Topo® XL PCR Cloning Kit) and mix well.

9. Transfer the solution to a 15 mL tube and shake horizontally for 1 h at 37 °C and 150 rpm.

10. Spread 25 µL of the suspension on LB plates containing 50 µg/mL kanamycin, 48 µg/mL IPTG, and 40 µg/mL X-gal.

11. Incubate the plates overnight at 37 °C.

12. Ensure that the plasmid library contains the desired insert size. Randomly pick several *E. coli* clones, grow each overnight in 5 mL LB broth supplemented with 50 µg/mL kanamycin, extract, digest, and analyze plasmid DNA by using standard techniques.

13. Count obtained clones and determine the blue–white ratio, which indicates the amount of insert-containing plasmids.

14. Extract total plasmid DNA by using standard techniques and store at –20 °C.

3.2 Generation of Large-Insert Metagenomic Libraries

3.2.1 Preparation of Host Cells

1. Streak the *E. coli* EPI300-T1® cells on a LB plate. The cells are included in the CopyControl™ Fosmid Library Production Kit. Incubate overnight at 37 °C. Seal the plate and store at 4 °C.

2. The day before performing the lambda packaging reaction (*see* Subheading 3.2.5) inoculate 5 mL of LB broth with a single colony of EPI300-T1® cells and incubate overnight at 37 °C and 150 rpm.

3.2.2 Shearing of Metagenomic DNA (See *Note 8*)

1. Randomly shear the environmental DNA by passing it several times through a small bore pipette tip.

2. Load 1–2 µL of the DNA on an agarose gel and check if more than 50% of the DNA fragments display the desired insert size. If not, repeat **step 1** until sufficiently sheared DNA is obtained.

3.2.3 Size Fractionation of the Insert DNA (See *Note 9*)

1. Size-select the sheared metagenomic DNA as described in Subheading 3.1.6 with the following modifications:

2. Run the DNA on a 1% LMP agarose gel prepared with 1× TBE buffer using pulsed field gel electrophoresis. We use a Biometra Rotaphor with voltage and ramp times as recommended by the manufacturer. Load 100 ng of fosmid control DNA into each of the outside lanes of the gel with the environmental DNA.

3. Heat the GELase buffer (50×) (included in the CopyControl™ Fosmid Library Production Kit) to 45 °C and melt the LMP

agarose by incubating the tube at 70 °C for 10–15 min. Transfer the tube to 45 °C.

4. Add the preheated GELase buffer (50×) to 1× final concentration. Per 100 μL of molten agarose add 1 U of GELase and gently mix. Incubate for 1 h. Proceed with **steps 8–11** in Subheading 3.1.6.

3.2.4 End-Repair of Insert DNA

1. Add the following reagents, which are all included in the CopyControl™ Fosmid Library Production Kit, to the 50 μL resuspended size-fractionated DNA from Subheading 3.2.3, **step 4**: 8 μL end-repair buffer (10×), 8 μL 2.5 mM dNTP Mix, 8 μL 10 mM ATP, 4 μL end-repair enzyme mix. Add H_2O to a final volume of 80 μL.

2. Incubate at room temperature for 2 h.

3. Inactivate the enzyme mix at 70 °C for 10 min.

4. Purify the blunt-ended DNA with SureClean (*see* Subheading 3.1.1, **step 2**).

5. Resuspend the DNA in 20–30 μL H_2O (*see* **Note 7**).

3.2.5 Ligation

1. Add the following reagents, which are also included in the CopyControl™ Fosmid Library Production Kit, to the end-repaired insert DNA (approx 600 ng): 1 μL Fast-Link ligation buffer (10×), 1 μL 10 mM ATP, 1 μL CopyControl™ pCC1FOSVector (0.5 μg/μL), 1 μL Fast-Link DNA ligase (2 U/μL). Add H_2O to a final volume of 10 μL.

2. Incubate overnight at 16 °C.

3. Add 0.5 μL Fast-Link DNA ligase to the reaction mix and incubate for another 1.5 h at room temperature.

4. Stop the reaction at 70 °C for 10 min.

3.2.6 Packaging of Fosmids

1. Inoculate 50 mL LB broth supplemented with 10 mM $MgSO_4$ with 5 mL of an overnight culture of the EPI300-T1® cells (*see* Subheading 3.2.1, **step 2**). Incubate the culture at 37 °C and 150 rpm until an OD_{600} of 0.8–1.0. Store the cells at 4 °C for up to 72 h when required.

2. Thaw one tube of the MaxPlax Lambda Packaging Extracts (included in the CopyControl™ Fosmid Library Production Kit) on ice.

3. Immediately transfer 25 μL of the packaging extract to a new microcentrifuge tube on ice. Store the remaining 25 μL of the MaxPlax Packaging Extract to –70 °C until use. Do not expose the packaging extracts to CO_2 sources such as dry ice.

4. Add the ligation reaction to the thawed packaging extracts on ice. Mix the solution without producing air bubbles. Briefly centrifuge the tube.

5. Incubate the reaction mix for 90 min at 30 °C.

6. Thaw the remaining packaging extract from **step 3** and add it to the reaction mix.

7. Incubate for an additional 90 min at 30 °C.

8. Add phage dilution buffer to a final volume of 1 mL and mix gently. Add 25 μL chloroform and mix gently. Store at 4 °C for up to 2 days.

3.2.7 Transduction of Host Cells

1. Add 10, 20, 30, 40, and 50 μL of the packaged phage particles individually to 100 μL of the prepared EPI300-T1® cells from Subheading 3.2.6, **step 1**.

2. Incubate for 45 min at 37 °C.

3. Spread the infected EPI300-T1® cells on a LB plate supplemented with 12.5 μg/mL chloramphenicol and incubate overnight at 37 °C.

4. Count colonies and mix the remaining packaged phage particles with the host cells in the ratio, which yielded the highest amount of fosmid-containing *E. coli* clones.

5. Incubate for 45 min at 37 °C.

6. Ensure that the fosmid library contains the desired insert size. For this purpose, pick randomly several *E. coli* clones, grow each in 5 mL LB broth supplemented with 12.5 μg/mL chloramphenicol overnight at 37 °C and 150 rpm.

7. To induce a high copy number of the fosmids in the host cells combine 500 μL of the overnight culture from **step 6**, 5 μL of the CopyControl™ Induction Solution (1.000×), and 4.5 mL LB broth supplemented with 12.5 μg/mL chloramphenicol in a 15 mL tube.

8. Shake the tubes at 37 °C horizontally for 5 h vigorously as aeration is critical for induction of a high copy number.

9. Extract, digest, and analyze the fosmid DNA by standard techniques to ensure that the fosmid library contains metagenomic DNA.

10. Store the fosmid library in microtiter plates containing LB broth supplemented with 12.5 μL chloramphenicol at −70 °C.

4 Notes

1. If the DNA pellet is difficult to resuspend, add another 20 μL of H_2O and heat to 37 °C for 30 min.

2. WGA of DNA results in a hyperbranched structure, which has to be resolved prior to cloning. By incubating the amplified

DNA with phi29 polymerase without primers the density of branching junctions is reduced. Resulting 3′ single-stranded overhangs are removed by S1 nuclease treatment. Nicks in the resulting double-stranded DNA are removed by incubation with DNA polymerase I, which can be performed during end-repair of the insert DNA (see Subheading 3.1.5).

3. Shearing of the metagenomic DNA can be done either mechanically using a Nebulizer or a HydroShear® (Zinsser Analytic, Frankfurt, Germany), or by partial restriction endonuclease digestion using, e.g., Bsp143I (Fermentas, St. Leon-Rot, Germany). Note that restriction endonuclease digestion will lead to more biased libraries than mechanical shearing of DNA.

4. If environmental DNA was not subjected to WGA, instead of DNA polymerase I the Klenow fragment should be added to the reaction mix. DNA polymerase I exhibits not only polymerase and proofreading activity, but also 5′–3′ exonuclease activity, which is important for removal of nicks, which originate from the S1 nuclease treatment described in Subheading 3.1.3.

5. Size fractionation of the insert DNA can also be done by gel extraction via columns, e.g., by using the QIAquick Gel Extraction Kit (Qiagen, Hilden, Germany). Gel purification via columns is less time-consuming but may result in breaking of the prepared DNA strands.

6. The oligosaccharides produced by GELase digestion are more soluble in ethanol in the presence of ammonium. When other salts are used for precipitation, co-precipitation of oligosaccharides may occur.

7. If the DNA concentration is too low after complete resuspension of the DNA pellet the DNA solution can be concentrated by freeze-drying. We use a Savant SpeedVac Plus SC110A (Thermo Fisher Scientific, Waltham, MA).

8. In some cases, this step can be omitted as DNA extraction from environmental samples frequently results in sufficiently sheared DNA. Therefore, prior to cloning the molecular weight of the isolated DNA should be checked by agarose gel electrophoresis.

9. Alternatively, if only a small amount of environmental DNA is available, the size fractionation step can be omitted. Only DNA fragments of approx. 40 kb will be packaged. However, without size fractionation chimeras may form. Size fractionation of the insert DNA is recommended when large contiguous DNA fragments are needed.

References

1. Handelsman J (2004) Metagenomics: application of genomics to uncultured microorganisms. Microbiol Mol Biol Rev 68:669–685

2. Simon C, Daniel R (2009) Achievements and new knowledge unraveled by metagenomic approaches. Appl Microbiol Biotechnol 85:265–276

3. Daniel R (2005) The metagenomics of soil. Nat Rev Microbiol 3:470–478

4. Simon C, Daniel R (2011) Metagenomic analyses: past and future trends. Appl Environ Microbiol 77:1153–1161

5. Daniel R (2004) The soil metagenome – a rich resource for the discovery of novel natural products. Curr Opin Biotechnol 15:199–204

6. Nacke H, Engelhaupt M, Brady S, Fischer C, Tautzt J, Daniel R (2012) Identification and characterization of novel cellulolytic and hemicellulolytic genes and enzymes derived from German grassland soil metagenomes. Biotechnol Lett 34:663–675

7. Placido A, Hai T, Ferrer M, Chernikova TN, Distaso M, Armstrong D et al (2015) Diversity of hydrolases from hydrothermal vent sediments of the Levante Bay, Vulcano Island (Aeolian archipelago) identified by activity-based metagenomics and biochemical characterization of new esterases and an arabinopyranosidase. Appl Microbiol Biotechnol 99(23):10031–10046

8. Simon C, Herath J, Rockstroh S, Daniel R (2009) Rapid identification of genes encoding DNA polymerases by function-based screening of metagenomic libraries derived from glacial ice. Appl Environ Microbiol 75:2964–2968

9. Cohen LJ, Kang HS, Chu J, Huang YH, Gordon EA, Reddy BV et al (2015) Functional metagenomic discovery of bacterial effectors in the human microbiome and isolation of commendamide, a GPCR G2A/132 agonist. Proc Natl Acad Sci U S A 112:E4825–E4834

10. Zhang K, Martiny AC, Reppas NB, Barry KW, Malek J, Chisholm SW, Church GM (2006) Sequencing genomes from single cells by polymerase cloning. Nat Biotechnol 24:680–686

11. GE Healthcare Life Sciences. Illustra™ GenomiPhi V2 DNA Amplification Kit: instruction manual. GE Healthcare Europe GmbH, Freiburg. https://www.gelifesciences.com/

12. Bioline. SureClean: instruction manual. Bioline, Luckenwalde. http://www.bioline.com/.

Chapter 2

Extraction of Total DNA and RNA from Marine Filter Samples and Generation of a cDNA as Universal Template for Marker Gene Studies

Dominik Schneider*, Franziska Wemheuer*, Birgit Pfeiffer, and Bernd Wemheuer

Abstract

Microbial communities play an important role in marine ecosystem processes. Although the number of studies targeting marker genes such as the 16S rRNA gene has been increased in the last few years, the vast majority of marine diversity is rather unexplored. Moreover, most studies focused on the entire bacterial community and thus disregarded active microbial community players. Here, we describe a detailed protocol for the simultaneous extraction of DNA and RNA from marine water samples and for the generation of cDNA from the isolated RNA which can be used as a universal template in various marker gene studies.

Key words Metagenomics, Metatranscriptomics, Marker gene studies, Microbial diversity, Microbial functions

1 Introduction

Sequencing of marker genes has been widely used for the investigation of microbial communities in many environments including water [1] or microbial biofilms [2]. However, the vast majority of investigations focused on assessing entire community structures by 16S rRNA gene analysis and thus did not consider the active microbial community members. In the last few years, RNA-based studies have received more attention. These studies provided first insights into community structure and diversity of the potentially active microbes and their functions (for example [1, 3–5]).

Here, we describe a standard protocol for the simultaneous extraction of DNA and RNA from marine water samples. The extraction is based on the protocol described by Weinbauer et al. [6]. It is

---

*Both Authors contributed equally.

Wolfgang R. Streit and Rolf Daniel (eds.), *Metagenomics: Methods and Protocols*, Methods in Molecular Biology, vol. 1539, DOI 10.1007/978-1-4939-6691-2_2, © Springer Science+Business Media LLC 2017

a combined mechanical and chemical extraction method utilizing a pH shift for the simultaneous extraction of RNA and DNA from individual membrane filters. Purified DNA-free RNA is subsequently converted to cDNA which can be used as a universal template in subsequent marker gene studies or for direct sequencing. The protocol has been already applied to investigate the response of marine archaeal and bacterial communities in the German Bight towards phytoplankton spring blooms [1, 4, 7]. Here, the cDNA served as template in PCRs targeting the archaeal and bacterial 16S rRNA transcripts. The provided method of cDNA generation can be applied to samples collected in a wide range of environments as long as high-quality environmental RNA is available.

2   Materials

Prepare all solutions using diethylpyrocarbonate (DEPC)-treated water and analytical grade reagents. For DEPC treatment, add 1 mL DEPC to 1 L ultrapure water. Stir for at least 1 h and remove residual DEPC by autoclaving at 121 °C for 20 min. Prepare and store all reagents at room temperature (unless indicated otherwise).

2.1   Bacterioplankton Samples

The basis for the simultaneous DNA and RNA extraction are membrane filter samples obtained as follows: seawater samples are prefiltered through a 10-μm-mesh-size nylon net and a precombusted (4 h at 450 °C) 47 mm-diameter glass fiber filter (Whatman® GF/D; Whatman, Maidstone, UK). The free-living bacterioplankton is subsequently harvested by filtration of 1 L prefiltered seawater through a filter sandwich consisting of a glass fiber filter (Whatman® GF/F) and a 47-mm-diameter (pore-size 0.2 μm) polycarbonate filter (Nuclepore®, Whatman).

2.2   Simultaneous DNA and RNA Extraction

1. Approximately 2 g of each 2 and 3 mm precombusted (4 h at 450 °C) glass beads (Carl Roth, Karlsruhe, Germany).

2. Sterile scissors and forceps.

3. Extraction buffer: 50 mM Sodium acetate and 10 mM EDTA, pH 4.2. Add about 800 mL water to a 1-L graduated cylinder or a glass beaker. Add 4.1 g sodium acetate and 3.72 g EDTA (disodium salt). Mix and adjust pH with acetic acid. Fill up to 1 L with DEPC-treated water.

4. SLS-solution: *N*-lauroylsarcosine sodium salt solution, 20%, for molecular biology (Sigma-Aldrich, St. Louis, USA).

5. Buffer-saturated phenol: Roti®-Aqua-Phenol (Carl Roth, Karlsruhe, Germany). Supplemented with 8-hydroxyquinoline, final concentration 1 mg/mL (*see* **Note 1**).

6. A high-speed cell disrupter such as the FastPrep®-24 Instrument (MP Biomedicals, Eschwege, Germany).

7. Greiner tubes, volume 50 mL (Greiner Bio-One, Frickenhausen, Germany).

8. 1 M Tris-base buffer, pH 10.5: Add 121 g Tris base to 900 mL water, adjust with HCl and fill up to 1 L.

9. 3 M sodium acetate, pH 4.8: Add 24.61 sodium acetate to a small amount of water. Mix and adjust pH with acetic acid. Fill with water to a final volume of 100 mL.

10. 24:1 chloroform–isoamyl alcohol (Carl Roth, Karlsruhe, Germany).

11. Isopropanol.

12. 35 mg/mL glycogen (Peqlab, Erlangen, Germany).

13. 96–100% ethanol.

14. 80% ethanol.

15. 1× TE buffer: mix 10 mL 1 M Tris-base, pH 8 adjusted with HCl, and 10 mL 0.5 M EDTA, pH 8 adjusted with NaOH with 980 mL DEPC-treated water.

2.3 Purification of Extracted DNA and RNA

1. 10 mg/mL Thermo Scientific™ RNase A (Thermo Fisher Scientific, Waltham, USA).

2. PeqGold Cycle-Pure Kit (Peqlab, Erlangen, Germany).

3. DEPC-treated water.

4. RNeasy MiniKit (Qiagen, Hilden, Germany).

5. 80% ethanol.

6. ß-mercaptoethanol (Carl Roth, Karlsruhe, Germany).

7. Thermo Scientific™ 2× RNA loading dye (Thermo Fisher Scientific, Waltham, USA).

2.4 DNA Digestion and Control PCR

1. Ambion™ TURBO DNA-*free*™ Kit (Thermo Fisher Scientific, Waltham, USA) (*see* **Note 2**).

2. Thermo Scientific™ *Taq* DNA polymerase, recombinant (1 U/μL), reaction buffer with $(NH_4)_2SO_4$ (10×) and 25 mM $MgCl_2$ (Thermo Fisher Scientific, Waltham, USA).

3. Thermo Scientific™ 10 mM dNTP Mix (Thermo Fisher Scientific, Waltham, USA).

4. Thermo Scientific™ Ribolock RNase Inhibitor (40 U/μL) (Thermo Fisher Scientific, Waltham, USA).

5. Ten micromolar solutions of each of the following oligonucleotides: 8F (5′-AGAGTTTGATCCTGGCTCAG-3′) [8], 518R (5′-ATTACCGCGGCTGCTGG-3′) [9], 1055F (5′-ATGGCT GTCGTCAGCT-3′) [10] and 1378R (5′-CGGTGTGTA CAAGGCCCGGGAACG-3′) [11] (*see* **Note 3**).

6. DEPC-treated water.

7. Phenol–chloroform–isoamyl alcohol (Carl Roth, Karlsruhe, Germany).

2.5 First and Second Strand Synthesis	1. Random hexamer primers (Roche, Penzberg, Germany).
	2. Invitrogen™ SuperScript® Double-Stranded cDNA Synthesis Kit (Thermo Fisher Scientific, Waltham, USA).
	3. DEPC-treated water.

3   Methods

Carry out all procedures at room temperature unless otherwise indicated. Use filter tips. Autoclave solutions (except SLS, phenol, phenol–chloroform–isoamyl alcohol and chloroform–isoamyl alcohol) and microtubes twice before use to avoid contamination with DNases, RNases, or nucleic acids. Wear gloves while working and take proper laboratory safety measures, i.e., work under a hood when dealing with phenol. Make sure to wear safety glasses and protective gloves, since phenol is highly toxic and corrosive. Diligently follow all waste disposal regulations when disposing of waste materials. Please read the notes added at the end of this protocol carefully.

3.1   Simultaneous DNA and RNA Extraction from Marine Filter Samples

3.1.1   Co-extraction of DNA and RNA

1. To prepare the extraction mixture for one extraction, mix 7.5 mL extraction buffer with 0.2 mL 20 % SLS-solution. Scale up as needed.

2. Place glass beads in a fresh 50 mL Greiner tube.

3. Use sterile scissor and forceps to cut the frozen filter sandwich in short pieces. Place the filter pieces in the Greiner tube.

4. Add 5 mL of the extraction mixture.

5. Add 5 mL of buffer-saturated phenol.

6. Vibrate the mixture with 4 m/s for 60 s using a FastPrep®-24 Instrument.

7. Centrifuge for 20 min at $7200 \times g$ and 4 °C. During centrifugation, the mixture separates into a lower phenol phase with glass beads, an interphase and an upper aqueous phase.

8. Transfer the upper aqueous phase containing the RNA to a fresh Greiner tube.

9. Add 2 mL of the extraction mixture and 2 mL of buffer-saturated phenol to the phenolic phase for repeated phenol extraction.

10. Mix thoroughly by vortexing the capped tube and centrifuge again for 20 min at $7200 \times g$ and 4 °C.

11. Transfer the upper aqueous phase to the already collected aqueous phase from **step 8**. The volume of the pooled aqueous phases is about 5 mL.

12. For DNA isolation, add 5 mL Tris-base to the phenolic phase and mix well. Store at 4 °C for at least 40 min but not longer than 3 h.

13. Continue with RNA isolation.

3.1.2 RNA Isolation

1. Add 0.1 volumes of 3 M sodium acetate to the Greiner tube containing the pooled aqueous phases from the extraction and phase separation procedure (*see* Subheading 3.1.1, **step 11**).

2. Add 5 mL of chloroform–isoamyl alcohol (*see* **Note 4**).

3. Mix vigorously by vortexing and centrifuge for 10 min at $9000 \times g$ and 4 °C to separate the phases.

4. Transfer the aqueous phase to a fresh Greiner tube and repeat **steps 2** and **3**.

5. Transfer the aqueous phase to a fresh Greiner tube and add a 1/700 volume of glycogen (*see* **Note 5**).

6. Mix vigorously and add 1 volume of isopropanol to precipitate the RNA.

7. Mix vigorously and incubate samples at –20 °C overnight (*see* **Note 6**).

8. Continue with DNA isolation.

3.1.3 DNA Isolation

1. Mix the Greiner tube containing the extracted DNA vigorously from Subheading 3.1.1, **step 12** and centrifuge for 15 min at $2000 \times g$ and 4 °C.

2. Transfer upper aqueous phase to a fresh Greiner tube.

3. Add 2 mL 1 M Tris-base to the lower phenolic phase and repeat mixing and centrifugation for 15 min at $2000 \times g$ and 4 °C.

4. Transfer upper aqueous phase to the aqueous phase already collected in **step 2**. Add 5 mL of chloroform–isoamyl alcohol to the Greiner tube.

5. Mix by vortexing and centrifuge for 10 min at $9000 \times g$ and 4 °C to separate the phases.

6. Transfer upper phase to a fresh Greiner tube and repeat **steps 4** and **5**.

7. Add 1/10 volume of 3 M sodium acetate and 1/700 volume of glycogen (*see* **Note 5**).

8. Mix vigorously. Add 2.5 volumes of ice-cold pure ethanol to precipitate the DNA.

9. Mix vigorously and incubate samples at –20 °C overnight (*see* **Note 6**).

3.1.4 Washing and Resuspension of RNA and DNA

1. Pellet the precipitated nucleic acids (*see* Subheading 3.1.2, **step 7** and Subheading 3.1.3, **step 9**) by centrifugation at maximum speed for 30 min and 4 °C.

2. Wash the pellets twice with 1 mL of ice-cold 80% ethanol. Centrifuge at maximum speed for 10 min and 4 °C.

3. Dry pellet for about 10 min at room temperature (*see* **Note 7**).

4. Dissolve the DNA or RNA in 200 μL 1× TE buffer.

3.2 DNA and RNA Purification

3.2.1 Removal of Residual RNA from DNA Samples

1. Add 1 µL RNase A to the extracted DNA (*see* Subheading 3.1.4, **step 4**).

2. Incubate at 37 °C for 1 h.

3. Purify the DNA using the peqGold Cycle-Pure Kit.

4. Elute DNA with 100 µL pre-warmed DEPC-treated water.

5. Repeat DNA elution with 100 µL Tris buffer (supplied with the Kit).

3.2.2 RNA Purification with the Qiagen RNeasy MiniKit

1. Add 700 µL RLT buffer and 7 µL ß-mercaptoethanol to the RNA from Subheading 3.1.4, **step 4**. Mix well.

2. Add 500 µL of 96–100 % ethanol to the diluted RNA. Mix well. Do not centrifuge. Proceed immediately to **step 3**.

3. Transfer 700 µL of the sample to an RNeasy Mini spin column placed in a 2 mL collection tube (supplied). Close the lid gently, and centrifuge for 15 s at >8000×g. Discard the flow-through.

4. Repeat **step 3** once.

5. Place the RNeasy Mini spin column in a new 2 mL collection tube (supplied).

6. Add 500 µL Buffer RPE (supplied) to the spin column.

7. Close the lid gently and centrifuge for 15 s at >8000×g. Discard the flow-through.

8. Add 500 µL of 80 % ethanol to the RNeasy Mini spin column. Close the lid gently, and centrifuge for 2 min at 8000×g.

9. Place the RNeasy Mini spin column in a new 2 mL collection tube (supplied). Open the lid of the spin column, and centrifuge at full speed for 5 min. Discard the flow-through and collection tube.

10. Place the RNeasy Mini spin column in a new 1.5 mL collection tube (supplied). Elute RNA two times with 50 µL DEPC-treated H_2O (~95 µL eluate).

11. Mix 5 µL of the purified RNA with 5 µL 2× RNA loading dye and control the success of the RNA extraction and purification by agarose gel electrophoresis.

3.2.3 DNA Digestion

1. If nucleic acid solution concentration is higher than 200 ng/µL, dilute with DEPC-treated water.

2. Add 1/10 volume of 10× TURBO DNase Buffer (supplied) to RNA sample.

3. Add 1/40 volume of Ribolock RNase Inhibitor (final concentration 1 U/µL).

4. Add 1 µL TURBO DNase (2 U) per 10 µg of RNA (*see* **Note 2**).

5. Incubate at 37 °C for 30 min.

6. Add 0.5 μL TURBO DNase (1 U) for every 10 μg of RNA.

7. Incubate at 37 °C for additional 15 min.

8. Add 0.1 volumes of DNase Inactivation Reagent (supplied) and mix well.

9. Incubate at room temperature for 5 min. Mix occasionally.

10. Centrifuge at $10,000 \times g$ for 1.5 min and transfer the RNA to a fresh tube.

11. Perform 16S rRNA control PCR (*see* Subheading 3.2.4). Repeat **steps 3–9** if necessary.

12. Add 1 volume of 25:24:1 phenol–chloroform–isoamyl alcohol and mix thoroughly.

13. Centrifuge at $14,000 \times g$ and 4 °C for 5 min.

14. Carefully transfer the upper aqueous layer to a fresh tube.

15. Add an equal volume of chloroform–isoamyl alcohol (24:1) and mix thoroughly.

16. Centrifuge at $14,000 \times g$ and 4 °C for 5 min.

17. Carefully transfer the upper aqueous layer to a new tube.

18. Add 1/10 volume of sodium acetate and 1 μL glycogen (10 mg/mL) and mix.

19. Add 2.5 volumes of ice-cold absolute ethanol and mix by vortexing.

20. Incubate overnight at –20 °C.

21. Centrifuge at 4 °C for 30 min at $14,000 \times g$.

22. Remove the supernatant carefully, avoid to lose the pellet.

23. Overlay the pellet with 0.5 mL of ice-cold 70 % ethanol.

24. Centrifuge for 10 min at $14,000 \times g$.

25. Remove the supernatant carefully; avoid to lose the pellet.

26. Dry the pellet at RT for 10 min to remove residual ethanol.

27. Dissolve the pellet in a small volume of DEPC-treated water (~12 μL per filter).

3.2.4 Control PCR for Residual DNA

1. Combine the following ingredients in a sterile DNA-free 0.2 mL PCR tube: 2.5 μL 10× *Taq* buffer, 1 μL dNTP mix, 2 μL 25 mM MgCl$_2$, 1 μL of each of the four oligonucleotides, and 1 μL *Taq* DNA polymerase (1 U/μL). Add up to a final volume of 24 μL with H$_2$O. The reaction mix can be scaled up as needed.

2. Add 1 μL of DNase-treated RNA from Subheading 3.2.3, **step 10** to the mixture.

3. Perform negative controls using the reaction mixture without template.

4. Use the following thermal cycling scheme: initial denaturation at 94 °C for 2 min, 28 cycles of denaturation at 94 °C for 1.5 min, annealing at 55 °C for 1 min, followed by extension at 72 °C for 40 s. Final extension at 72 °C for 10 min.

5. Control the success of the DNA digestion by running 5 µL of the PCR reaction on a 2% agarose gel.

3.3 First and Second Strand Synthesis

1. Add 1 µL of random hexamer primers to 10.5 µL of DNA-free RNA from Subheading 3.2.3, **step 27**.

2. Incubate at 70 °C for 10 min.

3. Quick-chill on ice.

4. Add in the following order: 4 µL first strand buffer, 0.5 µL Ribolock, 2 µL 100 mM DTT and 1 µL dNTP mixture.

5. Vortex gently and collect the reaction by brief centrifugation.

6. Incubate at 25 °C for 2 min to equilibrate the temperature.

7. Add 1 µL SuperScript™ II RT (200 U).

8. Incubate at 25 °C for 10 min.

9. Incubate at 45 °C for 1 h.

10. Place on ice.

11. On ice, add the following reagents in the order shown to the first-strand reaction tube: 94 µL DEPC-treated water, 30 µL second strand buffer (5×), 3 µL dNTPs, 0.5 µL *E. coli* DNA ligase (10 U/µL), 2 µL *E. coli* DNA polymerase I (10 U/µL), 0.5 µL *E. coli* RNase H (2 U/µL) (*see* **Note 8**).

12. Vortex gently to mix and incubate for 2 h at 16 °C. Do not allow the temperature to rise above 16 °C.

13. Add 1 µL (10 U) of T4 DNA Polymerase and continue to incubate at 16 °C for 5 min (*see* **Note 8**).

14. Place the tube on ice and add 10 µL of 0.5 M EDTA.

15. Purify with Bioline SureClean Plus Solution as recommended by the manufacturer (*see* **Note 9**).

4 Notes

1. 8-hydroxyquinoline works as an antioxidant. In addition, it has a helpful side effect: the phenol turns yellow. Thus, it simplifies the phase separation as the aqueous phase is colorless whereas the phenol phase is yellow.

2. DNases are sensitive to mechanical forces. Therefore, handle all solution containing a DNase carefully. Do not mix by vortexing.

3. The four oligonucleotides target two regions of the bacterial 16S rRNA gene. Hence, two PCR products are formed during

multiplex PCR (~500 bp and ~310 bp). If your desired PCR product is shorter than 300 bp, please use the same oligonucleotides you are planning to use in your marker gene study.

4. The chloroform–isoamyl alcohol is used to remove any residual phenol which is crucial for any downstream application.

5. Adding glycogen to any precipitation mix has two advantages. Firstly, the glycogen forms a visible pellet with the DNA. Secondly, the precipitation efficiency is increased.

6. DNA and RNA can be stored in precipitation mixtures for several months up to 1 or 2 years.

7. It is important not to let the pellet dry completely as this will greatly decrease its solubility.

8. The amounts of enzymes used in the second strand synthesis are halved compared to the manufacture's protocol but sufficient for cDNA synthesis. Additional second strand buffer and SuperScript™ II RT can be ordered from the supplier.

9. A PEG-solution (20% PEG 8000, 2.5 M NaCl) can be used as an alternative to Bioline SureClean Plus Solution. Add 1 volume PEG-solution to the reaction mixture from Subheading 3.3, **step 15**. Incubate at room temperature for 15 min followed by centrifugation at $14,000 \times g$. Wash the pellet with ethanol (80%) and centrifuge at $14,000 \times g$ for 5 min. Repeat the washing step. Dry the pellet at room temperature for 10 min and resuspend the cDNA in 50 μL DEPC-treated water or TE-buffer (1×).

References

1. Wemheuer B, Wemheuer F, Daniel R (2012) RNA-based assessment of diversity and composition of active archaeal communities in the German Bight. Archaea 2012:695826

2. Schneider D, Arp G, Reimer A, Reitner J, Daniel R (2013) Phylogenetic analysis of a microbialite-forming microbial mat from a hypersaline lake of the Kiritimati Atoll, Central Pacific. PLoS One 8:e66662

3. Wemheuer B, Wemheuer F, Hollensteiner J, Meyer F-D, Voget S, Daniel R (2015) The green impact: bacterioplankton response towards a phytoplankton spring bloom in the southern North Sea assessed by comparative metagenomic and metatranscriptomic approaches. Front Microbiol 6:805

4. Wemheuer B, Güllert S, Billerbeck S, Giebel H-A, Voget S, Simon M et al (2014) Impact of a phytoplankton bloom on the diversity of the active bacterial community in the southern North Sea as revealed by metatranscriptomic approaches. FEMS Microbiol Ecol 87:378–389

5. Schneider D, Reimer A, Hahlbrock A, Arp G, Daniel R (2015) Metagenomic and metatranscriptomic analyses of bacterial communities derived from a calcifying karst water creek biofilm and tufa. Geophys J 32:316–331

6. Weinbauer MG, Fritz I, Wenderoth DF, Höfle MG (2002) Simultaneous extraction from bacterioplankton of total RNA and DNA suitable for quantitative structure and function analyses. Appl Environ Microbiol 68:1082–1087

7. Voget S, Wemheuer B, Brinkhoff T, Vollmers J, Dietrich S, Giebel H-A et al (2015) Adaptation of an abundant *Roseobacter* RCA organism to pelagic systems revealed by genomic and transcriptomic analyses. ISME J 9:371–384

8. Miteva VI, Sheridan PP, Brenchley JE (2004) Phylogenetic and physiological diversity of microorganisms isolated from a deep greenland glacier ice core. Appl Environ Microbiol 70:202–213

9. Muyzer G, de Waal EC, Uitterlinden AG (1993) Profiling of complex microbial populations by denaturing gradient gel electrophoresis analysis of polymerase chain reaction-amplified genes

coding for 16S rRNA. Appl Environ Microbiol 59:695–700

10. Amann RI, Ludwig W, Schleifer KH (1995) Phylogenetic identification and *in situ* detection of individual microbial cells without cultivation. Microbiol Rev 59:143–169

11. Heuer H, Krsek M, Baker P, Smalla K, Wellington EM (1997) Analysis of actinomycete communities by specific amplification of genes encoding 16S rRNA and gel-electrophoretic separation in denaturing gradients. Appl Environ Microbiol 63:3233–3241

Chapter 3

Construction and Screening of Marine Metagenomic Large Insert Libraries

Nancy Weiland-Bräuer, Daniela Langfeldt, and Ruth A. Schmitz

Abstract

The marine environment covers more than 70% of the world's surface. Marine microbial communities are highly diverse and have evolved during extended evolutionary processes of physiological adaptations under the influence of a variety of ecological conditions and selection pressures. They harbor an enormous diversity of microbes with still unknown and probably new physiological characteristics. In the past, marine microbes, mostly bacteria of microbial consortia attached to marine tissues of multicellular organisms, have proven to be a rich source of highly potent bioactive compounds, which represent a considerable number of drug candidates. However, to date, the biodiversity of marine microbes and the versatility of their bioactive compounds and metabolites have not been fully explored. This chapter describes sampling in the marine environment, construction of metagenomic large insert libraries from marine habitats, and exemplarily one function based screen of metagenomic clones for identification of quorum quenching activities.

Key words Isolation of metagenomic DNA, 16S rDNA phylogenetic analysis, Construction of fosmid libraries, Function-based screen, Quorum quenching

1 Introduction

The oceans are the largest ecological system on earth [1] harboring marine microorganisms with an average cell density of approximately 5×10^5 cells/mL, leading to the estimation that the oceans are a living space for approximately 3.6×10^{28} microorganisms [2]. Marine microbial communities are highly diverse and have evolved during extended evolutionary processes of physiological adaptations under the influence of a variety of ecological conditions and selection pressures. They harbor an enormous diversity of metabolically complex microbes with still unknown and probably new physiological characteristics and are thus rich sources for isolating novel bioactive compounds and genes [3, 4]. Microbes are also known to form symbiotic relationships with various marine invertebrates, e.g., sponges, corals, and squids, and are thus suspected to produce particular biologically active and pharmacologically valuable natural products [5, 6].

Wolfgang R. Streit and Rolf Daniel (eds.), *Metagenomics: Methods and Protocols*, Methods in Molecular Biology, vol. 1539, DOI 10.1007/978-1-4939-6691-2_3, © Springer Science+Business Media LLC 2017

Marine natural products constantly play a crucial role in biomedical research and drug development, either directly as drugs or as templates for chemical drug synthesis [7, 8]. Research on chemistry of natural products derived from marine microorganisms more and more came into the focus in recent years [9, 10]. In contrast to marine eukaryotes, microorganisms represent promising sources for natural compounds with the advantage of feasible and sustainable production of large quantities of secondary metabolites with low cost, partially based on their rich secondary metabolism [11]. Moreover, aiming to adapt and survive in the marine ecosystem, several marine microorganisms have been shown to accumulate structurally unique bioactive compounds not found in other organisms [12]. This is documented in a number of reports dealing with secondary metabolites from marine bacteria [13–17]. In year 2015 a total of 4.033 compounds were described from marine microorganisms [18] reflecting an increase of 82% during one decade. In particular, the microbial consortia attached to marine multicellular organisms are attractive model systems to understand the complex interplay between the microbiota and their host. These host-microbe interactions may be also relevant to the human barrier organ and its microbiota providing insight into the development of human diseases and identification of new drug targets.

Current estimates indicate that more than 99% of the microorganisms present in many natural environments are not readily cultivable with conventional approaches [19]. To overcome the difficulties and limitations associated with cultivation techniques, several DNA-based molecular methods have been developed in order to explore the diversity and potential of microbial communities [20–23]. The rapidly developing field of so-called "metagenomics" aims to analyze the complex genomes and genomic information of microbial communities present in different environmental habitats. Today, metagenomic methods are often used to characterize the composition and the dynamics within microbial communities, e.g., by amplicon sequencing using novel high-troughput techniques. On the other hand, metagenomic approaches are not limited to phylogenetic analyses; additionally they provide the unique opportunity to gain information on the functional role of the different microbes within a community; for example the identification of novel enzymes for biotechnological applications [21, 24–28]. Examples are the discovery of a new bacterial rhodopsin, proteorhodopsin [29–32] and the insights into symbiosis between a marine oligochaete and its microbial community [33]. In recent years, efficient DNA isolation techniques have been established for various habitats and vector systems to clone large metagenomic DNA fragments (such as cosmids, fosmids, or BACs). Large clone libraries allow screening for functional activities and construction kits are available as commercial kits [34, 35], where heterologous expression is mostly performed in the host *Escherichia coli*. Recently, novel expression tools and alternative host organisms which can be useful for highly successful metagenomic library construction and screening were described [36].

2 Materials

2.1 Sampling

2.1.1 Marine Water Sampling

1. Membrane pump with respective membranes (polycarbonate or polyvinylidene fluoride membrane filters of 10 and 0.22 μm pore size) or a Conductivity Temperature Depth sensor (CTD) equipped with a 24 Niskin 10 L bottle rosette.

2. Peristaltic pump to accelerate the filtration.

3. In situ pumps for marine deep water sampling.

4. Liquid nitrogen to freeze the filters for long term storage at −80 °C.

2.1.2 Sampling from Marine Invertebrates

1. Equipment for sampling marine organisms, e.g., clean buckets, bottles, a dip net.

2. Autoclaved seawater to wash away loosely attached microorganisms.

3. Sterile petri dishes and sterile cotton-tipped applicators to swab microorganisms from the surfaces of the marine eukaryote.

4. Sterile pistils or mortars to homogenize whole animals of small size.

5. Liquid nitrogen to freeze the samples for long term storage at −80 °C.

2.2 Isolation of Metagenomic DNA

1. 37 °C and 65 °C incubator, centrifuge.

2. DNA extraction buffer: 100 mM Tris–HCl pH 8.0, 100 mM sodium-EDTA, 100 mM sodium-phosphate, 1.5 M NaCl, 1% CTAB (vol/vol).

3. TE buffer: 10 mM Tris/pH 8.0, 1 mM EDTA.

4. 20 mg/mL Proteinase K (Fermentas, St. Leon-Rot), 50 mg/mL Lysozyme (Roth, Karlsruhe), RNase A (Qiagen, Hilden), 20% SDS, chloroform, 100% isopropanol, 70% ethanol.

2.3 16S rDNA Phylogenetic Analysis

1. Reaction tubes, pipettes, thermocycler.

2. Universal primer Pyro_27F (5′-*CTATGCGCCTTGCCAG CCCGCT* CAGTC*AGAGTTTGATCCTGGCTCAG*-3′) and barcoded reverse primer 338R (5′-*CGTATCGCCTCCCTC GCGCCA*TCAGXXXXXX XXXXCA*TGCTGCCTCCCGTAG GAGT*-3′).

3. Phusion Hot Start DNA Polymerase (Thermo Fisher Scientific, Waltham, MA).

4. MinElute Gel Extraction Kit (Qiagen, Hilden).

5. Quant-iT PicoGreen Kit (Invitrogen, Darmstadt), NanoDrop 3300 fluorometer.

6. GS FLX Titanium series Kit (Sequencing Kit XLR70, Pico Titer Plate Kit 70×75, SV emPCR Kit/Lib-A, Maintenance Wash Kit; Roche, Mannheim).

7. 454 GS245 FLX Titanium Sequencer (Roche, Branford, CT).

2.4 Construction of a Metagenomic Large Insert Library

1. CopyControl™ Fosmid Library Production Kit (Epicentre, Madison, WI).

2. TE buffer: 10 mM Tris pH 8.0, 1 mM EDTA.

3. 0.025 μm cellulose filters type VS from Millipore (Schwalbach).

4. Phage-dilution buffer: 10 mM Tris–HCl pH 8.3, 100 mM NaCl, 10 mM $MgCl_2$.

5. LB containing 10 mM $MgSO_4$ for growth of EPI300-T1R host cells.

6. LB plates supplemented with 12.5 μg/mL chloramphenicol.

7. Microtiter plates (96 wells) containing 150 μL LB supplemented with 12.5 μg/mL chloramphenicol.

8. Dimethyl sulfoxide (DMSO).

2.5 Screening Metagenomic Libraries for Quorum Quenching Activities

1. 0.5 mL 0.2 μm centrifugal filter units (Carl Roth, Karlsruhe), Geno/Grinder 2000 (BT&C/OPS Diagnostics, Bridgewater, NJ).

2. LB plates.

3. Topagar containing 0.8 % agar supplemented with final concentrations of 100 μM N-(β-ketocaproyl)-L-homoserine lactone (3-oxo-C6-HSL) (Sigma-Aldrich, Munich), 100 μg/mL ampicillin, 30 μg/mL kanamycin, and 10 % (vol/vol) growing culture of the reporter strain AI1-QQ.1 [37].

4. Topagar containing 0.8 % agar supplemented with final concentrations of 50 mM 4-hydroxy-5-methyl-3-furanone (Sigma-Aldrich, Munich), 100 μg/mL ampicillin, 30 μg/mL kanamycin, and 5 % (vol/vol) growing culture of the reporter strain AI2-QQ.1 [37].

5. 50 mM Tris–HCl pH 8.0.

6. 0.1 and 2.5 mm glass beads (Carl Roth, Karlsruhe).

3 Methods

3.1 Sampling Procedures

3.1.1 Marine Surface Water Sampling

Surface water can be collected either by membrane pumps or any other highly effective clean pumping system on board. Further, samples can also be taken by a Conductivity Temperature Depth sensor (CTD), equipped with a 24 Niskin 10 L bottle rosette (Fig. 1).

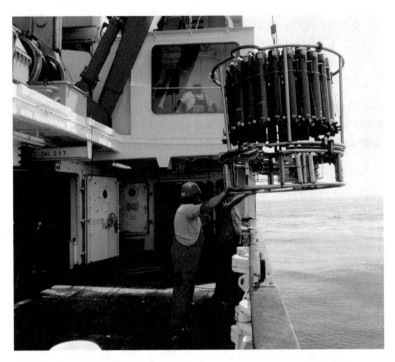

Fig. 1 CTD equipped with a 24 Niskin 10 L bottle rosette on German research vessel Meteor

Samples from the potentially high productive surface layer around chlorophyll maxima should exceed a volume of 100 L but do not necessarily need to be larger than 200 L, due to the high abundance of microorganisms there. After collecting, pre-filtration with filters of 10 μm pore size is performed directly followed by a consecutive filtration with polycarbonate or polyvinylidene fluoride membrane filters of 0.22 μm pore size (*see* **Note 1**). To carry out this large volume filtration in an appropriate time frame, an efficient pumping system is requested, for example a peristaltic pump (*see* **Note 2**). Filters are immediately frozen and stored at −80 °C (*see* **Note 3**).

3.1.2 Marine Deep Water Sampling

Samples from below the euphotic zone, where not much cell material is present, should be collected in larger volumes of at least 200 L. A CTD equipped with a 24 Niskin 10 L bottle rosette can be used for the collection of such samples; filtration is then carried out as described above. As this sampling method is limited to a certain volume, mostly 240 L, it is highly time consuming, and may lead to stress responses due to dramatically changing environmental conditions during the filtration time on board (light, temperature, pressure). In this case, a sample collection by in situ pumps should be preferred. Those pumps can be set at the depth of interest, depending on the cable length of the ships' winch

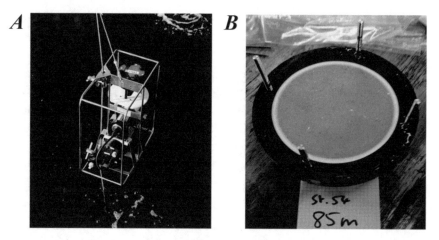

Fig. 2 Deployment of an in situ pump from RV Meteor, (**a**) filter-holder with filter of an in situ pump (**b**)

(Fig. 2a); this method further allows simultaneous deployment of several pumps at different depths. Therefore, the use of in situ pumps is highly time saving, and additionally leads to a higher conservation and consequently to a more realistic image of the microbial community (*see* **Note 4**). Moreover, a filtration of higher volumes of water is possible, depending on the pump type up to 5000 L. Filtration is also conducted using carbonate membrane filters of 0.22 μm pore size redundantizing further pre-filtration. After recovering the pumps, filters are immediately removed from the pumps (Fig. 2b), frozen and stored as described above.

3.1.3 Sampling from Marine Invertebrates

After sampling, the marine organisms are thoroughly rinsed with filtered (0.22 μm) and autoclaved seawater to remove loosely attached microorganisms. If possible the organisms are then placed in sterile petri dishes and an area of approximately 2–5 cm² (depending on the amounts of microbes and downstream applications) is swabbed with a sterile cotton-tipped applicator. In case of a fragile organism, the complete animal can be homogenized with a pistil or mortar, if necessary under liquid nitrogen, to extract DNA resulting in a mixture of prokaryotic and eukaryotic DNA of unknown ratio. In this case, enrichment of prokaryotic cells for example by fractionated centrifugation can be applied prior to DNA extraction. For comparative phylogenetic analysis, ambient seawater should be sampled and filtered as described above.

3.2 Isolation of Metagenomic DNA

DNA from filters, swabs or whole animals is commonly extracted by a direct lysis of the microorganisms. Additional steps prior to the lysis may be required to isolate DNA from inhibitor-contaminated habitats or enrich prokaryotic cells in order to minimize co-extraction of eukaryotic DNA [38]. The following modified protocol of Henne *et al.* [39] describes the genomic DNA isolation based on direct lysis of the microorganisms from filter, swab and tissue samples. The volumes are appropriate for 2.5 cm² of a filter and should be adjusted according to the filter or sample size.

1. 1.35 mL DNA extraction buffer (*see* **Note 5**), supplemented with 20 µL Proteinase K (20 mg/mL) and 200 µL lysozyme (50 mg/mL) are added to the sample followed by an incubation at 37 °C for 30 min; optional shaking (150 rpm).

2. 1.5 µL (17,000 U) RNase A are added followed by further incubation at 37 °C for 30 min.

3. 150 µL 20% SDS are added followed by an incubation for 2 h at 65 °C and subsequent centrifugation at 4500 × g for 10 min.

4. Chloroform extraction of the supernatant followed by precipitation of the nucleic acids with isopropanol (0.7 vol) for 1 h at room temperature and subsequent centrifugation for 45 min at 16,000 × g and 4 °C.

5. The DNA precipitate is washed with 70% ethanol, dried and solved in 25 µL TE buffer.

This extraction protocol uses enzymatic methods to remove cell walls, resulting in sphaeroplasts or protoplasts. The use of sodium dodecyl sulfate (SDS) disrupts mainly tertiary or quaternary protein structures; cetyl trimethylammonium bromide (CTAB) additionally removes polysaccharides and remaining proteins. An increase from 1 to 5% CTAB in the DNA extraction buffer allows an improved lysis of archaeal cell walls which significantly differ from the bacterial cell walls [40, 41] (*see* **Note 6**). In some cases, e.g., DNA extraction of samples containing high amounts of gram-positive bacteria, initial mechanical cell lyses might be necessary, e.g., using a bead beater with small glass, ceramic, zirconium, or steel beads [42] (*see* **Note 7**). Finally, the isolated metagenomic DNA is analyzed by gel electrophoresis and should contain large fragments (Fig. 3) in case of constructing a metagenomic large insert library.

3.3 16S Amplicon Sequencing

The establishment of next-generation sequencing techniques has revolutionized the study of microorganisms in natural environments [43]. Nowadays, 16S rRNA gene based amplicon sequencing is used to taxonomically identify and classify bacteria present in a habitat. Small hypervariable regions like the V1–V2 hypervariable region of the bacterial 16S rRNA gene present in the metagenomic DNA are PCR amplified with barcoded primers (Fig. 4). The hypervariable regions V1–2 are amplified using universal primer Pyro_27F (5′-*CTATGCGCCTTGCCAGCCCGC* TCAGTC<u>AGA GTTTGATCCTGGCTCAG</u>-3′) and barcoded reverse primer 338R (5′-*CGTATCGCCTCCCTCGCGCCAT*CAGXXXXXXXXX XCA*TG CTGCCTCCCGTAGGAGT*-3′). The primers contain the 454 Life Sciences forward Adaptor B and reverse A (*italics*) and the broadly conserved bacterial primers 27F and 338R (<u>underlined</u>). A

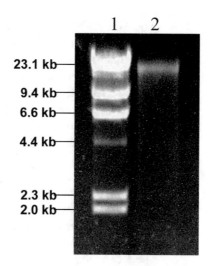

Fig. 3 Gel electrophoretic analysis of metagenomic high molecular weight DNA

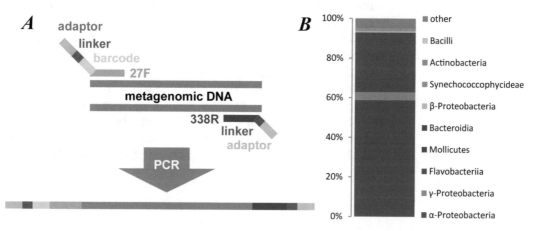

Fig. 4 Phylogenetic analysis of a marine habitat using 16S rRNA amplicon sequencing. (**a**) GS FLX Titanium series amplicon sequencing. (**b**) Respective phylogenetic composition of the marine habitat based on 16S rDNA sequencing analysis

unique 10mer multiplex identifier (designated X) is added to every reverse primer to tag each PCR product.

10–100 ng of extracted DNA (*see* **Note 8**) are applied in a standard amplification protocol including Phusion Hot Start DNA Polymerase: e.g., 30 s at 98 °C followed by 35 cycles of 9 s at 98 °C, 30 s at 55 °C, and 30 s at 72 °C; and 10 min at 72 °C. Amplicons are size-checked and purified using MinElute Gel Extraction Kit. Purified amplicons are quantified using Quant-iT PicoGreen Kit using a NanoDrop 3300 fluorometer.

Pyro-sequencing is carried out according to the manufacturer's instructions using the GS FLX Titanium series Kit. The library is sequenced using the 454 GS245 FLX Titanium Sequencer [44, 45].

The 16S rDNA analysis not only allows insight into present community structure of the respective habitat, it also points out the likely potential of the habitat to detect new biotechnological relevant enzymes. In addition to the knowledge gained on the actual microbial diversity, additional PCR amplifications can be performed using specific primer sets in order to analyze the presence of functional genes, e.g., the *nifH* gene for diazotrophs, encoding a structural gene of nitrogenase, the key enzyme of nitrogen fixation [46, 47].

3.4 Construction of a Metagenomic Large Insert Library

Fosmid and Bacterial Artificial Chromosome (BAC) vectors have been developed to clone large genomic DNA fragments of up to 40 kb and ~120 kb, respectively. These vectors replicate using the single-copy F-factor replicon and show high stability carrying large inserts [48]. Meanwhile, novel large insert vectors have been developed carrying both, the single-copy and an additional inducible high copy number origin of replication [34, 49]. This ensures on the one hand insert stability and successful cloning of encoded and expressed toxic proteins and unstable DNA sequences, and on the other hand allows increased DNA yields in vector preparations and functional screens of clone libraries by induction to high copy numbers [50, 51]. Thus, BACs and fosmids have become standard tools for constructing genomic clone libraries.

Genomic library construction kits are commercially available that pursue blunt-end cloning strategies resulting in complete and unbiased libraries. The "Copy Control™ Fosmid Library Production Kit" (e.g., with pCC1FOS) combines all advantages to stable insert large DNA fragments into the vector with little expenditure of time (Fig. 5).

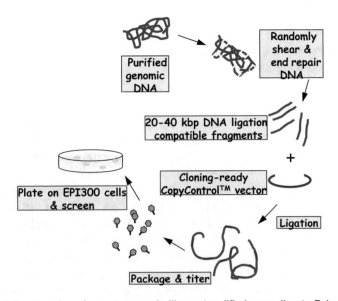

Fig. 5 Construction of a metagenomic library (modified according to Epicentre, Madison, WI)

In the following the corresponding protocol according to the manufacturer's instructions is presented:

1. *Preparation of DNA*: High molecular weight (meta)genomic DNA is isolated as described above and diluted in TE buffer at a concentration of ~500 ng/μL (*see* **Note 9**).

2. *Shearing*: DNA fragments in the range of 20–40 kb are obtained by multiple pipetting the DNA solution using a 200 μL pipette tip.

3. *End-Repair of the DNA fragments*: The end-repair reaction described below (Table 1) generates blunt-ended, 5′-phosphorylated DNA fragments and can be scaled up or down depending on the amount of available DNA, followed by incubation at room temperature (RT) for 45 min (*see* **Note 10**).

4. *Dialysis*: The End-Repair reaction mix is dialyzed for 30 min at RT against sterile water to remove interfering salts. This step can be performed for example by using 0.025 μm cellulose filters type VS from Millipore placed on the surface of sterile water in a petri dish, on which the reaction mix is placed.

5. *Ligation*: The ligation reaction is mixed in a 10:1 M ratio of CopyControl pCC1FOS vector to insert DNA and incubated for 2 h at RT followed by overnight incubation at 16 °C (*see* **Note 11**). The following reagents are combined in the order listed (Table 2).

6. *Packaging reaction*: 10 μL of the ligation reaction are added to one-half of the provided *MaxPlax Lambda Packaging extract* (25 μL) in a reaction tube being kept on ice. The packaging reaction is incubated at 30 °C. After 90 min the remaining 25 μL of *Lambda Packaging extract* are added and the reaction is incubated for additional 90 min at 30 °C. Following the incubation, the Phage-Dilution buffer is added to 1 mL final volume and mixed gently. For storage at 4 °C, 25 μL of chloroform are added.

Table 1
End-repair of DNA fragments

Sterile water	x μL
10× End-Repair buffer	8 μL
2.5 mM dNTPs	8 μL
10 mM ATP	8 μL
Up to 20 μg sheared DNA	x μL
End-Repair enzyme mix	4 μL
Total reaction volume	80 μL

Table 2
Ligation reaction

Sterile water	x µL
10× Fast-Link ligation buffer	1 µL
10 mM ATP	1 µL
CopyControl pCC1FOS vector (0.5 mg/mL)	1 µL
insert DNA (0.25 µg of 40 kb DNA)	x µL
Fast-Link DNA ligase	1 µL
Total reaction volume	10 µL

7. *Titration of the packaged CopyControl fosmid library.* Prior to transducing the complete packaging reaction, it is recommended to determine the phage particle titer (e.g., CopyControl Fosmid clones). 10 µL of the packaging reaction is added to 100 µL of exponentially growing EPI300-T1R host cells (LB containing 10 mM MgSO$_4$) followed by incubation at 37 °C for 20 min. Aliquots of the transduced EPI300-T1R cells are plated on LB plates supplemented with 12.5 µg/mL chloramphenicol and incubated overnight at 37 °C to select for the CopyControl Fosmid clones. Colonies are counted and the phage particles titer is calculated.

8. *Transduction and plating the CopyControl fosmid library.* According to the titration and the estimated number of clones required, the volume of the packing reaction, (fosmid library) required for the construction of the respective clone library is calculated. The transduction into EPI300-T1R host cells is performed as described above in several parallel reactions using the volumes mentioned above. Appropriate aliquots of the infected bacteria are plated on LB plates supplemented with 12.5 µg/mL chloramphenicol for selection and incubated overnight at 37 °C. Fosmid clones obtained are grown in microtiter plates (96 wells) and subsequently stored at −80 °C in the presence of 8 % DMSO.

9. *Induction to higher copy numbers.* The fosmid clones of a library can be induced to reach higher fosmid copy numbers in order to achieve high fosmid DNA yields for sequencing, fingerprinting or other downstream applications. Induction to higher copy numbers is also recommended for direct function-based screening assays of the clone library for example on plates. The induction can be achieved in any desired culture volume depending on the downstream application. In general, LB medium is supplemented with chloramphenicol and 2 µL/mL of autoinduction solution and the respective fosmid clone followed by incubation at 37 °C with agitation overnight.

3.5 Sequence-Based Screens of Metagenomic Libraries Using a PCR-Amplification Approach

A sequence-based analysis of metagenomic DNA can be performed by monitoring the presence of respective key genes by PCR amplification in order to identify genes and metabolic pathways. The primers are designed based on the sequences known for the respective gene with the primers binding to conserved regions of the genes. PCR-amplification is performed using the metagenomic DNA, fosmid pools or single fosmids of the metagenomic library. The respective amplified PCR fragment is cloned (e.g., into a TA cloning vector) followed by sequence analysis of randomly chosen clones. An example is the identification of a gene encoding a novel cytochrome P450 monooxygenase with a robust catalytic activity in a soil metagenomic library [52]. Another example is the unexpected high diversity and distribution of the *nifH*-gene, one of the functional key genes for nitrogen fixation, discovered in the surface water of the Pacific Ocean [46, 47, 53].

Large scale sequencing projects such as the one initiated by Craig Venter for the metagenome of the Saragossa Sea resulted in the identification of numerous novel genes and is a famous example of sequence-based metagenome analyses [54]. More than one billion base pairs of DNA were sequenced, representing approximately 1.800 genomes. From these data, several nearly complete genomes were assembled. Sequence analysis predicted that 1,214,207 novel proteins were encoded in this environmental DNA. One of the most important advantages of next-generation sequencing is the wealth of sequence information it can produce. Deep sequencing refers to the sequencing of a genomic region multiple times—typically hundreds or even thousands of times. This makes it possible to detect organisms that exist in very low abundance within complex populations [55]. The development of fast, accurate, and inexpensive sequencing technologies, coupled with significant improvements in bioinformatics enabled that the sequencing of microbial genomes has become routine [56]. Recent technical improvements allow nearly complete genome assembly from individual microbes directly from environmental samples, without the need of cultivation [57]. This development will enhance our understanding of microbial diversity in nature. Sequence-based metagenomics has the potential to revolutionize our understanding of microbial diversity and function on earth. It is obvious that further advances in bioinformatics are needed to manage the vast quantities of data derived from such sequencing projects [58].

3.6 Function-Based Screens of Metagenomic Libraries

Functional screens for novel genes in metagenomic libraries explore the genetic potential of a habitat by directly monitoring products or enzymatic activities of the metagenomic clones. Metagenomic libraries have been screened for various biomolecules, such as biotechnologically relevant enzymes. So far, functional screens of metagenomic libraries have identified for example several novel antibiotics, e.g., turbomycin A and B [59], aminoacylated antibiotics [60] or small antimicrobial molecules [61, 62] from soil metagenomes, exoenzymes such as lipases [63–65] and marine chitinases [66, 67], or membrane proteins [68]. In the following, the screen for quorum quenching activities will be described exemplarily.

3.6.1 Screening Metagenomic Libraries for Natural Quorum Quenching Compounds

The bacterial cell-cell communication based on small signal molecules (autoinducers), so-called quorum sensing (QS), is a cell density-dependent process effecting gene regulation in bacteria. Accumulation and perception of autoinducers enables the bacteria to detect an increasing cell density by sensing the signal molecule concentration and thus allows changing their gene expression to coordinate behaviors that require high cell densities, e.g., pathogenicity and biofilm formation [69–71]. Well known and studied autoinducers are acyl-homoserine lactones (AHL) in Gram-negative bacteria, oligopeptide signals in Gram-positive bacteria, and furan molecules known as autoinducer-2 (AI-2) in both groups [72]. In addition, several other autoinducers like AI-3 of enterohemorrhagic *E. coli* (EHEC) [73, 74] and CAI-1 of *Vibrio cholerae* [75] were recently identified which are proposed to be interkingdom signaling systems between microbes and their hosts.

QS is known to play a crucial role in bacterial biofilm formation [69]. Undesired biofilms can cause material degradation, fouling, contamination, or even infections [76, 77]. Since biofilm formation crucially depends on QS, one attractive strategy considered to prevent biofilm formation is to interfere with the signaling mechanisms (quorum quenching, QQ) [78–80]. Novel naturally occurring quorum quenching compounds or mechanisms can be identified using cultivation-independent methods, e.g., metagenomic approaches, and can be applied as novel therapeutic agents combating resistant microorganisms [81–85]. Recently, we established two reporter strains AI1-QQ.1 and AI2-QQ.1 [37] to identify such quorum quenching compounds interfering with AHL- and AI-2 based cell-cell communication. The *E. coli*-based reporter strains contain the gene encoding the lethal protein CcdB under the control of the AHL-(P*luxI*) or AI-2-(P*lsrA*) inducible promoter. Consequently, *E. coli* strains carrying such a reporter fusion are unable to grow in the presence of the respective signal molecules, unless nontoxic interfering molecules are present. Both, cell extracts and culture supernatants of single clones or clone pools (up to 96 single clones equivalent to one microtiter plate) can be rapidly and easily screened for quorum quenching activities. The following protocol describes (I) the preparation of cell extracts and cell-free culture supernatants and (II) the quorum quenching assay (Fig. 6).

(I) PREPARATION OF CELL EXTRACTS AND CELL-FREE CULTURE SUPERNATANTS FROM METAGENOMIC FOSMID CLONES

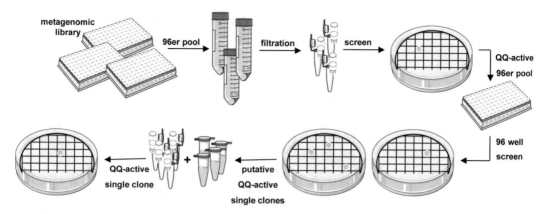

Fig. 6 Flowchart of screening for quorum quenching activities in cell extracts and cell-free culture supernatants of metagenomics fosmid clones

1. Individual fosmid clones are grown separately in a well of a MTP containing 150 μL medium (*see* **Note 12**). Separately grown cutures are combined to a pool (up to 96 individual clones) and harvested by centrifugation at $4000 \times g$ and 4 °C for 30 min to prepare cell-free culture supernatants and cell extracts.

2. Culture supernatants are subsequently filtered using 0.2 μm centrifugal filter units and stored at 4 °C.

3. The residual cell pellets are resuspended in 500 μL 50 mM Tris–HCl (pH 8.0) and mechanically disrupted in the presence of 0.1 and 2.5 mm glass beads using a Geno/Grinder 2000 for 6 min at 1300 strokes/min at RT.

4. Samples are centrifuged at $10,000 \times g$ and 4 °C for 25 min and subsequently filtered with 0.2 μm filter units.

5. Cell-free culture supernatants and cell extracts of pools of 96 clones are screened in three independent replicates to verify their quorum quenching activity.

6. Following, individual clones of quorum quenching positive 96er pools are cultivated in 3 mL LB medium. Cell-free supernatants and cell extracts are prepared as described above.

(II) QUORUM QUENCHING ASSAY

1. LB agar plates are covered with 3 mL supplemented top agar containing final concentrations of 100 μM *N*-(β-Ketocaproyl)-L-homoserine lactone (3-oxo-C6-HSL), 100 μg/mL ampicillin, 30 μg/mL kanamycin, and 10 % (vol/vol) growing culture of the reporter strain AI1-QQ.1.

2. AI-2 quorum quenching plates are prepared in the same manner, but the top agar is supplemented with final concentrations of 50 mM 4-hydroxy-5-methyl-3-furanone, 100 μg/mL ampicillin, 30 μg/mL kanamycin, and 5 % (vol/vol) growing culture of the reporter strain AI2-QQ.1.

3. Plates are dried under a clean bench for 20 min at RT.

4. 5 µL of test substances (cell extract and supernatant) are applied.

5. Plates are incubated overnight at 37 °C.

6. QQ activities are visualized by growth of the respective reporter strain (Fig. 7).

7. QQ activities are verified in at least three biological replicates starting with clone pools (up to 96 combined individual clones) to single clones.

In order to identify the respective open reading frame (ORF) of a confirmed fosmid conferring QQ activity, two alternative methods can be used (*III*) subcloning or (*IV*) in vitro transposon mutagenesis, e.g., using the EZ-Tn5™ <oriV/KAN-2> Insertion kit from Epicentre (Madison/USA).

(III) Subcloning

Fosmid-DNA is isolated and restricted with an appropriate restriction endonuclease to completeness. The respective DNA fragments are analyzed on an agarose gel; selected fragments excised, and purified using for example the NucleoSpin ExtractII kit (Macherey-Nagel, Düren). The purified fragments are cloned into the restricted cloning vector (using the same restriction endonuclease) and the ligation reaction is transformed in appropriately processed host cells (mainly *E. coli* derivate [86]). The resulting clones can be analyzed to determine QQ activities (see above), and after recovery the vector inserts of positive clones are sequenced.

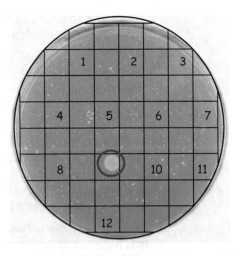

Fig. 7 Original test plate illustrates growth re-establishment of the reporter strain AI1-QQ. 1 by interference with the present signal molecule (*circled*)

(IV) In vitro transposon mutagenesis

ORFs are identified using the EZ-Tn5™ <oriV/KAN-2> Insertion kit (Epicentre, Madison, WI) for in vitro transposon mutagenesis. After the in vitro transposon mutagenesis of the fosmids followed by transformation into *E. coli*, the transformant-clones are screened for loss of QQ activity. Fosmid DNA of clones that lost the activity are prepared using Presto™ Mini Plasmid kit (GeneAid, Taiwan) and sequenced using primers hybridizing to the 5′ and 3′ end of the transposon reading into the flanking metagenomic regions. The obtained DNA sequences flanking the transposon are assembled in order to identify the respective QQ-ORF, which can be cloned in an expression vector to purify the protein in high amounts.

4   Notes

1. Based on the higher number of pores polyvinylidene fluoride filters are preferred to filter high water volumes through a single filter especially when working with small filter diameters.

2. The filtration should be realized as fast as possible with a supporting peristaltic pump in a cold room or for large volumes preferentially using an in situ pump at the respective conditions at the sampling site.

3. For long time storage filters have to be frozen at −80 °C in practicable dimensions. Before liquid nitrogen treatment, the filters have to be cut into convenient pieces to rule out needless freeze–thaw cycles.

4. The sampling procedures have to be performed rapidly because of the changing environmental conditions.

5. Sometimes extracted metagenomic DNA shows a high degradation because of DNases present in the sample. In this case, addition of EDTA to the DNA extraction buffer helps suppressing the damage of DNA (EDTA is used for scavenging metal ions to deactivate metal-dependent enzymes).

6. The standard DNA extraction protocol has to be modified when the samples contain high amounts of polysaccharides and glycoproteins. In this case, the sample should be treated with higher percentages of CTAB to support disintegration of samples.

7. In some cases, an additional mechanical cell lyses step might be necessary as some bacteria/archaea may not be cracked with enzymatic methods.

8. The crucial step of the 16S rDNA PCR amplification is to amplify the bacterial/archaeal 16S rDNA fragments from the optimal amount of template DNA, which can differ from 1 pg to 1 μg.

9. If the extracted metagenomic DNA will be used for library construction, the DNA should routinely be analyzed for degradation to decide if shearing is necessary or this step might be skipped.

10. Before preparing the End-Repair reaction, the DNA concentration has to be determined precisely by measuring the absorbance at 260/280 nm, as in the following dNTPs are added and all following steps and calculations are based on this DNA quantification.

11. A size selection of 20–40 kb End-repaired fragments can be performed to ensure that only large inserts are ligated into the pCC1FOS vector. In special cases the molar ratio 10:1 of fosmid vector to insert DNA can be optimized (5:1 or 7.5:1) to increase the clone number. Autoinduction solution (Epicentre, Madison, WI) can be added prior to culture inoculation to cause induction from single-copy number to a higher-copy number of fosmids of approximately 50 fosmids per cell. The Fosmid Autoinduction solution induces expression of a mutant *trfA* gene contained in the TransforMax EPI300 host cells. Expression of *trfA* gene results in initiation of replication from the *oriV* high copy origin of replication and subsequent amplification of the CopyControl clones to high copy number. In addition, CopyControl Autoinduction solution also contains ingredients which enhance cell growth, leading to higher culture densities, and subsequently higher DNA yields as well as huger amounts of gene products.

12. 150 µL culture medium is filled per MTP well. Fosmid clones are transferred from storage MTPs using sterile metal stamps and sealed with lids. MTPs are incubated at 37 °C overnight in a container with moisturized paper towels to prevent evaporation of medium.

References

1. Kodzius R, Gojobori T (2015) Marine metagenomics as a source for bioprospecting. Mar Genomics 24(Pt 1):21–30

2. DeLong EF, Karl DM (2005) Genomic perspectives in microbial oceanography. Nature 437:336–342

3. Karl DM (2007) Microbial oceanography: paradigms, processes and promise. Nat Rev Microbiol 5:759–769

4. Reen FJ, Gutiérrez-Barranquero JA, Dobson ADW, Adams C, O'Gara F (2015) Emerging concepts promising new horizons for marine biodiscovery and synthetic biology. Mar Drugs 13:2924–2954

5. Kennedy J, Marchesi JR, Dobson AD (2007) Metagenomic approaches to exploit the biotechnological potential of the microbial consortia of marine sponges. Appl Microbiol Biotechnol 75:11–20

6. Zhang X, Wei W, Tan R (2015) Symbionts, a promising source of bioactive natural products. Sci China Chem 58:1097

7. Bowman JP (2007) Bioactive compound synthetic capacity and ecological significance of marine bacterial genus *Pseudoalteromonas*. Mar Drugs 5:220–241

8. Jaiganesh R, Sampath Kumar NS (2012) Marine bacterial sources of bioactive compounds. Adv Food Nutr Res 65:389–408

9. Singh AJ, Field JJ, Atkinson PH, Northcote PT, Miller JH (2015) From marine organism to potential drug: using innovative techniques to identify and characterize novel compounds - a bottom-up approach. In: Bioactive natural products, chemistry and biology. Wiley-Blackwell, London, pp 443–472

10. Machado H, Sonnenschein EC, Melchiorsen J, Gram L (2015) Genome mining reveals unlocked bioactive potential of marine Gram-negative bacteria. BMC Genomics 16:158

11. Molina G, Pelissari FM, Pessoa MG, Pastore GM (2015) Bioactive compounds obtained through biotechnology. In: Biotechnology of bioactive compounds: sources and applications. Wiley-Blackwell, London, p 433

12. Bhakuni DS, Rawat DS (2005) Bioactive metabolites of marine algae, fungi and bacteria. In: Bioactive marine natural products. Springer, Netherlands, pp 1–25

13. Sidebottom AM, Carlson EE (2015) A reinvigorated era of bacterial secondary metabolite discovery. Curr Opin Chem Biol 24:104–111

14. Blunt JW, Copp BR, Keyzers RA, Munro MHG, Prinsep MR (2014) Marine natural products. Nat Prod Rep 31:160–258

15. Newman DJ, Hill RT (2006) New drugs from marine microbes: the tide is turning. J Ind Microbiol Biotechnol 33:539–544

16. Roussis V, King RL, Fenical W (1993) Secondary metabolite chemistry of the Australian brown alga Encyothalia cliftonii: evidence for herbivore chemical defence. Phytochemistry 34:107–111

17. Kobayashi J, Ishibashi M (1993) Bioactive metabolites of symbiotic marine microorganisms. Chem Rev 93:1753–1769

18. Blunt JW, Copp BR, Keyzers RA, Munro MH, Prinsep MR (2015) Marine natural products. Nat Prod Rep 32:116–211

19. Amann RI, Ludwig W, Schleifer K-H (1995) Phylogenetic identification and in situ detection of individual microbial cells without cultivation. Microbiol Rev 59:143–169

20. Streit WR, Schmitz RA (2004) Metagenomics--the key to the uncultured microbes. Curr Opin Microbiol 7:492–498

21. Lorenz P, Eck J (2005) Metagenomics and industrial applications. Nat Rev Microbiol 3:510–516

22. Pham VD, Palden T, DeLong EF (2007) Large-scale screens of metagenomic libraries. J Vis Exp 201.

23. DeLong EF (2009) The microbial ocean from genomes to biomes. Nature 459:200–206

24. Fu J, Leiros H-KS, de Pascale D, Johnson KA, Blencke H-M, Landfald B (2013) Functional and structural studies of a novel cold-adapted esterase from an Arctic intertidal metagenomic library. Appl Microbiol Biotechnol 97:3965–3978

25. Xing M-N, Zhang X-Z, Huang H (2012) Application of metagenomic techniques in mining enzymes from microbial communities for biofuel synthesis. Biotechnol Adv 30:920–929

26. Wang Q, Qian C, Zhang X-Z, Liu N, Yan X, Zhou Z (2012) Characterization of a novel thermostable ß-glucosidase from a metagenomic library of termite gut. Enzyme Microb Technol 51:319–324

27. Nimchua T, Uengwetwanit T, Eurwilaichitr L (2012) Metagenomic analysis of novel lignocellulose-degrading enzymes from higher termite guts inhabiting microbes. J Microbiol Biotechnol 22:462–469

28. Steele HL, Jaeger KE, Daniel R, Streit WR (2009) Advances in recovery of novel biocatalysts from metagenomes. J Mol Microbiol Biotechnol 16:25–37

29. Beja O, Suzuki MT, Koonin EV, Aravind L, Hadd A, Nguyen LP et al (2000) Construction and analysis of bacterial artificial chromosome libraries from a marine microbial assemblage. Environ Microbiol 2:516–529

30. Beja O, Spudich E, Spudich J, Leclerc M, DeLong E (2001) Proteorhodopsin phototrophy in the ocean. Nature 411:786–789

31. de la Torre JR, Christianson LM, Beja O, Suzuki MT, Karl DM, Heidelberg J, DeLong EF (2003) Proteorhodopsin genes are distributed among divergent marine bacterial taxa. Proc Natl Acad Sci U S A 100:12830–12835

32. O'Malley MA (2007) Exploratory experimentation and scientific practice: metagenomics and the proteorhodopsin case. Hist Philos Life Sci 29:337–360

33. Woyke T, Teeling H, Ivanova NN, Huntemann M, Richter M, Gloeckner FO et al (2006) Symbiosis insights through metagenomic analysis of a microbial consortium. Nature 443:950–955

34. Wild J, Hradecna Z, Szybalski W (2002) Conditionally amplifiable BACs: switching from single-copy to high-copy vectors and genomic clones. Genome Res 12:1434–1444

35. Shizuya H, Kouros-Mehr H (2001) The development and applications of the bacterial artificial

chromosome cloning system. Keio J Med 50:26–30

36. Liebl W, Angelov A, Juergensen J, Chow J, Loeschcke A, Drepper T et al (2014) Alternative hosts for functional (meta) genome analysis. Appl Microbiol Biotechnol 98:8099–8109

37. Weiland-Bräuer N, Pinnow N, Schmitz RA (2015) Novel reporter for identification of interference with acyl homoserine lactone and autoinducer-2 quorum sensing. Appl Environ Microbiol 81:1477–1489

38. Gabor EM, de Vries EJ, Janssen DB (2003) Efficient recovery of environmental DNA for expression cloning by indirect extraction methods. FEMS Microbiol Ecol 44:153–163

39. Henne A, Daniel R, Schmitz RA, Gottschalk G (1999) Construction of environmental DNA libraries in *Escherichia coli* and screening for the presence of genes conferring utilization of 4-hydroxybutyrate. Appl Environ Microbiol 65:3901–3907

40. Sogin ML, Morrison HG, Huber JA, Mark Welch D, Huse SM, Neal PR et al (2006) Microbial diversity in the deep sea and the underexplored "rare biosphere". Proc Natl Acad Sci U S A 103:12115–12120

41. De Corte D, Yokokawa T, Varela MM, Agogue H, Herndl GJ (2009) Spatial distribution of Bacteria and Archaea and amoA gene copy numbers throughout the water column of the Eastern Mediterranean Sea. ISME J 3:147–158

42. Treusch AH, Kletzin A, Raddatz G, Ochsenreiter T, Quaiser A, Meurer G et al (2004) Characterization of large-insert DNA libraries from soil for environmental genomic studies of Archaea. Environ Microbiol 6:970–980

43. Metzker ML (2010) Sequencing technologies - the next generation. Nat Rev Genet 11:31–46

44. Langfeldt D, Neulinger SC, Heuer W, Staufenbiel I, Kunzel S, Baines JF et al (2014) Composition of microbial oral biofilms during maturation in young healthy adults. PLoS One 9:e87449

45. Weiland-Bräuer N, Neulinger SC, Pinnow N, Künzel S, Baines JF, Schmitz RA (2015) Composition of bacterial communities associated with *Aurelia aurita* changes with compartment, life stage, and population. Appl Environ Microbiol 81:6038–6052

46. Langlois RJ, LaRoche J, Raab PA (2005) Diazotrophic diversity and distribution in the tropical and subtropical Atlantic Ocean. Appl Environ Microbiol 71:7910–7919

47. Langlois RJ, Hummer D, LaRoche J (2008) Abundances and distributions of the dominant nifH phylotypes in the Northern Atlantic Ocean. Appl Environ Microbiol 74:1922–1931

48. Wild J, Hradecna Z, Posfai G, Szybalski W (1996) A broad-host-range in vivo pop-out and amplification system for generating large quantities of 50- to 100-kb genomic fragments for direct DNA sequencing. Gene 179:181–188

49. Aakvik T, Degnes KF, Dahlsrud R, Schmidt F, Dam R, Yu L et al (2009) A plasmid RK2-based broad-host-range cloning vector useful for transfer of metagenomic libraries to a variety of bacterial species. FEMS Microbiol Lett 296:149–158

50. Sektas M, Szybalski W (1998) Tightly controlled two-stage expression vectors employing the Flp/FRT-mediated inversion of cloned genes. Mol Biotechnol 9:17–24

51. Westenberg M, Bamps S, Soedling H, Hope IA, Dolphin CT (2010) *Escherichia coli* MW005: lambda Red-mediated recombineering and copy-number induction of oriV-equipped constructs in a single host. BMC Biotechnol 10:27

52. Kim BS, Kim SY, Park J, Park W, Hwang KY, Yoon YJ et al (2007) Sequence-based screening for self-sufficient P450 monooxygenase from a metagenome library. J Appl Microbiol 102:1392–1400

53. Langlois R, Großkopf T, Mills M, Takeda S, LaRoche J (2015) Widespread distribution and expression of gamma A (UMB), an uncultured, diazotrophic, y-proteobacterial *nifH* phylotype. PLoS One 10:e0128912

54. Venter JC, Remington K, Heidelberg JF, Halpern AL, Rusch D, Eisen JA et al (2004) Environmental genome shotgun sequencing of the Sargasso Sea. Science 304:66–74

55. Gonzalez A, Knight R (2012) Advancing analytical algorithms and pipelines for billions of microbial sequences. Curr Opin Biotechnol 23:64–71

56. Caporaso JG, Lauber CL, Walters WA, Berg-Lyons D, Huntley J, Fierer N et al (2012) Ultra-high-throughput microbial community analysis on the Illumina HiSeq and MiSeq platforms. ISME J 6:1621–1624

57. Lasken RS (2013) Single-cell sequencing in its prime. Nat Biotechnol 31:211–212

58. Hicks MA, Prather KL (2014) Bioprospecting in the genomic age. Adv Appl Microbiol 87(87):111–146

59. Gillespie DE, Brady SF, Bettermann AD, Cianciotto NP, Liles MR, Rondon MR et al (2002) Isolation of antibiotics turbomycin a and B from a metagenomic library of soil microbial DNA. Appl Environ Microbiol 68:4301–4306

60. Brady SF, Chao CJ, Clardy J (2002) New natural product families from an environmental DNA (eDNA) gene cluster. J Am Chem Soc 124:9968–9969

61. Banik JJ, Brady SF (2010) Recent application of metagenomic approaches toward the discovery of antimicrobials and other bioactive small molecules. Curr Opin Microbiol 13:603–609

62. MacNeil IA, Tiong CL, Minor C, August PR, Grossman TH, Loiacono KA et al (2001) Expression and isolation of antimicrobial small molecules from soil DNA libraries. J Mol Microbiol Biotechnol 3:301–308

63. Madalozzo AD, Martini VP, Kuniyoshi KK, de Souza EM, Pedrosa FO, Glogauer A et al (2015) Immobilization of LipC12, a new lipase obtained by metagenomics, and its application in the synthesis of biodiesel esters. J Mol Catal B: Enzym 116:45–51

64. Selvin J, Kennedy J, Lejon DPH, Kiran GS, Dobson ADW (2012) Isolation identification and biochemical characterization of a novel halo-tolerant lipase from the metagenome of the marine sponge *Haliclona simulans*. Microb Cell Fact 11:72

65. Henne A, Schmitz RA, Bomeke M, Gottschalk G, Daniel R (2000) Screening of environmental DNA libraries for the presence of genes conferring lipolytic activity on *Escherichia coli*. Appl Environ Microbiol 66:3113–3116

66. Cretoiu MS, Kielak AM, Al-Soud WA, Sörensen SJ, van Elsas JD (2012) Mining of unexplored habitats for novel chitinases - *chiA* as a helper gene proxy in metagenomics. Appl Microbiol Biotechnol 94:1347–1358

67. Cottrell MT, Moore JA, Kirchman DL (1999) Chitinases from uncultured marine microorganisms. Appl Environ Microbiol 65:2553–2557

68. Majernik A, Gottschalk G, Daniel R (2001) Screening of environmental DNA libraries for the presence of genes conferring Na(+)(Li(+))/H(+) antiporter activity on Escherichia coli: characterization of the recovered genes and the corresponding gene products. J Bacteriol 183:6645–6653

69. Dickschat JS (2010) Quorum sensing and bacterial biofilms. Nat Prod Rep 27:343–369

70. Shrout JD, Tolker-Nielsen T, Givskov M, Parsek MR (2011) The contribution of cell-cell signaling and motility to bacterial biofilm formation. MRS Bull 36:367–373

71. Landini P, Antoniani D, Burgess JG, Nijland R (2010) Molecular mechanisms of compounds affecting bacterial biofilm formation and dispersal. Appl Microbiol Biotechnol 86:813

72. Liu L, Tan X, Jia A (2012) Relationship between bacterial quorum sensing and biofilm formation--a review. Wei Sheng Wu Xue Bao 52:271–278

73. Moreira CG, Sperandio V (2010) The epinephrine/norepinephrine/autoinducer-3 interkingdom signaling system in Escherichia coli O157:H7. In: Lyte M, Cryan JF (eds) Microbial endocrinology. Springer, New York, NY, pp 213–227

74. Zohar B-A, Kolodkin-Gal I (2015) Quorum sensing in Escherichia coli: interkingdom, inter-and intraspecies dialogues, and a suicide-inducing peptide. In: Quorum sensing vs quorum quenching: a battle with no end in sight. Springer, New York, NY, pp 85–99

75. Higgins DA, Pomianek ME, Kraml CM, Taylor RK, Semmelhack MF, Bassler BL (2007) The major *Vibrio cholerae* autoinducer and its role in virulence factor production. Nature 450:883–886

76. Donlan RM, Costerton JW (2002) Biofilms: survival mechanisms of clinically relevant microorganisms. Clin Microbiol Rev 15:167–193

77. Elias S, Banin E (2012) Multi-species biofilms: living with friendly neighbors. FEMS Microbiol Rev 36:990

78. Dong YH, Zhang LH (2005) Quorum sensing and quorum-quenching enzymes. J Microbiol 43(Spec No):101–109

79. Hoiby N, Bjarnsholt T, Givskov M, Molin S, Ciofu O (2010) Antibiotic resistance of bacterial biofilms. Int J Antimicrob Agents 35:322–332

80. Romero M, Acuna L, Otero A (2012) Patents on quorum quenching: interfering with bacterial communication as a strategy to fight infections. Recent Pat Biotechnol 6:2–12

81. Dong YH, Wang LH, Xu JL, Zhang HB, Zhang XF, Zhang LH (2001) Quenching quorum-sensing-dependent bacterial infection by an N-acyl homoserine lactonase. Nature 411:813–817

82. Hentzer M, Wu H, Andersen JB, Riedel K, Rasmussen TB, Bagge N et al (2003) Attenuation of *Pseudomonas aeruginosa* virulence by quorum sensing inhibitors. EMBO J 22:3803–3815

83. Zhang LH (2003) Quorum quenching and proactive host defense. Trends Plant Sci 8:238–244

84. Zhang LH, Dong YH (2004) Quorum sensing and signal interference: diverse implications. Mol Microbiol 53:1563–1571

85. Kalia VC, Purohit HJ (2011) Quenching the quorum sensing system: potential antibacterial drug targets. Crit Rev Microbiol 37:121–140

86. Inoue H, Nojima H, Okayama H (1990) High efficiency transformation of *Escherichia coli* with plasmids. Gene 96:23–28

Chapter 4

Constructing and Screening a Metagenomic Library of a Cold and Alkaline Extreme Environment

Mikkel A. Glaring, Jan K. Vester, and Peter Stougaard

Abstract

Natural cold or alkaline environments are common on Earth. A rare combination of these two extremes is found in the permanently cold (less than 6 °C) and alkaline (pH above 10) ikaite columns in the Ikka Fjord in Southern Greenland. Bioprospecting efforts have established the ikaite columns as a source of bacteria and enzymes adapted to these conditions. They have also highlighted the limitations of cultivation-based methods in this extreme environment and metagenomic approaches may provide access to novel extremophilic enzymes from the uncultured majority of bacteria. Here, we describe the construction and screening of a metagenomic library of the prokaryotic community inhabiting the ikaite columns.

Key words Extreme environments, Extremophilic enzymes, Cell extraction, Metagenome, Function-based screen, Biotechnology

1 Introduction

Extremophiles are organisms that grow and reproduce optimally at or near the extreme ranges of environmental variables. This can be extremes of temperature, pH, pressure, salinity, or aridity and biospheres representing one or more of these variables are common on Earth. Permanently cold areas, such as polar and alpine regions and the deep sea, make up the largest fraction of extreme biospheres [1]. Naturally occurring alkaline environments are much less frequent, but are distributed globally in the form of soda lakes and deserts, and alkaline ground water. There is significant interest in the biotechnological potential of microorganisms and enzymes from cold and alkaline environments and numerous studies have focused on isolation of novel enzymes for low temperature and high pH applications [2–4]. Enzymes from psychrophiles are generally cold-active and heat-labile. This allows industrial processes to be run at low or ambient temperature, which reduces energy and production costs. It also permits selective inactivation by moderate heating, which is an advantage in the food industry [4].

Wolfgang R. Streit and Rolf Daniel (eds.), *Metagenomics: Methods and Protocols*, Methods in Molecular Biology, vol. 1539, DOI 10.1007/978-1-4939-6691-2_4, © Springer Science+Business Media LLC 2017

Enzymes from alkaliphiles find use in several high pH applications, particularly in detergent formulations and the paper and leather industries [2].

Bioprospecting efforts in extreme environments may be faced with several practical challenges. First of all, obtaining biological material may be difficult due to limited access to sampling sites, difficult sampling procedures, logistical issues with storage and transport of biological material, and environmental protection laws. Once in the laboratory, insufficient knowledge on the microbial community and on growth requirements may limit the output of conventional cultivation techniques and thus hide the true biotechnological potential of the environment. Metagenome sequencing and functional screening of metagenomic libraries circumvent the problems with cultivating extremophiles, but may be hampered by low amounts of environmental DNA and difficulties in finding suitable hosts for heterologous expression of extremophilic enzymes.

Permanently cold, stable alkaline environments are a very rare occurrence and only a few such environments have been described. The unique submarine ikaite tufa columns located in the Ikka Fjord in Southern Greenland (Fig. 1) represent a permanently cold

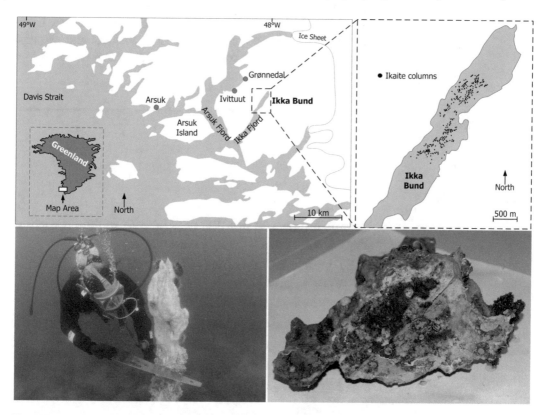

Fig. 1 *Top;* location of the Ikka Fjord in Southern Greenland. *Bottom;* images of a diver harvesting a small ikaite column and a cross-sectional view of the top of an older column

(less than 6 °C) and alkaline (pH above 10) environment with a salinity of less than 10‰ [5–7]. The columns are composed of a metastable hexahydrate of calcium carbonate, called ikaite, a rare low-temperature mineral named after the location where it was first described. Previous reports have shown that the ikaite columns are home to a surprisingly diverse bacterial community and bioprospecting for cold- and alkaline-adapted enzyme has been carried out over the last decade [8–12]. The unique polyextreme nature of the ikaite columns makes them an obvious target for studies aimed at identifying low temperature versions of industrial alkaline enzymes.

Based on high-throughput sequencing of 16S rRNA genes and cultivation experiments, it has been determined that only a minor fraction of the total bacterial diversity in the ikaite columns can be cultivated using standard methods [11]. Extended incubation of mixed cultures from ikaite columns has been shown to increase the diversity of cultivable bacteria [13], but these cultivation attempts are inherently biased towards certain phylogenetic groups, which makes metagenomic approaches to enzyme discovery an attractive alternative. These approaches, however, are hampered by low cell numbers and difficulties in extracting DNA directly from ikaite material. The following protocol describes the construction of a metagenomic library from low-biomass ikaite material using a prokaryotic cell extraction protocol and presents a screening procedure for cold- and alkaline-active enzymes in a standard *E. coli* strain.

2   Materials

2.1   Extraction of Intact Cells and DNA Extraction

1. 0.9 % NaCl.

2. 0.1 % NaN_3.

3. Methanol.

4. Detergent mix: 100 mM EDTA, 100 mM sodium pyrophosphate ($Na_4O_7P_2$), 1 % (v/v) Tween 80.

5. STET-buffer: 50 mM Tris-HCl, 50 mM EDTA, 8 % (w/v) sucrose, 5 % (v/v) Triton X-100.

6. Lysozyme (chicken egg white, Sigma-Aldrich).

7. 20 % sodium dodecyl sulfate (SDS).

8. Phenol–chloroform–isoamyl alcohol (25:24:1).

9. Sterile deionized water.

10. 5 M NaCl.

11. Isopropanol.

12. 70 % ethanol.

13. TE buffer: 10 mM Tris-HCl pH 8.0, 1 mM EDTA.

14. Standard agarose.

15. 0.5× Tris-acetate-EDTA (TAE) buffer: 20 mM Tris-acetate pH 8.3, 0.5 mM EDTA.

16. QIAquick Gel Extraction kit (Qiagen).

2.2 Library Construction

1. REPLI-g Mini Kit (Qiagen) for multiple displacement amplification (MDA).

2. Restriction enzymes $ApaLI$ (10 U/μL) and $NsiI$ (10 U/μL) (New England Biolabs, Ipswich, MA, USA).

3. 0.5× TAE buffer.

4. Low melting point SeaPlaque Agarose (Lonza Bioscience, Basel, Switzerland).

5. Ethidium bromide staining solution: 0.5 μg/mL in 0.5× TAE.

6. GELase Agarose Gel-Digesting Preparation (Epicentre, Madison, WI, USA).

7. 3 M sodium acetate, pH 5.2.

8. 96 and 70% ethanol.

9. GFX PCR DNA and Gel Band Purification Kit (GE Healthcare Europe GmbH, Brondby, Denmark).

10. Shrimp alkaline phosphatase (rSAP; New England Biolabs).

11. T4 DNA ligase (New England Biolabs).

12. MF-Millipore membrane filter, pore size 0.025 μm (Merck Millipore).

13. MegaX DH10B T1^R electrocompetent $E.$ $coli$ cells (Life Technologies, Thermo Fisher Scientific).

14. Standard plasmid preparation kit for purification of plasmid DNA from liquid cultures of $E.$ $coli$ transformants.

2.3 Enzyme Activity Screening

1. Square screening plates, e.g., Nunc Square BioAssay Dishes, 241×241×20 mm (Thermo Scientific).

2. LB agar medium.

3. 12.5 mg/mL chloramphenicol stock.

4. 10% (w/v) arabinose stock, filter-sterilized.

5. Tributyrin (1,3-di(butanoyloxy)propan-2-yl butanoate).

6. 5-bromo-4-chloro-3-indolyl-β-D-galactopyranoside (X-β-gal).

7. 5-bromo-4-chloro-3-indolyl-α-D-galactopyranoside (X-α-gal).

8. Azurine-crosslinked (AZCL) insoluble chromogenic substrates (Megazyme, Wicklow, Ireland).

3   Methods

3.1   Obtaining DNA from Ikaite Samples

The ikaite columns are composed of a calcium carbonate mineral called ikaite. While newly formed ikaite is soft and porous, older material is affected by recrystallization of ikaite into monohydrocalcite and calcite, which forms a hardened cement-like material (Fig. 1). This matrix and the high concentration of positively charged calcium ions, which may cause adsorption of DNA to ikaite surfaces, pose a significant challenge to direct DNA extraction. Low levels of biomass and the presence of significant numbers of microscopic eukaryotes further complicates the preparation of metagenomic libraries. Direct extraction of DNA from such an environment would yield metagenomes dominated by DNA of eukaryotic origin, which would significantly complicate the subsequent functional screening of libraries in bacterial hosts by lowering the frequency of useful coding regions.

In order to produce libraries useful for functional screening, a cell extraction protocol is used to enrich for the smaller prokaryotic cells present in the ikaite matrix. Isolation of intact cells also minimizes interference from extracellular DNA present in the environment, such as that derived from biofilm [14]. To avoid extensive cell lysis before extraction, we recommend using unfrozen environmental material. In the case of ikaite, samples can be stored at 4 °C for extended periods, but this may severely affect the microbial community composition and therefore the final metagenomic library [13]. The cell extraction protocol is a modified version of a previously published method [15] and is suitable for 100–150 g of ikaite material. All steps are performed at 4 °C.

3.1.1   Extraction of Intact Cells from the Ikaite Matrix

1. Mix the harvested ikaite material with 450 mL 0.9 % NaCl and homogenize in a Waring blender at low speed. Centrifuge the slurry at $3000 \times g$ for 5 min.

2. Wash the pellet twice by resuspending in 100 mL 0.9 % NaCl and centrifuging at $3000 \times g$ for 5 min (*see* **Note 1**).

3. Resuspend the pelleted material in a mixture containing 100 mL 0.9 % NaCl with 0.1 % NaN_3, 17 mL methanol and 17 mL detergent mix and detach cells by vortexing at 1400 rpm for 60 min.

4. Separate the detached cells from ikaite particles and the larger eukaryotic cells by low-speed centrifugation at $500 \times g$ for 2 min.

5. Collect the smaller prokaryotic cells present in the supernatant by centrifugation at $10,000 \times g$ for 10 min.

3.1.2   DNA Extraction from Intact Cells

1. Resuspend the cell pellet in 1.5 mL STET-buffer with 2 mg/mL lysozyme and incubate at 37 °C for 30 min.

2. Add SDS to a final concentration of 2 % and incubate for 30 min at 37 °C followed by 30 min at 65 °C. DNA is extracted from the lysed cells using traditional phenol/chloroform extraction.

3. Add 1 volume of phenol–chloroform–isoamyl alcohol (25:24:1) to the sample and mix vigorously by vortexing or shaking for 20 s. Centrifuge at room temperature for 5 min at 16,000×g.

4. Transfer the upper aqueous phase to a new tube. Be careful not to carry over any phenol. Re-extract the lower phenol phase by adding 1 volume of sterile water, mixing and centrifuging as above, and transferring the new aqueous phase to the tube containing the first extraction.

5. Add 1/10 volume of 5 M NaCl and mix carefully.

6. Add 1 volume of isopropanol and mix. If a large amount of DNA is present, this will show as precipitating white threads. Centrifuge at room temperature for 5 min at 16,000×g.

7. Wash the DNA pellet three times with 70 % ethanol. Air-dry the pellet and resuspend it in TE buffer.

8. Load the purified DNA on a 0.5× TAE 1 % agarose gel and gel-purify high molecular weight DNA (>8 kb) using a QIAquick Gel Extraction kit.

3.2 Library Construction

The ikaite cell extraction protocol yields high quality metagenomic DNA enriched in prokaryotic sequences, but does not solve the problem of low biomass, which limits the amount of DNA that can be obtained from ikaite material. While the cell extraction protocol could in theory be scaled up to increase the yield of DNA, the protected nature of the ikaite columns, the difficult sampling procedure, and problems with transporting and storing ikaite material locally, makes this solution unappealing. To obtain sufficient amounts of DNA for subsequent cloning an amplification step may therefore be necessary. Multiple displacement amplification (MDA) with the φ29 DNA polymerase is a whole genome amplification technique which can rapidly amplify minute amounts of DNA. However, MDA introduces a significant amount of bias in the DNA template, which will ultimately influence the final diversity of the library [11, 16].

Unlike alkaline-adapted bacteria, which generally maintain a near-neutral intracellular pH [17], enzymes from cold-adapted bacteria may also require a cold-adapted expression system for efficient protein production. Several systems based on engineered *E. coli* strains or naturally cold-adapted expression hosts are available [18]. A commercially available system is the Arctic Express *E. coli* strain (Agilent Technologies, Santa Clara, CA, USA) carrying chaperones from the psychrophilic bacterium *Oleispira antarctica* to facilitate proper folding of proteins at low temperature.

Alternatively, the psychrophilic Gram-negative bacterium *Pseudoalteromonas haloplanktis* TAC125 has been established as a host for expression and secretion of recombinant proteins [19].

The choice of expression vector will depend on the screening target and the community composition of the metagenome. Screening for single enzyme activities can be carried out using relatively small insert sizes in plasmid vectors, as these are suitable for single gene products and are easy to handle. If the screen does not rely on vector-based promoters, a larger insert size in fosmid/cosmid or bacterial artificial chromosome (BAC) vectors can be used to increase the metagenome coverage without increasing the library size. Shuttle vectors carrying multiple origins of replication can be used to move the library between different expression hosts and since metagenomic libraries are inherently based on mixed communities, this can be particularly useful for increasing the hit-rate in functional screens.

The vector pGNS-BAC is a broad-host-range shuttle vector for Gram-negative bacteria with an arabinose-inducible copy number, which has been successfully used in six different γ-Proteobacteria [20]. This vector was chosen for a metagenomic library of the ikaite community primarily because it is a BAC-vector allowing insertion of larger fragments than a conventional expression vector and as a broad-host-range shuttle vector it enables conjugal transfer to alternative Gram-negative hosts. The molecular work and initial screening can therefore be conducted in *E. coli* and if necessary, the vector can be transferred to a more suitable host for expression and screening of cold- or alkaline-active enzymes, e.g., a psychrophilic bacterium (*see* **Note 2**). In our hands, the pGNS-BAC vector continued to show a high frequency of self-ligation and it was consequently modified to include a multiple cloning site with four unique restriction sites inserted into the *Hind*III site of the original vector (mod. pGNS-BAC, *see* **Note 3**) [11].

3.2.1 Preparation of High Molecular Weight DNA for Cloning

1. The purified high molecular weight DNA is used as a template for MDA using the REPLI-g Mini Kit following the manufacturer's protocol.

2. Mix approximately 100 µg of the resulting DNA with restriction enzyme buffer in a total volume of 120 µL on ice.

3. Divide the DNA mixture into three tubes with a volume of 60 µL (tube 1), 40 µL (tube 2), and 20 µL (tube 3).

4. Keep the three tubes on ice and add 1.5 µL *Apa*LI (10 U/µL) and 1.5 µL *Nsi*I (10 U/µL) to tube 1 and mix carefully.

5. Transfer 20 µL from tube 1 to tube 2 and mix carefully.

6. Transfer 20 µL from tube 2 to tube 3 and mix carefully. All three tubes should now contain 40 µL. Keep on ice.

7. The three tubes are incubated for exactly 10 min at 37 °C and then transferred to ice (*Apa*LI cannot be heat inactivated).

8. Analyze 1 μL from each tube by gel electrophoresis on a 1% agarose gel to verify the partial digestion of DNA (*see* **Note 4**).

9. Mix the digested DNA from the three tubes and load the DNA on a long (minimum 20 cm) 0.5× TAE 1% low melting point SeaPlaque Agarose gel and run overnight at 30 V. Avoid the use of DNA dyes in the loading buffer and DNA ladder.

10. Stain the gel in ethidium bromide and excise DNA fragments longer than 8 kb under long-wavelength UV (365 nm).

11. DNA is extracted from the gel using the GELase Agarose Gel-Digesting Preparation following the manufacturer's protocol.

12. For concentrating the gel-purified DNA add 1/10 volume of 3 M sodium acetate (pH 5.2) and 3 volumes of 96% ethanol. Incubate on ice for at least 15 min. For dilute DNA samples an overnight incubation at 5 °C gives the best results.

13. Centrifuge at $14,000 \times g$ for 30 min at 4 °C and discard the supernatant.

14. Rinse the pellet with 70% ethanol and centrifuge again for 15 min.

15. Discard the supernatant and dissolve the DNA pellet in a desired buffer. Be aware that a significant portion of the DNA pellet may be deposited on the tube walls.

3.2.2 Preparation of the Modified pGNS-BAC Vector

1. Digest 10 μg mod.pGNS-BAC plasmid with 2 μL each of *Apa*LI (10 U/μL) and *Nsi*I (10 U/μL) in a total volume of 50 μL. Heat the vector DNA to 65 °C and then cool on ice before adding it to the restriction enzyme mixture. Incubate at 37 °C for minimum 1 h.

2. Purify the digested mod.pGNS-BAC using a GFX PCR DNA and Gel Band Purification Kit.

3. Treat the digested, purified vector DNA with shrimp alkaline phosphatase following the manufacturer's protocol. Inactivate the phosphatase by heating the mixture to 65 °C for 5 min.

4. Perform a test transformation of relevant competent cells to confirm that the background from undigested vector is minimal.

3.2.3 Construction of a Metagenomic Library in E. coli

1. Mix the partially digested metagenomic DNA with the digested mod.pGNS-BAC vector in an approximate molar ratio of 10:1. Ligate using T4 DNA ligase following the manufacturer's protocol with overnight incubation at 15 °C.

2. Inactivate the ligase at 65 °C for 20 min.

3. Desalt the ligation mixture by drop dialysis by spotting 25 μL drops on a membrane filter (pore size 0.025 μm) floating on deionized water in a petri dish. Dialyze for 30 min and collect the drops with a pipette [21].

4. Transform the ligation mixture into MegaX DH10B T1^R electrocompetent *E. coli* cells. A test transformation is recommended for scaling the ligation and transformation protocols to the desired library size.

5. Spread onto LB agar library plates supplemented with 12.5 μg/mL chloramphenicol.

6. The average insert size of the library can be determined by plasmid DNA purification from liquid cultures of 20–30 randomly picked colonies, followed by restriction enzyme digestion with *Apa*LI and *Nsi*I and agarose gel electrophoresis (*see* **Note 3**).

7. Pick colonies into liquid LB medium with 12.5 μg/mL chloramphenicol and 10% glycerol. Grow overnight at 37 °C with shaking and store at –80 °C. Libraries can be arranged by manual picking of clones, but since this can be extremely laborious for even small libraries, it is strongly advised to use robotic assistance for colony picking and organization of the library.

3.3 Screening for Enzymes Active at Low Temperature and High pH

Low temperature as an environmental condition affects both intracellular and extracellular enzymes and screening for cold-adapted enzymes is therefore relevant for both types. Screening for high pH enzymes on the other hand, is mostly relevant for extracellular enzymes since bacteria maintain a near-neutral intracellular pH. Screening for intracellular activities are commonly performed on soluble 5-bromo-4-chloro-3-indolyl-linked (also called X-linked) substrates. Extracellular enzymes can be screened on azurine-cross-linked (AZCL) insoluble chromogenic substrates or other substrates where degradation forms a visible halo around the active colony. Some substrates may require secondary staining to visualize enzyme activity, such as Congo red staining of carboxymethyl cellulose (CMC) plates to detect cellulase activity [22] and cetyl pyridinium chloride (CPC) staining of alginate plates to detect alginate lyase activity [23], but these are generally destructive assays, which prevent the reuse of screening plates (*see* **Note 5**).

E. coli does not generally grow well at temperatures below 20 °C, which can be an issue in screening for cold-active enzymes. It is however, possible to build biomass at 37 °C before transferring to a lower temperature for screening. Expression and stability of some cold-active enzymes may also depend on the shift to a lower temperature and as mentioned above, there is also the option of using engineered *E. coli* strains for increased low-temperature expression.

For small libraries, clones can be arranged using a 96-well pin replicator. By offsetting the position of the replicator, so that clones from the second plate is positioned within the space between the clones from the first plate, it is possible to fit up to twelve 96-well plates (1152 clones) in one large screening plate (24×24 cm). Due to the close spacing, active clones should be re-streaked and screened to verify the observed activity.

<table>
<tr><td>

3.3.1 Functional
Screening of E. coli Clones
at Low Temperature

</td><td>

1. Transfer the library to square screening plates containing LB agar supplemented with 12.5 μg/mL chloramphenicol, 0.01% (w/v) arabinose and an appropriate substrate as follows.

   (a) Lipase: 1% tributyrin.

   (b) β- and α-galactosidase: 20 μg/mL X-β-gal or X-α-gal, respectively.

   (c) Extracellular enzyme activities: 0.05% (w/v) AZCL substrate, such as AZCL-casein for protease and ACZL-amylose for α-amylase screening.

2. Grow colonies overnight at 37 °C.

3. Transfer plates to 20 °C for 2 days and score for activity.

4. Transfer plates to 15 °C and score for activity continuously for at least 14 days.

</td></tr>
<tr><td>

3.3.2 Functional
Screening of E. coli Clones
at High pH

</td><td>

1. Transfer the library to square screening plates containing LB agar supplemented with 12.5 μg/mL chloramphenicol and 0.01% (w/v) arabinose. Grow colonies overnight at 37 °C.

2. Prepare an agar screening-overlay with 0.8% agar buffered to pH 10 with 50 mM carbonate-bicarbonate buffer and containing an appropriate substrate as described above.

3. Cool the library plates at 4 °C.

4. Cool the overlay to approximately 50 °C and gently pour a thin layer over the library plates.

5. Return the library plates to 4 °C immediately and keep cold until the overlay has cooled.

6. Incubate the overlaid library plates at an appropriate temperature for screening, such as 15 °C for cold-active enzymes, and score for activity continuously for at least 14 days.

</td></tr>
<tr><td>

3.4 Investigating Metagenome Bias and Enzyme Potential

</td><td>

Each step involving manipulation of environmental material, cells, or DNA runs the risk of introducing bias in the composition of the metagenome compared to the original environmental sample. This bias and the composition of the input material used for library construction can be evaluated by studying the microbial diversity in the metagenomic DNA based on the presence of 16S rRNA genes. The primers 27F (AGAGTTTGATCMTGGCTCAG) and 1492R (TACGGYTACCTTGTTACGACTT) amplify bacterial 16S rRNA genes and the resulting PCR products can be cloned and sequenced, and the results compared to a 16S rRNA gene database, such as the Ribosomal Database Project (RDP; http://rdp.cme.msu.edu/). Another option is to use high-throughput sequencing of 16S rRNA genes for determination of total microbial diversity. The increasing availability of next-generation sequencing solutions makes this an attractive option even for small-scale analysis of few samples. The primers 341F (CCTAYGGGRBGCASCAG)

</td></tr>
</table>

and 806R (GGACTACNNGGGTATCTAAT) amplify the V3-V4 hypervariable regions of both bacterial and archaeal 16S rRNA genes [24]. This region is suitable for community analysis and can be covered by both pyrosequencing and paired-end Illumina sequencing.

Metagenomic sequencing of the cloned library can be used as a tool to evaluate the enzymatic potential of the library. For smaller libraries, DNA can be obtained by growing *E. coli* clones individually in liquid culture in 96-well format, followed by pooling and extraction of plasmid DNA [11]. The final output will include sequences coming from the vector, but these can be easily filtered out before further analysis.

4 Notes

1. It is advisable to follow the effectiveness of the cell extraction procedure by microscopic analysis. Small aliquots of supernatants and resuspended cell material can be stained by SYBR Green (Molecular Probes) and inspected by fluorescence microscopy to determine the efficiency of each extraction step and provide a rough estimate of the ratio between eukaryotic and prokaryotic cells.

2. Before attempting to transfer the library to an alternative expression host, it is important to be aware of the following characteristics of the new host.

   (a) Natural antibiotic resistances that interfere with vector selection.

   (b) Growth characteristics, e.g., pH and temperature ranges.

   (c) The ability to participate in triparental mating for transfer of the library.

   (d) Plasmid stability in the new host.

   (e) Preservation abilities, i.e., does it survive freezing at −80 °C.

   (f) Any endogenous enzymatic activities that may give rise to background activity.

3. As mentioned above, the observed frequency of self-ligation with the original pGNS-BAC vector was 30–40% in our experiments. A high frequency of empty clones reduces the hit rate and a larger library would therefore be required for effective screening. Modification of the vector reduced the frequency to approximately 15% [11]. It is advisable to investigate both the average insert size and the frequency of empty clones before proceeding with library organization in order to evaluate whether the library is suitable for large-scale screening.

4. Tube 1 should show the highest degree of digestion with a significant DNA smear from the genomic DNA at the top and down to a few hundred base pairs. Tubes 2 and 3 should show a progressive decrease in digestion. In case of insufficient digestion, incubate the tubes for an additional 5 min at 37 °C and reanalyze the digests.

5. Screening a metagenomic library on multiple substrates and under multiple conditions can become impractical due to the number of plates required even for small libraries. To simplify the screening procedure, it is possible to reuse plates for screening multiple conditions. For example, plates used for low temperature screening at neutral pH can be overlaid with high pH agar for a second screen of the same plate. In addition to this, mixing of multiple substrates in one plate can significantly lower the number of required screening plates. Since the hit rate in functional metagenomics is usually very low, the precise activity of positive clones can be verified by subsequent re-streaking on the individual substrates.

References

1. Siddiqui KS, Williams TJ, Wilkins D, Yau S, Allen MA, Brown MV et al (2013) Psychrophiles. Annu Rev Earth Planet Sci 41:87–115

2. Fujinami S, Fujisawa M (2010) Industrial applications of alkaliphiles and their enzymes - past, present and future. Environ Technol 31:845–856

3. Margesin R, Feller G (2010) Biotechnological applications of psychrophiles. Environ Technol 31:835–844

4. Cavicchioli R, Charlton T, Ertan H, Omar SM, Siddiqui KS, Williams TJ (2011) Biotechnological uses of enzymes from psychrophiles. Microbial Biotechnol 4:449–460

5. Buchardt B, Seaman P, Stockmann G, Vous M, Wilken U, Duwel L et al (1997) Submarine columns of ikaite tufa. Nature 390:129–130

6. Buchardt B, Israelson C, Seaman P, Stockmann G (2001) Ikaite tufa towers in Ikka Fjord, southwest Greenland: their formation by mixing of seawater and alkaline spring water. J Sediment Res 71:176–189

7. Hansen MO, Buchardt B, Kuhl M, Elberling B (2011) The fate of submarine ikaite tufa columns in Southwest Greenland under changing climate conditions. J Sediment Res 81:553–561

8. Schmidt M, Larsen DM, Stougaard P (2010) A lipase with broad temperature range from an alkaliphilic gamma-proteobacterium isolated in Greenland. Environ Technol 31:1091–1100

9. Glaring MA, Vester JK, Lylloff JE, Abu Al-Soud W, Sorensen SJ, Stougaard P (2015) Microbial diversity in a permanently cold and alkaline environment in Greenland. PLoS One 10:e0124863

10. Vester JK, Glaring MA, Stougaard P (2015) An exceptionally cold-adapted alpha-amylase from a metagenomic library of a cold and alkaline environment. Appl Microbiol Biotechnol 99:717–727

11. Vester JK, Glaring MA, Stougaard P (2014) Discovery of novel enzymes with industrial potential from a cold and alkaline environment by a combination of functional metagenomics and culturing. Microb Cell Fact 13:72

12. Schmidt M, Stougaard P (2010) Identification, cloning and expression of a cold-active β-galactosidase from a novel Arctic bacterium, *Alkalilactibacillus ikkense*. Environ Technol 31:1107–1114

13. Vester JK, Glaring MA, Stougaard P (2013) Improving diversity in cultures of bacteria from an extreme environment. Can J Microbiol 59:581–586

14. Okshevsky M, Meyer RL (2015) The role of extracellular DNA in the establishment, maintenance and perpetuation of bacterial biofilms. Crit Rev Microbiol 41:341–352

15. Kallmeyer J, Smith DC, Spivack AJ, D'Hondt S (2008) New cell extraction procedure applied to deep subsurface sediments. Limnol Oceanogr Methods 6:236–245

16. Yilmaz S, Allgaier M, Hugenholtz P (2010) Multiple displacement amplification compromises quantitative analysis of metagenomes. Nat Methods 7:943–944

17. Horikoshi K (1999) Alkaliphiles: some applications of their products for biotechnology. Microbiol Mol Biol Rev 63:735–750

18. Vester JK, Glaring MA, Stougaard P (2015) Improved cultivation and metagenomics as new tools for bioprospecting in cold environments. Extremophiles 19:17–29

19. Parrilli E, De Vizio D, Cirulli C, Tutino ML (2008) Development of an improved *Pseudoalteromonas haloplanktis* TAC125 strain for recombinant protein secretion at low temperature. Microb Cell Fact 7:2

20. Kakirde KS, Wild J, Godiska R, Mead DA, Wiggins AG, Goodman RM et al (2011) Gram negative shuttle BAC vector for heterologous expression of metagenomic libraries. Gene 475:57–62

21. Saraswat M, Grand RS, Patrick WM (2013) Desalting DNA by drop dialysis increases library size upon transformation. Biosci Biotechnol Biochem 77:402–404

22. Teather RM, Wood PJ (1982) Use of Congo red-polysaccharide interactions in enumeration and characterization of cellulolytic bacteria from the bovine rumen. Appl Environ Microbiol 43:777–780

23. Gacesa P, Wusteman FS (1990) Plate assay for simultaneous detection of alginate lyases and determination of substrate specificity. Appl Environ Microbiol 56:2265–2267

24. Sundberg C, Al-Soud WA, Larsson M, Alm E, Yekta SS, Svensson BH et al (2013) 454 pyrosequencing analyses of bacterial and archaeal richness in 21 full-scale biogas digesters. FEMS Microbiol Ecol 85:612–626

Chapter 5

DNA-, RNA-, and Protein-Based Stable-Isotope Probing for High-Throughput Biomarker Analysis of Active Microorganisms

Eleanor Jameson, Martin Taubert, Sara Coyotzi, Yin Chen, Özge Eyice, Hendrik Schäfer, J. Colin Murrell, Josh D. Neufeld, and Marc G. Dumont

Abstract

Stable-isotope probing (SIP) enables researchers to target active populations within complex microbial communities, which is achieved by providing growth substrates enriched in heavy isotopes, usually in the form of ^{13}C, ^{18}O, or ^{15}N. After growth on the substrate and subsequent extraction of microbial biomarkers, typically nucleic acids or proteins, the SIP technique is used for the recovery and analysis of isotope-labeled biomarkers from active microbial populations. In the years following the initial development of DNA- and RNA-based SIP, it was common practice to characterize labeled populations by targeted gene analysis. Such approaches usually involved fingerprint-based analyses or sequencing of clone libraries containing 16S rRNA genes or functional marker gene amplicons. Although molecular fingerprinting remains a valuable approach for rapid confirmation of isotope labeling, recent advances in sequencing technology mean that it is possible to obtain affordable and comprehensive amplicon profiles, metagenomes, or metatranscriptomes from SIP experiments. Not only can the abundance of microbial groups be inferred from metagenomes, but researchers can bin, assemble, and explore individual genomes to build hypotheses about the metabolic capabilities of labeled microorganisms. Analysis of labeled mRNA is a more recent advance that can provide independent metatranscriptome-based analysis of active microorganisms. The power of metatranscriptomics is that mRNA abundance often correlates closely with the corresponding activity of encoded enzymes, thus providing insight into microbial metabolism at the time of sampling. Together, these advances have improved the sensitivity of SIP methods and allow the use of labeled substrates at ecologically relevant concentrations. Particularly as methods improve and costs continue to drop, we expect that the integration of SIP with multiple omics-based methods will become prevalent components of microbial ecology studies, leading to further breakthroughs in our understanding of novel microbial populations and elucidation of the metabolic function of complex microbial communities. In this chapter we provide protocols for obtaining labeled DNA, RNA, and proteins that can be used for downstream omics-based analyses.

Key words Stable-isotope probing, DNA, RNA, Protein, Metagenomics, Metatranscriptomics, Proteomics

Wolfgang R. Streit and Rolf Daniel (eds.), *Metagenomics: Methods and Protocols*, Methods in Molecular Biology, vol. 1539, DOI 10.1007/978-1-4939-6691-2_5, © Springer Science+Business Media LLC 2017

1   Introduction

Our ability to quantify and characterize microbial diversity and function in the environment has been accelerated by circumventing traditional limitations inherent to classical cultivation strategies. Although millions of small subunit (SSU) rRNA genes have been collected through cultivation-independent surveys, the physiology and metabolic functions of most of these uncultivated microorganisms cannot be determined reliably from ribosomal gene sequences alone. One successful strategy for unraveling the function of uncultivated microbes is metagenomics, which involves the retrieval and analysis of genome fragments from all community members in an environmental sample simultaneously [1]. Metagenomic DNA contains regions corresponding to housekeeping genes, including the 16S rRNA gene, which can reveal the phylogenetic affiliation of associated microorganisms, in addition to their adjacent enzyme-encoding genes, especially following the assembly of sequences from metagenomes. These enzyme-coding "functional" genes help us to deduce the potential metabolic and biogeochemical roles of these microorganisms in the environment.

Conventional metagenomic approaches involve cloning of DNA extracted from the environment, followed by sequence-based and/or function-based screens. Increasingly, extracted community DNA is sequenced directly, circumventing the need to capture nucleic acids in a vector for propagation within a surrogate host. Either way, a challenge is that massive shotgun sequencing of environmental DNA routinely focuses on the most abundant species in a sample. Given the relative rarity of most microbial community members, comprising the "rare biosphere" of most environmental habitats [2], sequencing of bulk DNA extracted from the environment can overlook extensive phylogenetic novelty and the potentially important roles of keystone members of the microbial community. For example, assuming an underlying community structure for the Global Ocean Sampling expedition dataset [3], only ~50% of total community DNA was captured, despite substantial sequencing effort. Nearly five times the sequencing reads collected in this study would have been required to access 90% of the species diversity of these samples [4]. Furthermore, function-based screening for enzymes of relevance to industry, biotechnology, and pharmaceutics may be challenging because of extremely low target gene frequency. An alternative approach is cultivation of microorganisms using defined or complex media, especially given that such approaches capture rare biosphere members [5]. However, cultivation represents an indiscriminate approach for recovering microbial community members, as far as it relates to the functional contributions of cultivated microorganisms within the context of the original environmental sample. In other words, no direct evidence implicates cultivated organisms as relevant to a function of interest in the environment being studied. Similarly, classical enrichment of individual populations, and thereby the enrichment of genes of interest prior to metagenomic analysis, often results in the selection of r-selected microorganisms that may be irrelevant to the natural environment but are nonetheless best adapted to imposed enrichment conditions.

Stable-isotope probing of DNA (DNA-SIP DNA Stable-Isotope probing) is a cultivation-independent method that can selectively label microorganisms that assimilate a specific stable-isotope labeled substrate (e.g., ^{13}C, ^{15}N; [6]). Since its inception, DNA-SIP has been used widely to study microorganisms involved in particular bioprocesses (reviewed in refs. 7–10). When carried out under near-natural conditions, SIP has unparalleled potential to select for labeled genomes of active populations while minimizing the potential for enrichment bias [11, 12]. In combination with metagenomics, DNA-SIP facilitates the selective isolation of DNA from functionally relevant microorganisms to construct metagenomic libraries in a directed manner that has not been possible previously [7, 11–18]. The goal of capturing labeled DNA within metagenomic libraries was first achieved by exposing a soil sample to ^{13}CH$_4$, retrieving high-quality labeled DNA within a bacterial artificial chromosome (BAC) library for the discovery of multiple clones with *pmoA*-containing operons [19]. Since then, several studies have collected labeled nucleic acids for generating metagenomic libraries for sequence-based analyses or functional screens (as reviewed in ref. 20). Although differential abundance binning [21] has not yet been used for the recovery of individual assembled genomes from sequenced heavy DNA, the coupling of low-diversity labeled DNA, from multiple time points or samples, would theoretically be an ideal approach in the future.

Alongside the development of SIP and related metagenomic applications, a major concern when combining DNA-SIP with metagenomics has been the challenge of obtaining sufficient ^{13}C-labeled heavy DNA template for construction of metagenomic libraries while minimizing substrate concentrations for corresponding SIP incubations (i.e., reducing the risk of enrichment bias). Technological developments for sequencing platforms, in particular Illumina, have largely overcome this problem. Together with low substrate/template concentrations and the widespread availability and affordability of high-throughput sequencing approaches, DNA-SIP is now ideally suited to help assign functions to microbial community members from complex microbial communities.

The extension of SIP to mRNA and protein greatly expands the functional relevance of data derived from SIP methodology (*see* Fig. 1). Studies have demonstrated mRNA-SIP [22–24] and its combination with metatranscriptomic analysis [25], but this remains a relatively unexplored approach. SIP-proteomics (reviewed in refs. 26–28) is more mature, in comparison, and the

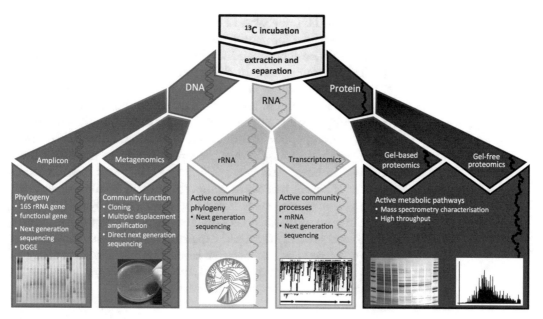

Fig. 1 Graphical overview of stable-isotope probing approaches, coupled to metagenomic, transcriptomic, or proteomic analyses

detection of heavy isotope incorporation in proteins for investigation of elemental fluxes in microbial communities has been described [29–32]. Metaproteomic analysis involves proteolytic cleavage of proteins into peptides followed by analysis of these peptides via mass spectrometry (MS). The determination of the molecular masses of peptides and their MS/MS fragmentation patterns allows identification of the peptide's sequence using a reference database. Contemporary high resolution MS, in combination with ultra-high pressure liquid chromatography (UHPLC) allow for high-throughput identification of tens of thousands of proteins from the microbial community.

Because peptide masses are changed by incorporation of heavy isotopes, MS also offers an ideal tool to investigate heavy isotope incorporation into peptides isolated from a SIP incubation. The general workflow is comparable to a conventional metaproteomic analysis, with the additional step of detection and quantification of heavy isotope abundance during data analysis [26, 27]. The sensitivity and accuracy of current MS instruments allows the detection of small changes in the isotopic composition of peptides. For example, a difference of 0.1 at.% for ^{13}C or ^{15}N can be detected [33, 34]. This also enables the detection of low levels of heavy isotope incorporation, which is more challenging with DNA- and RNA-based approaches. In addition to carbon and nitrogen, the use of other elements present in peptides for SIP experiments has been described, including sulfur (^{33}S, ^{34}S, ^{36}S) or hydrogen (^{2}D) [35, 36].

One of the drawbacks of SIP-proteomics is its reliance on reference sequences for peptide identification, thus reducing the proportion of identified peptides when derived from novel microbial species. A combination of SIP-proteomics with DNA- or RNA-SIP, coupled with metagenomics or metatranscriptomics approaches to acquire sequence data directly from the microbial community being investigated, is thus highly desirable. Furthermore, peptide identification is based on the masses of unlabeled peptides, complicating the investigation of material highly enriched in heavy isotopes. Different methods and bioinformatics tools have been introduced to infer the identity of labeled peptides, but no standardized analysis pipeline exists currently [29, 37, 38].

Here we provide protocols and technical notes for DNA-, RNA-, and protein-based SIP experimentation, which will enable a user to recover and characterize labeled biomarkers for a range of subsequent molecular techniques, including metagenomics, metatranscriptomics, and metaproteomics.

2 Materials

2.1 Reagents and Equipment for DNA-SIP, RNA-SIP, and Protein-SIP

In addition to being described below, reagents and equipment required have been described in detail elsewhere and we recommend that readers refer to these protocols for additional information [26, 39, 40].

2.2 Reagents and Equipment for Nucleic Acid Purification

1. Bead beater.
2. 2 mL screw-cap tubes.
3. 0.1-mm zirconia-silica beads (Roth), baked 16 h at 180 °C.
4. Nucleic acid extraction buffer (2.5 g SDS (sodium dodecyl sulfate detergent), 20 mL 1 M sodium phosphate (pH 8.0), 2 mL 5 M NaCl, 10 mL 0.5 M EDTA (pH 8.0), Water to 100 mL).
5. Precipitation solution: 30% polyethylene glycol 6000, 1.6 M NaCl.
6. Phenol–choloroform–isoamyl alcohol (25:24:1, pH 8.0).
7. Chloroform–isoamyl alcohol (24:1).
8. 2-mL non-stick microcentrifuge tubes (Ambion).
9. 75% ethanol.
10. RNase-free DNase Set (Qiagen).
11. RNeasy kit (Qiagen).
12. Nuclease-free water.

2.3 DNA/RNA Ultracentrifugation

1. Ultracentrifuge and vertical (or near vertical) rotor, such as the Vti 65.2 (Beckman Coulter).
2. CsCl stock solution (7.163 M; density is 1.890 g/mL in water) for DNA, or Illustra CsTFA (VWR) for RNA.

3. Deionised formamide.

4. Gradient buffer (GB): 0.1 M Tris–HCl, 0.1 M KCl, 1 mM EDTA, pH 8.0.

5. Ethanol.

6. RNAse inhibitor.

7. DNA precipitation solution: 30% polyethylene glycol 6000, 1.6 M NaCl.

8. Linear polyacrylamide (LPA; e.g., co-precipitant pink [Bioline]) (*see* **Note 1**).

9. Suitable device for gradient fractionation. For example, the Multi-Speed Syringe Pump (BSP) works well with a 60-mL syringe for gradient fractionation.

10. Digital refractometer (e.g., Reichert AR200) for determining gradient density.

2.4 16S rRNA Gene Sequencing

16S rRNA gene amplicon sequencing primers and methods are described in several publications, such as [41] or [42].

2.5 Metagenome/ Metatranscriptome Sequencing

Sequencing of amplicons or metagenomic DNA with a MiSeq (Illumina) is currently the most common choice as it offers highest throughput per run and fewest consensus errors [43]. Below are listed several kits that we have used, but we recommend adopting the most current methodology, discussing options with your sequencing service provider when appropriate.

1. NEBNext Ultra II DNA Library Prep Kit for Illumina (*see* **Note 2**).

2. TruSeq RNA Library Preparation Kit.

3. NEBNext Multiplex Oligos for Illumina.

4. MiSeq Reagent Kit v3 (600 cycle) Illumina.

2.6 Reagents and Equipment for Protein Purification

1. 100 mM phenylmethanesulfonyl fluoride (PMSF) dissolved in pure isopropanol.

2. 0.1 M ammonium acetate dissolved in pure methanol.

3. 80% acetone.

4. 70% ethanol.

5. Equipment for sodium dodecyl sulfate-polyacrylamide gel electrophoresis (SDS-PAGE).

6. SDS sample buffer (e.g., 60 mM Tris–HCl pH 6.8, 10% glycerol, 2% SDS, 5% β-mercaptoethanol, 0.01% bromophenol blue).

2.7 In-Gel Tryptic Digestion of Proteins

1. Acetonitrile.

2. Wash solution: 40% acetonitrile, 10% acetic acid.

3. 5 mM ammonium bicarbonate.

4. 10 mM ammonium bicarbonate.

5. 10 mM 1,4-dithiothreitol (DTT) in 10 mM ammonium bicarbonate.

6. 100 mM 2-iodoacetamide in 10 mM ammonium bicarbonate.

7. Trypsin-buffer: dissolve 20 µg Trypsin Proteomics Sequencing Grade in 20 µL 1 mM HCl. Add 5 µL of dissolved trypsin to 495 µL of 5 mM ammonium bicarbonate directly before use.

8. Peptide extraction buffer: 50% acetonitrile, 5% formic acid.

3 Methods

The initial steps of any DNA-, RNA-, or protein-SIP protocol involve numerous experimental design considerations, including the choice of environmental sample, substrate, substrate concentration, replication, controls, and incubation times. In particular, the inclusion of experimental replicates and control incubations with unlabeled substrate are essential for generating reliable and informative results. Control samples (i.e., with the corresponding unlabeled substrate) must be processed throughout the entire procedure to help confirm labeled DNA in the samples receiving stable isotopes, and this is especially necessary with low biomass/slow metabolism samples.

Sample incubations ideally mimic in situ environmental conditions and disrupt the sample as little as possible. However, including a starvation period as a pre-incubation step (e.g., carbon compound deprivation) prior to feeding the labeled compound can be helpful for reducing the content of native compounds in the sample and favor isotopic labeling during the incubation with added substrate. Substrate concentration for incubation and optimum incubation time can be determined through "titration" incubations to ensure DNA labeling without compromising the ecological relevance of the experiment. Conversely, in biotechnology-oriented research, for example, when the purpose is enzyme discovery, high substrate concentrations and short incubation times might help find ideal gene candidates for industrial processes.

Although we have highlighted a few experimental considerations here, additional details are beyond the scope of this protocol and will be highly variable based on individual samples and substrates. Please refer to ref. 39 for additional discussion of appropriate incubation conditions for labeling target organisms in environmental samples.

3.1 Nucleic Acid Extraction from Labeled Soil or Sediment Samples

The following protocol will retrieve total nucleic acids from an environmental sample; please refer to Subheading 3.5 on how to adapt this procedure to recover proteins.

In practice, it is unnecessary to remove RNA from the extract for DNA-SIP because RNA typically does not interfere with any downstream analysis steps. In contrast, careful removal of DNA is required for RNA-SIP. If only DNA-SIP is being conducted, then DNA extraction can be done with the PowerSoil DNA Isolation Kit (MO BIO Laboratories) according to the manufacturer's protocol (*see* **Note 3**).

1. Add 200 μL of glass beads into a sterile 2-mL screw-cap tube.

2. Add soil or sediment sample to the tube, to a maximum of 0.5 g of material. Add more for sediment or soils with high water contents.

3. Centrifuge and remove the supernatant, leaving the pellet (~0.5 mL tube volume).

4. Add 1 mL of nucleic acid extraction buffer and bead beat for 45 s at 6 m/s.

5. Centrifuge at maximum speed for 5 min at 20 °C.

6. Place supernatant in a 2 mL microcentrifuge tube and add 850 μL of phenol–chloroform–isoamyl alcohol (25:24:1). Mix well. To the soil/sediment pellet, add another 900 μL of nucleic acid extraction buffer and repeat bead beating and spin. Place the supernatant from the second extraction in a 2-mL microcentrifuge tube. Add 850 μL of phenol–chloroform–isoamyl alcohol and mix well. Spin the first and second round extractions for 5 min at maximum speed in a microcentrifuge (~13,000×g; 20 °C).

7. Recover the aqueous phase from the tubes and place in a 2-mL tube. If the solution is cloudy, repeat the phenol–chloroform extraction step. If the extract is clear, proceed to the next step.

8. Add 800 μL of chloroform, mix well, and centrifuge again.

9. Place the aqueous supernatant into a 2-mL non-stick tube. Add 1 mL of precipitation solution and mix thoroughly. Leave for at least 1 h on bench.

10. Centrifuge for 30 min at maximum speed (4 °C).

11. Aspirate the supernatant and add 800 μL of cold 75 % ethanol to the pellet. Mix well and centrifuge 10 min at maximum speed (4 °C).

12. Aspirate the ethanol wash, ensuring that the last drops of liquid have been removed around the pellet.

13. Allow the pellet to just-dry (do not over-dry) for 30 min on the bench. Dissolve each pellet in 50 μL of nuclease free water and pool the first and second round extracts for a total of 100 μL of total nucleic acids. Continue to the next step to obtain purified RNA, or store the extract at −80 °C.

14. To half of the nucleic acid extract (50 μL), add 37.5 μL of water, 10 μL of buffer RDD (Qiagen), and 2.5 μL of DNase.

Mix gently and leave on the bench for 10 min. Store the remainder of your extract at –80 °C.

15. Continue with the RNA purification protocol using the RNeasy kit. Elute RNA from column by adding 30 μL of water twice (you will obtain 50–60 μL of RNA eluate).

16. Verify that your RNA is free of contaminating DNA by a PCR targeting the 16S rRNA gene. Set-up a reverse transcription PCR assay, but include a control without added reverse transcriptase enzyme (i.e., substitute with an equivalent volume of water). Repeat the DNase treatment if a product is obtained without added reverse transcriptase.

17. Store RNA in non-stick microcentrifuge tubes (e.g., Ambion) at –80 °C. It is also recommended to store in multiple aliquots to avoid freeze-thawing the stock solution.

3.2 Isolation of Labeled DNA by CsCl Gradient Centrifugation

1. Calculate the total volume of DNA sample and GB to mix with 4.9 mL of CsCl stock solution for a 1.725 g/mL gradient solution desired density, as follows:

2. $\text{GB / DNA volume} = (\text{CsCl stock solution density} - 1.725) \times 4.9 \times 1.52$

3. Add the appropriate DNA and GB volumes required to achieve the volume determined before at the bottom of a sterile 15-mL tube and gently tap to mix. Aim to add between 0.5 and 5 μg of DNA to each gradient. If possible, maximizing DNA addition to the gradient, within the specified range, is ideal for yielding sufficient labeled material for downstream analyses.

4. Add 4.9 mL of CsCl to the tube containing DNA/GB and gently mix by inversion. Prepare a GB control without DNA to evaluate possible contamination. If possible, include a second control combining pure culture ^{12}C-DNA and ^{13}C-DNA to verify gradient formation.

5. Fill the ultracentrifuge tubes slowly with the resulting solution up to the tube neck base using a Pasteur pipette, avoiding bubble formation.

6. Pair the tubes by weight and adjust as necessary (±0.01 g) for balance during ultracentrifugation.

7. Seal the tubes, verifying the absence of leakage by applying gentle pressure to the tube between two fingers. Confirm that each tube pair remains balanced.

8. Load the rotor and centrifuge for 36–40 h at $177,000 \times g$ (average; 44,100 rpm for a Vti65.2 rotor) at 20 °C. Program the ultracentrifuge with vacuum, maximum acceleration, and without brake for the final deceleration.

9. Remove the rotor from the ultracentrifuge and carefully remove each tube sequentially for fractionation. Do not allow

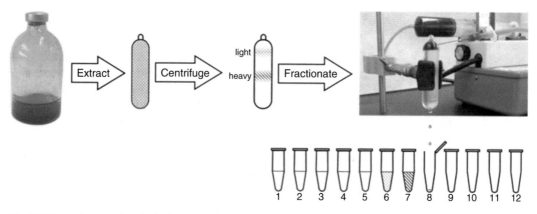

Fig. 2 Schematic overview including a visual example of gradient fractionation using a syringe pump and a burette stand in order to hold the gradient during the fractionation process

tubes to fall over or become inverted. Fractionate all tubes within 2–3 h.

10. Fractionate the contents of each tube into 12 fractions by displacing from the top with water that contains a few mg of bromophenol blue, which assists with visualization of the displaced gradient (Fig. 2).

11. Use a 23-gauge 1″ length needle to pierce the top of the tube for injecting the aqueous solution. Ensure that the water is already in the tube and needle when piercing the top to avoid air being injected into the tube. Then, pierce the bottom of the tube with a second needle. Displace the tube contents at approximately 425 μL/min using a syringe pump. At this rate, change the sterile 1.5 mL collection tube every minute until all 12 fractions have been collected. Measure the refractive index of the gradient fractions, at least for the control (no DNA) gradient. Using a calibrated refractometer, it is possible to convert the refractive index of the gradients into density. Once calibrated, a digital refractometer provides consistent data for several years.

12. Precipitate the DNA from each fraction by adding 4 μL of LPA and 850 μL of DNA precipitation solution. Mix by inversion after each addition and leave at room temperature from 2 h to overnight to ensure maximal precipitation.

13. Centrifuge at $13,000 \times g$ at 15–20 °C for 30 min. Aspirate and discard the supernatant. Add 500 μL of 70% ethanol to wash the pellet. Centrifuge at $13,000 \times g$ at 15–20 °C for 10 min. Aspirate and discard the supernatant. Allow to dry for 15 min at room temperature.

14. Dissolve the DNA in 30 μL of TE buffer on ice. Visually check DNA from each fraction using 5 μL aliquots on 1% agarose gels.

15. Quantify DNA through absorbance at 260 nm (e.g., NanoDrop or Qubit), or by qPCR of the 16S rRNA gene.

16. Confirming that labeling was successful is done by comparing microbial community profiles from light and heavy fractions of the isotope-labeled gradients and the corresponding native substrate controls. In addition, it is important to verify that results from replicate incubations were consistent. The use of fingerprinting of 16S rRNA genes by denaturing gradient gel electrophoresis (DGGE) or high-throughput sequencing can be alternative or complementary approaches for this step. In addition, such profiling helps verify that the pure culture control generated appropriate physical separation of labeled and unlabeled DNA (i.e., ^{12}C-DNA and ^{13}C-DNA control), and also verify the absence of contamination in the control (no DNA) gradient.

3.3 Isolation of Labeled RNA by CsTFA Gradient Centrifugation

Many of the procedures for isopycnic banding and isolation of labeled DNA (Subheading 3.2) are the same for labeled RNA, with some important differences indicated here. Total RNA can be used or it is possible to perform an mRNA enrichment step before loading the RNA into the gradient (*see* **Note 4**).

1. For each gradient, combine 4.9 mL of CsTFA (2.0 g/mL) with 1 mL of gradient buffer (GB), vortexing thoroughly. If necessary, adjust the refractive index to 1.3702 by small additions of either CsTFA or GB. Add 210 μL of deionised formamide and vortex thoroughly. The refractive index should be approximately 1.3725.

2. Add 0.5 μg of RNA to each gradient (*see* **Note 5**). Ensure that the tubes are balanced (±0.01 g) and properly sealed.

3. Centrifuge for 65 h at 130,000 × g and at 20 °C, using ultracentrifuge vacuum, acceleration, and deceleration conditions specified for DNA-SIP above.

4. Fractionate the gradients by displacing from the top with nuclease-free water (Fig. 2). Twelve fractions per gradient are usually sufficient, but more fractions can be collected to obtain a higher resolution. Measure the refractive index of the gradient fractions.

5. Precipitate the RNA by adding 4 μL LPA to each fraction, 1/10th volume of 3 M sodium acetate (pH 5.2), and 2.5 volumes of ethanol. Vortex thoroughly and leave 1 h at −20 °C, then spin 30 min at maximum speed (~13,000 × g) on a benchtop microcentrifuge at 4 °C. Remove the supernatant and add 1 mL of 70% ethanol. Spin in microcentrifuge, aspirate and discard the ethanol. Remove the last drops of ethanol with a small pipette tip and allow the pellet to just dry. Add 6 μL of

nuclease-free water containing 1 unit/μL of RNAse inhibitor. Vortex briefly and store at –80 °C.

6. Quantify the amount of RNA in each gradient fraction. It is often helpful to do this by quantitative PCR of 16S rRNA, but this can also be done by absorbance at 260 nm or by using a fluorometric RNA detection method.

7. Send RNA samples to a sequencing service to perform the library preparation and Illumina sequencing.

3.4 Analysis of Metagenomes and Metatranscriptomes

There are several bioinformatic tools that provide approaches to analyzing community composition directly based on metagenomic read data or assembled metagenome data, such as Kraken [44], metaphlan [45], Kaiju [46], MG-RAST [47], and others. Due to reliance on databases containing sequenced genomes of relevant microorganisms, which often do not include representatives of uncultivated lineages that are relevant in a given environment, these bioinformatics tools may generate a biased perspective of microbial community functional profiles compared to those based on ribosomal gene amplicons. However, these tools have the advantage of assessing community composition across all domains of life (and also include viruses) in a single assessment, without requiring PCR amplification of ribosomal RNA genes.

Although it is beyond the scope of this chapter to describe the methods and approaches available to analyze metagenomes and metatranscriptomes, such methods have been reviewed extensively elsewhere.

3.5 Protein Extraction from Labeled Samples

The following protocol is designed for researchers performing a DNA/RNA-SIP experiment who also want to investigate the proteomes of their samples, and is based on the protocol for nucleic acid extraction (Subheading 3.1), thus allowing simultaneous protein extraction (*see* **Note 6**).

1. Add PMSF (a protease inhibitor) to the nucleic acid extraction buffer to a final concentration of 1 mM. Perform bead beating and phenol–chloroform–isoamyl alcohol extraction as described in Subheading 3.1. Proteins will be dissolved in the organic (phenol-containing) phase.

2. Combine the phenol–chloroform–isoamyl alcohol phases (but not the organic phase from the chloroform extraction step). Add fivefold volume of ice-cold 0.1 M ammonium acetate in methanol. Incubate overnight at –20 °C to precipitate protein.

3. Centrifuge for 30 min at $13,000 \times g$ (4 °C, use of a swing-out rotor is recommended), remove supernatant.

4. Wash pellet five times by resuspending in 1 mL of the following solvents (ice-cold), followed by 20 min of incubation at –20 °C

and centrifugation at $13,000 \times g$ (4 °C) for each washing step: 2× 0.1 M ammonium acetate in methanol, 2× 80 % acetone, 1× 70 % ethanol. After removal of supernatant on last washing step, let the pellet to air-dry.

5. Perform a sodium dodecyl sulfate–polyacrylamide gel electro-phoresis (SDS-PAGE) following standard laboratory proce-dures. Prepare samples by resuspending and boiling for 10 min in 20–50 µL SDS sample buffer. Stop electrophoresis when the samples have entered the gel by about 2–3 cm. This step is used for further purification of proteins and a rough pre-separation.

3.6 In-Gel Tryptic Digestion of Proteins

1. Cut gel horizontally into 2–4 pieces per lane and transfer the pieces into individual 0.5 mL tubes. Perform all following steps at room temperature unless indicated otherwise. Add 200 µL wash solution to each gel piece, shake for 1 h. Remove wash solution and add 200 µL acetonitrile, shake for 5 min.

2. Remove acetonitrile, dry gel pieces in a vacuum centrifuge for 5 min. Add 30 µL 10 mM DTT solution and shake for 30 min (reduction of proteins).

3. Remove DTT solution, add 30 µL 100 mM 2-iodoacetamide solution and shake for 30 min (alkylation of proteins).

4. Remove 2-iodoacetamide solution, add 200 µL acetonitrile, shake for 5 min.

5. Remove acetonitrile, add 200 µL 10 mM ammonium bicar-bonate solution, shake for 10 min.

6. Remove the ammonium bicarbonate solution, add 200 µL ace-tonitrile, shake for 5 min.

7. Remove acetonitrile, dry gel pieces in a vacuum centrifuge for 5 min.

8. Add 20 µL of trypsin-buffer and incubate at 37 °C over night.

9. Add 30 µL 5 mM ammonium bicarbonate solution and shake for 10 min.

10. Remove and collect the ammonium bicarbonate solution in separate tube for each gel piece.

11. Add 30 µL peptide extraction buffer to gel piece and shake for 10 min.

12. Remove peptide extraction buffer and add it to the collected ammonium bicarbonate solution.

13. Repeat **steps 11** and **12** once more.

14. For each gel piece from **step 7**, you now should have one tube containing the gel piece without any liquid (which can be dis-carded) and one tube containing the collected solutions (ammonium bicarbonate and peptide extraction buffer),

containing the tryptic peptides. Completely evaporate the solution in a vacuum centrifuge (this can take several hours).

15. Resuspend in 0.1 % formic acid and perform ZipTip (Millipore) purification and enrichment of peptides according to manufacturer's manual.

16. Dry the peptide containing eluate in a vacuum centrifuge and resuspend in an appropriate volume (10–20 μL) of 0.1 % formic acid for liquid chromatography-mass spectrometry (LC-MS) analysis. These samples can be stored at −20 °C until analysis.

3.7 SIP-Proteomics Analysis by High Resolution MS

The general procedure of a SIP-proteomics analysis is the same as a normal proteomics experiment, and thus should be done according to "in house" proteomics protocols. If a high resolution MS (e.g., Orbitrap) or the bioinformatics tools required for protein identification from mass spectral data and according computing power is unavailable in house, analysis could be performed in cooperation with a proteomics core facility.

In general, peptide identification relies on the presence of unlabeled peptides. If a sample is highly enriched in ^{13}C, peptides can no longer be identified and must then be inferred from the corresponding unlabeled samples (*see* **Note 7**). Here, a brief overview on the basic principle of estimation of heavy isotope incorporation is given.

1. Manual inspection of mass spectra of heavy isotope labeled samples can already be used to detect signals of ^{13}C labeled peptides, as these show a different pattern than the signals of unlabeled peptides (*see* Fig. 3). This is an easy way to determine if a SIP experiment has worked.

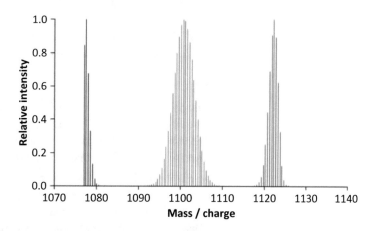

Fig. 3 Theoretical mass spectra of the peptide EAGLCTHEKINGLIVESIVK (charge = 2) with 1.1 % ^{13}C (*black*, natural abundance), 50 % ^{13}C (*blue*) and 95 % ^{13}C (*red*). Heavy isotope labeled peptides show a Poisson-like distribution of isotopic peaks with left- and right-tailing. Unlabeled peptides never show left-tailing of isotopic peaks

2. Perform phylogenetic classification on all peptides identified in unlabeled and labeled samples by determining the lowest common ancestor (e.g., using the tools available at unipept.ugent.be). Make a comparison of the number of identified peptides per taxonomic group between ^{12}C and ^{13}C samples. A drop in identifications from ^{12}C to ^{13}C samples is the first hint that a specific taxonomic group has been labeled because the labeled peptides are not identified anymore.

3. Verify the presence of ^{13}C in peptides of the taxonomic groups of interest. This can be done using the software tools stated above. Alternatively, if only a low number of peptides have to be investigated, manual analysis can be performed, as described previously [30]. Quantification of ^{13}C incorporation into 10 peptides per taxonomic group is usually sufficient to give a rough estimate of the extent of assimilation of carbon from the labeled carbon source.

4   Notes

1. Glycogen as a co-precipitant is a potential source of contamination with nucleic acids [48]. Therefore, we recommend using LPA as it is equally effective as co-precipitant, with less risk of introducing contamination to gradient fractions.

2. NEBNext Ultra II DNA Library Prep (NEB, Hitchin UK) provides a high library yield (~100 nM) from ≥500 pg input DNA.

3. Methods for DNA extraction from DNA-SIP incubated samples need to be selected carefully. For example, avoid methods that shear DNA (e.g., bead-beating protocols) when large-insert metagenomic libraries are desired. Purify the DNA before loading into CsCl gradients if humic contaminants are present, even though CsCl gradient can partially purify loaded DNA.

4. It is possible to perform mRNA enrichment at this stage by removing rRNA molecules (e.g., RiboZero Kit, Illumina). This can increase the proportion of sequence reads originating from mRNA in the metatranscriptome >10-fold.

5. Do not to add more than ~1 μg of total RNA to each gradient because it might precipitate in the gradient. The authors do not know of a way to prevent this from occurring with higher concentrations of RNA, nor how to recover RNA if it has precipitated.

6. Protocols for protein extraction depend strongly on the type of sample material available (e.g., water, sediment, soil), so this protocol cannot be guaranteed to work for every sample type.

Do not use any treatment requiring the addition of proteases or other proteins (e.g., lysozyme) to your sample. If this represents a change to your normal nucleic acid extraction protocol, check first that DNA/RNA extraction efficiency is not adversely affected.

7. This can be done by additional MS analysis of a mixture of the labeled and the unlabeled sample or by mapping of identifications from the unlabeled sample to the labeled sample via the software tools SIPPER or MetaProSIP [37, 38]. An alternative, but computationally expensive, approach also allows identification of labeled peptides [29].

Acknowledgments

Yin Chen acknowledges funding from NERC grant NE/I027061/1, and Yin Chen and J. Colin Murrell both acknowledge funding from the Gordon and Betty Moore Foundation Marine Microbiology Initiative Grant GBMF3303 and the Earth and Life Systems Alliance, Norwich Research Park, Norwich, UK. Josh D. Neufeld acknowledges a Discovery Grant from the Natural Sciences and Engineering Research Council of Canada (NSERC).

References

1. Handelsman J (2004) Metagenomics: application of genomics to uncultured microorganisms. Microbiol Mol Biol Rev 68:669–685

2. Lynch MD, Neufeld JD (2015) Ecology and exploration of the rare biosphere. Nat Rev Microbiol 13:217–229

3. Rusch DB, Halpern AL, Sutton G, Heidelberg KB, Williamson S, Yooseph S et al (2007) The sorcerer II global ocean sampling expedition: northwest Atlantic through eastern tropical Pacific. PLoS Biol 5:e77

4. Quince C, Curtis TP, Sloan WT (2008) The rational exploration of microbial diversity. ISME J 2:997–1006

5. Shade A, Hogan CS, Klimowicz AK, Linske M, McManus PS, Handelsman J (2012) Culturing captures members of the soil rare biosphere. Environ Microbiol 14:2247–2252

6. Radajewski S, Ineson P, Parekh NR, Murrell JC (2000) Stable-isotope probing as a tool in microbial ecology. Nature 403:646–649

7. Dumont MG, Murrell JC (2005) Stable isotope probing - linking microbial identity to function. Nat Rev Microbiol 3:499–504

8. Neufeld JD, Wagner M, Murrell JC (2007) Who eats what, where and when? Isotope-labelling experiments are coming of age. ISME J 1:103–110

9. Uhlik O, Leewis MC, Strejcek M, Musilova L, Mackova M, Leigh MB, Macek T (2013) Stable isotope probing in the metagenomics era: a bridge towards improved bioremediation. Biotechnol Adv 31:154–165

10. Grob C, Taubert M, Howat AM, Burns OJ, Chen Y, Murrell JC (2015) Generating enriched metagenomes from active microorganisms with DNA stable isotope probing. Hydrocarb Lipid Microbiol Protoc 10:1007

11. Friedrich MW (2006) Stable-isotope probing of DNA: insights into the function of uncultivated microorganisms from isotopically labeled metagenomes. Curr Opin Biotechnol 17:59–66

12. Neufeld JD, Dumont MG, Vohra J, Murrell JC (2007) Methodological considerations for the use of stable isotope probing in microbial ecology. Microb Ecol 53:435–442

13. Schloss PD, Handelsman J (2003) Biotechnological prospects from metagenomics. Curr Opin Biotechnol 14:303–310

14. Wellington EM, Berry A, Krsek M (2003) Resolving functional diversity in relation to

microbial community structure in soil: exploiting genomics and stable isotope probing. Curr Opin Microbiol 6:295–301

15. Martineau C, Whyte LG, Greer CW (2010) Stable isotope probing analysis of the diversity and activity of methanotrophic bacteria in soils from the Canadian high Arctic. Appl Environ Microbiol 76:5773–5784

16. Bell TH, Yergeau E, Martineau C, Juck D, Whyte LG, Greer CW (2011) Identification of nitrogen-incorporating bacteria in petroleum-contaminated arctic soils by using [15N] DNA-based stable isotope probing and pyrosequencing. Appl Environ Microbiol 77:4163–4171

17. Eyice Ö, Namura M, Chen Y, Mead A, Samavedam S, Schäfer H (2015) SIP metagenomics identifies uncultivated Methylophilaceae as dimethylsulphide degrading bacteria in soil and lake sediment. ISME J 9:2336–2348

18. Grob C, Taubert M, Howat AM, Burns OJ, Dixon JL, Richnow HH et al (2015) Combining metagenomics with metaproteomics and stable isotope probing reveals metabolic pathways used by a naturally occurring marine methylotroph. Environ Microbiol 17:4007–4018

19. Dumont MG, Radajewski SM, Miguez CB, McDonald IR, Murrell JC (2006) Identification of a complete methane monooxygenase operon from soil by combining stable isotope probing and metagenomic analysis. Environ Microbiol 8:1240–1250

20. Coyotzi S, Pratscher J, Murrell JC, Neufeld JD (2016) Targeted metagenomics of active microbial populations with stable-isotope probing. Curr Opin Biotechnol 41:1–8

21. Albertsen M, Hugenholtz P, Skarshewski A, Nielsen KL, Tyson GW, Nielsen PH (2013) Genome sequences of rare, uncultured bacteria obtained by differential coverage binning of multiple metagenomes. Nat Biotechnol 31:533–538

22. Dumont MG, Pommerenke B, Casper P, Conrad R (2011) DNA-, rRNA- and mRNA-based stable isotope probing of aerobic methanotrophs in lake sediment. Environ Microbiol 13:1153–1167

23. Haichar FZ, Roncato MA, Achouak W (2012) Stable isotope probing of bacterial community structure and gene expression in the rhizosphere of Arabidopsis thaliana. FEMS Microbiol Ecol 81:291–302

24. Huang WE, Ferguson A, Singer AC, Lawson K, Thompson IP, Kalin RM et al (2009) Resolving genetic functions within microbial populations: in situ analyses using rRNA and

mRNA stable isotope probing coupled with single-cell raman-fluorescence in situ hybridization. Appl Environ Microbiol 75:234–241

25. Dumont MG, Pommerenke B, Casper P (2013) Using stable isotope probing to obtain a targeted metatranscriptome of aerobic methanotrophs in lake sediment. Environ Microbiol Rep 5:757–764

26. Jehmlich N, Schmidt F, Taubert M, Seifert J, Bastida F, von Bergen M et al (2010) Protein-based stable isotope probing. Nat Protoc 5:1957–1966

27. Seifert J, Taubert M, Jehmlich N, Schmidt F, Volker U, Vogt C et al (2012) Protein-based stable isotope probing (protein-SIP) in functional metaproteomics. Mass Spectrom Rev 31:683–697

28. von Bergen M, Jehmlich N, Taubert M, Vogt C, Bastida F, Herbst FA et al (2013) Insights from quantitative metaproteomics and protein-stable isotope probing into microbial ecology. ISME J 7:1877–1885

29. Pan C, Fischer CR, Hyatt D, Bowen BP, Hettich RL, Banfield JF (2011) Quantitative tracking of isotope flows in proteomes of microbial communities. Mol Cell Proteomics 10(M110):006049

30. Taubert M, Vogt C, Wubet T, Kleinsteuber S, Tarkka MT, Harms H et al (2012) Protein-SIP enables time-resolved analysis of the carbon flux in a sulfate-reducing, benzene-degrading microbial consortium. ISME J 6:2291–2301

31. Lünsmann V, Kappelmeyer U, Benndorf R, Martinez-Lavanchy PM, Taubert A, Adrian L et al (2016) In situ protein-SIP highlights Burkholderiaceae as key players degrading toluene by para ring hydroxylation in a constructed wetland model. Environ Microbiol 18:1176

32. Herbst FA, Bahr A, Duarte M, Pieper DH, Richnow HH, von Bergen M et al (2013) Elucidation of in situ polycyclic aromatic hydrocarbon degradation by functional metaproteomics (protein-SIP). Proteomics 13:2910–2920

33. Taubert M, Baumann S, von Bergen M, Seifert J (2011) Exploring the limits of robust detection of incorporation of ^{13}C by mass spectrometry in protein-based stable isotope probing (protein-SIP). Anal Bioanal Chem 401:1975–1982

34. Taubert M, von Bergen M, Seifert J (2013) Limitations in detection of ^{15}N incorporation by mass spectrometry in protein-based stable isotope probing (protein-SIP). Anal Bioanal Chem 405:3989–3996

35. Jehmlich N, Kopinke FD, Lenhard S, Vogt C, Herbst FA, Seifert J et al (2012) Sulfur-^{36}S stable

isotope labeling of amino acids for quantification (SULAQ). Proteomics 12:37–42

36. Justice NB, Li Z, Wang Y, Spaudling SE, Mosier AC, Hettich RL et al (2014) ^{15}N- and ^{2}H proteomic stable isotope probing links nitrogen flow to archaeal heterotrophic activity. Environ Microbiol 16:3224–3237

37. Slysz GW, Steinke L, Ward DM, Klatt CG, Clauss TR, Purvine SO et al (2014) Automated data extraction from in situ protein-stable isotope probing studies. J Proteome Res 13:1200–1210

38. Sachsenberg T, Herbst FA, Taubert M, Kermer R, Jehmlich N, von Bergen M et al (2015) MetaProSIP: automated inference of stable isotope incorporation rates in proteins for functional metaproteomics. J Proteome Res 14:619–627

39. Neufeld JD, Vohra J, Dumont MG, Lueders T, Manefield M, Friedrich MW, Murrell JC (2007) DNA stable-isotope probing. Nat Protoc 2:860–866

40. Whiteley AS, Thomson B, Lueders T, Manefield M (2007) RNA stable-isotope probing. Nat Protoc 2:838–844

41. Bartram AK, Lynch MD, Stearns JC, Moreno-Hagelsieb G, Neufeld JD (2011) Generation of multimillion-sequence 16S rRNA gene libraries from complex microbial communities by assembling paired-end illumina reads. Appl Environ Microbiol 77:3846–3852

42. Caporaso JG, Lauber CL, Walters WA, Berg-Lyons D, Huntley J, Fierer N et al (2012) Ultra-high-throughput microbial community analysis on the Illumina HiSeq and MiSeq platforms. ISME J 6:1621–1624

43. Jünemann S, Sedlazeck FJ, Prior K, Albersmeier A, John U, Kalinowski J et al (2013) Updating benchtop sequencing performance comparison. Nat Biotechnol 31:294–296

44. Wood DE, Salzberg SL (2014) Kraken: ultra-fast metagenomic sequence classification using exact alignments. Genome Biol 15:R46

45. Segata N, Waldron L, Ballarini A, Narasimhan V, Jousson O, Huttenhower C (2012) Metagenomic microbial community profiling using unique clade-specific marker genes. Nat Methods 9:811–814

46. Menzel P, Ng KL, and Krogh A (2015) Kaiju: fast and sensitive taxonomic classification for metagenomics. bioRxiv. doi: 10.1101/031229.

47. Meyer F, Paarmann D, D'Souza M, Olson R, Glass EM, Kubal M et al (2008) The metagenomics RAST server - a public resource for the automatic phylogenetic and functional analysis of metagenomes. BMC Bioinformatics 9:386

48. Bartram A, Poon C, Neufeld J (2009) Nucleic acid contamination of glycogen used in nucleic acid precipitation and assessment of linear polyacrylamide as an alternative co-precipitant. Biotechniques 47:1019–1022

Chapter 6

Assessing Bacterial and Fungal Diversity in the Plant Endosphere

Bernd Wemheuer and Franziska Wemheuer

Abstract

Plants are colonized various microorganisms including endophytes. These microbes can play an important role in agricultural production as they promote plant growth and/or enhance the resistance of their host plant against diseases and environmental stress conditions. Although culture-independent molecular approaches such as DNA barcoding have greatly enhanced our understanding of bacterial and fungal endophyte communities, there are some methodical problems when investigating endophyte diversity. One main issue are sequence contaminations such as plastid-derived rRNA gene sequences which are co-amplified due to their high homology to bacterial 16S rRNA genes. The same is true for plant and fungal ITS sequences. The application of highly specific-primers suppressing co-amplification of these sequence contaminations is a good solution for this issue. Here, we describe a detailed protocol for assessing bacterial and fungal endophyte diversity in plants using these primers in combination with next-generation sequencing.

Key words Endophytic communities, DNA barcoding, Microbial diversity

1 Introduction

Endophytes are microorganisms that colonize healthy plant tissues intracellularly and/or intercellularly. Endophytic microorganisms including bacteria or fungi have been found in a wide range of plants [1]. Beneficial endophytes play an important role in agricultural production as they promote plant growth and health. In addition, these microbes can enhance the tolerance of their host plant against diseases and environmental stress conditions such as drought (as reviewed in refs. 1, 2). Consequently, it is crucial to understand the interactions between endophytes, their host plant and changing environmental conditions.

Culture-dependent approaches have been frequently applied to study bacterial and fungal communities in the plant endosphere. However, these approaches have provided only limited access to

Wolfgang R. Streit and Rolf Daniel (eds.), *Metagenomics: Methods and Protocols*, Methods in Molecular Biology, vol. 1539, DOI 10.1007/978-1-4939-6691-2_6, © Springer Science+Business Media LLC 2017

endophytic communities as most microorganisms cannot be cultivated using common laboratory techniques. As a consequence, the number of culture-independent molecular approaches investigating bacterial and fungal endophytes in different plant species has been increased during the last few years [3–5]. These studies have greatly enhanced our understanding of the diversity and community structure of endophytes. However, co-amplification of plastid and mitochondrial rDNA sequences or plant ITS sequences from mixed plant–endophytic DNA extracts can be particularly problematic in the analysis of bacterial or fungal endophytic communities, respectively.

Here, we describe a standard protocol for assessing bacterial and fungal community structure and diversity in the plant endosphere combining next-generation sequencing with DNA barcoding. The protocol is based on PCR reactions with highly specific primers targeting marker genes but suppressing the co-amplification of plastid, mitochondrial, and plant DNA. The protocol has been already applied to investigate the response of the bacterial endophytic community in different plants species towards management regimes [5]. As different plant compartments harbor distinct endophytic communities, the endophytic communities of different plant parts should be analyzed separately [1, 6].

2   Materials

Prepare all solutions using sterile-filtered as well as Diethylpyrocarbonate (DEPC)-treated water and analytical grade reagents. For DEPC treatment, add 1 mL DEPC to 1 L ultrapure water. Stir for at least 1 h and remove residual DEPC by autoclaving at 121 °C for 20 min. Prepare and store all reagents at room temperature (unless indicated otherwise).

2.1 Collection of Plant Samples

1. Sterile scissors.
2. Sterile-filtered and DEPC-treated water.

2.2 Processing of Plant Material

2.2.1 Surface Sterilization of Plant Samples

1. 70% ethanol.
2. 2% sodium hypochlorite.
3. Sterile-filtered and DEPC-treated water.
4. LB agar (Luria/Miller) (Carl Roth, Karlsruhe, Germany).
5. Potato extract glucose agar (Carl Roth, Karlsruhe, Germany).
6. Malt extract agar (Carl Roth, Karlsruhe, Germany).

2.2.2 Homogenization of Plant Material

1. Mortar and pestle.
2. Liquid nitrogen.

2.3 DNA Extraction from Powdered Plant Material

1. Proteinase K, 20 mg/mL (Applichem, Darmstadt, Germany).

2. Glass beads (A556.1; Carl Roth, Karlsruhe, Germany).

3. PeqGold Plant DNA Mini kit (Peqlab, Erlangen, Germany).

4. Sterile-filtered and DEPC-treated water.

2.4 Amplification of Marker Genes

2.4.1 Amplification of Fungal ITS Sequences

1. Phusion High-Fidelity DNA Polymerase (2 U/μL) with reaction buffer GC (5×), 100 % dimethyl sulfoxide (DMSO) and 50 mM MgCl₂ (Thermo Fisher Scientific, Waltham, USA).

2. Fermentas™ 10 mM dNTP Mix (Thermo Fisher Scientific, Waltham, USA).

3. Ten micromolar solutions of each of the following oligonucleotides: ITS1-F_KYO2 (5′-TAGAGGAAGTAAAAGT CGTAA-3′) [7], ITS4 (5′-TCCTCCGCTTATTGATATGC-3′) [8] (*see* **Note 1**) as well as ITS3_KYO2 (5′-GATGAAGAACGYA GYRAA-3′) [7], ITS4 (5′-TCCTCCGCTTATTGATATGC-3′) [8] (*see* **Notes 1** and **2**).

4. PeqGOLD Gel Extraction kit (Peqlab, Erlangen, Germany).

5. Sterile-filtered and DEPC-treated water.

2.4.2 Amplification of Bacterial 16S rRNA Genes

1. Fermentas™ *Taq* DNA polymerase (1 U/μL) and reaction buffer with (NH₄)₂SO₄ (10×) and 25 mM MgCl₂ (Thermo Fisher Scientific, Waltham, USA).

2. Phusion High-Fidelity DNA Polymerase (2 U/μL) with HF reaction buffer (5×) (Thermo Fisher Scientific, Waltham, USA).

3. Fermentas™ 10 mM dNTP Mix (Thermo Fisher Scientific, Waltham, USA).

4. Ten micromolar solutions of each of the following oligonucleotides: 799f (5′-AACMGGATTAGATACCCKG-3′) [9], 1492R (5′-GCYTACCTTGTTACGACTT-3′) [10] (*see* **Note 3**) and F968 (5′-AACGCGAAGAACCTTAC-3′) [11], R1401 (5′-CGGTGTGTACAAGACCC-3′) [11] (*see* **Notes 2** and **4**).

5. PeqGOLD Gel Extraction Kit (Peqlab, Erlangen, Germany).

6. Sterile-filtered and DEPC-treated water.

2.5 Processing of Obtained Sequence Data

1. A computer running a 64-bit version of Linux and having at least 4 GB of memory available.

2. A 64 bit version of USEARCH (current version 8.1.1861; [12]) (*see* **Note 5**).

3. Reference files for use in UCHIME: the latest UNITE/INSDC reference dataset (https://unite.ut.ee/repository.php) for fungi [13] and the latest RDP Classifier trainset (https://sourceforge. net/projects/rdp-classifier/) for bacteria [14] (*see* **Note 6**).

4. Reference files for OTU classification: the latest QIIME release of the UNITE/INSDC dataset (https://unite.ut.ee/repository.php) for fungi [13] and the latest qiime release for the SILVA SSURef database (http://tax4fun.gobics.de/) for bacteria [15] (*see* **Note 7**).

5. R [16] (*see* **Note 8**).

3   Methods

Carry out all procedures at room temperature unless otherwise indicated. Use filter tips to set up PCR reactions. Autoclave solutions, mortar, pestle, and microtubes twice before use to avoid contamination with DNases, RNases, or nucleic acids. Wear gloves while working and take proper laboratory safety measures. Make sure to wear safety glasses and protective gloves, especially when working with liquid nitrogen. Diligently follow all waste disposal regulations when disposing of waste materials. Please read the notes added at the end of this protocol carefully.

3.1   Collection of Plant Material

1. Collect samples from different plant compartments such as leaves or roots using sterile scissors.

2. Samples from different plant parts should be processed separately as they harbor distinct endophytic communities.

3. Shake root samples and subsequently wash them with sterile filtered and DEPC-treated water to remove the adhering rhizosphere soil.

4. Store plant material at 4 °C prior to surface sterilization.

3.2   Processing of Plant Material

Surface sterilization is performed as described by Araujo et al. [17] with slight modifications.

3.2.1   Surface-Sterilization

1. Rinse plant material with 70% ethanol for 2 min.

2. Rinse plant material with 2% sodium hypochlorite for 3 min.

3. Rinse plant material with 70% ethanol for 30 s.

4. Rinse plant material three times with water for 30 s.

5. To control the success of the applied disinfection process, plate 100 μL aliquots of water from the final wash used in **step 4** on different agar plates.

6. Incubate agar plates at 25 °C in the dark for at least 2 weeks.

7. Use wash water from **step 4** in the first PCR targeting either the 16S rRNA gene or the ITS region to control the success of DNA removal (*see* Subheading 3.4.1, **step 2** and Subheading 3.4.2, **step 2**, respectively).

3.2.2 Homogenization of Plant Material

1. Homogenize surface-sterilized plant material with liquid nitrogen using sterile mortar and pestle.

2. Store powdered plant material at −20 °C until DNA extraction.

3.3 DNA Extraction

1. Extract DNA using the peqGOLD Plant DNA Mini kit according to the manufacturer's instructions with two modifications to improve initial cell lysis: add glass beads and 10 μL Proteinase K to the first step of the DNA extraction protocol.

2. Elute DNA with sterile-filtered and DEPC-treated water.

3.4 Amplification and Sequencing of Marker Genes

3.4.1 Amplification of Fungal ITS rRNA Genes

1. For the first PCR reaction mixture, combine the following ingredients in a sterile DNA-free 0.2 mL PCR tube: 5 μL of 5× Phusion GC buffer, 1 μL of primer ITS1F-KYO2, 1 μL of primer ITS4, 1.25 μL DMSO, 0.75 μL $MgCl_2$, 0.5 μL dNTP mix, 0.25 μL Phusion polymerase (2 U/μL), and approximately 25 ng of the DNA from Subheading 3.3, **step 2**. Add water to a final volume of 25 μL.

2. To control the success of the surface sterilization, use the water from the final washing step of the surface sterilization (*see* Subheading 3.2.1, **step** 7 as template.

3. Perform negative controls using the reaction mixture without template.

4. Use the following thermal cycling scheme for amplification: initial denaturation at 98 °C for 30 s, 6 cycles of: 15 s at 98 °C, 30 s at 53 °C (−0.5 °C per cycle), and 30 s at 72 °C, 20 cycles of: 15 s at 98 °C, 30 s at 50 °C, and 30 s at 72 °C, and a final extension at 72 °C for 2 min.

5. Control the success of the PCR by gel electrophoresis.

6. For the second PCR reaction mixture, combine the following ingredients in a sterile DNA-free 0.2 mL PCR tube: 5 μL of 5× Phusion GC buffer, 1 μL of primer ITS3F-KYO2 containing the MiSeq adaptor, 1 μL of primer ITS4 containing the MiSeq adaptor, 1.25 μL DMSO, 0.75 μL $MgCl_2$, 0.5 μL dNTP mix, and 0.25 μL Phusion polymerase (2 U/μL). Add up to a final volume of 24 μL with H_2O. The reaction mix can be scaled up as needed.

7. Add 1 μL of the first PCR reaction mixture.

8. Perform negative controls using the reaction mixture without template.

9. Use the thermal cycling scheme for amplification as described in **step 4**.

10. Purify the resulting PCR products using the peqGOLD Gel Extraction kit (Peqlab) according to the manufacturer's instructions.

11. Determine the sequences using the MiSeq Reagent Kit v3 on a MiSeq sequencer (Illumina, San Diego, USA).

1. For the first PCR reaction mixture, combine the following ingredients in a sterile DNA-free 0.2 mL PCR tube: 2.5 μL of 10× Mg-free *Taq* polymerase buffer, 1.75 μL MgCl$_2$, 0.5 μL of primer 799f, 0.5 μL of primer 1492r, 0.5 μL dNTP mix, 1.25 μL DMSO, and 1.5 μL *Taq* DNA polymerase (1 U/μL) and approximately 25 ng of the DNA from Subheading 3.3, **step 2** to the mixture. Add water to a final volume of 25 μL.

2. To control the success of the surface sterilization, use the wash water from the final washing step of the surface sterilization (*see* Subheading 3.2.1, **step 7**) as template.

3. Perform negative controls using the reaction mixture without template.

4. Use the following thermal cycling scheme for amplification: initial denaturation at 95 °C for 5 min, 35 cycles of: 1 min at 95 °C, 1 min at 50 °C, and 1 min at 72 °C, and a final extension at 72 °C for 5 min.

5. Control the success of the PCR by gel electrophoresis.

6. Purify the bacterial-specific band by gel extraction using the peqGOLD Gel Extraction Kit according to the manufacturer's instructions (*see* **Note 4**). Elute DNA in 30 μL sterile-filtered and DEPC-treated water.

7. For the second PCR reaction mixture, combine the following ingredients: 5 μL of 5× Phusion HF buffer, 1 μL of primer F968 containing the MiSeq adaptor, 1 μL of primer R1401 containing the MiSeq adaptor, 0.5 μL dNTP mix, and 0.5 μL of Phusion polymerase (2 U/μL). Add up to a final volume of 24 μL with H$_2$O. The reaction mix can be scaled up as needed.

8. Add 1 μL of the purified PCR product from **step 6**.

9. Perform negative controls using the reaction mixture without template.

10. Use the following thermal cycling scheme for amplification: initial denaturation at 98 °C for 30 s, 30 cycles of: 15 s at 98 °C, 30 s at 53 °C, and 30 s at 72 °C, and a final extension at 72 °C for 2 min.

11. Purify obtained PCR products using the peqGOLD Gel Extraction kit according to manufacturer's instructions.

12. Determine the sequences using the MiSeq Reagent Kit v3 on a MiSeq sequencer (Illumina, San Diego, USA).

3.5 Processing of Obtained Sequence Data

*3.5.1 Preprocessing
of Sequence Data
(Sample-Wise)*

After sequencing, you will obtain at least two files per sample: one file from the forward run and the second one from the reverse run. In the first step, sequences must be merged prior to further processing. In addition, reads being too short or having a bad quality have to be removed. Afterwards, every sample is tagged: a label is added to the header of each sequence. This label is needed for later remapping of all sequences on the final OTU sequences and OTU table generation. Afterwards, sequences can be dereplicated to remove redundant sequences and to decrease file size and, consequently, memory demand (*see* Subheading 3.3.2, **step 2** and **Note 5**). After preprocessing, data can also be uploaded to SILVA-NGS (https://www.arb-silva.de/ngs/) or MG-RAST (http://metagenomics.anl.gov/) for further processing.

1. Merge paired-end reads and remove reads having low-quality or being too short
   usearch -fastq_mergepairs SampleX_forward.fastq -reverse /
   SampleX_reverse.fastq   -fastqout   SampleX_merged_filtered.fastq /
   -fastq_minmergelen 300 -fastq_merge_maxee 1.0

2. Convert fastq to fasta and label all sequences for later remapping

usearch -fastq_filter SampleX_merged_filtered.fastq –fastaout /

SampleX_merged_filtered.fasta -sample "SampleX"

3.5.2 Processing of Preprocessed Data

The initial step is to join all preprocessed sequences from all investigated samples. Do not mix 16S rRNA gene and ITS data. They need to be processed separately. Afterwards, sequences are dereplicated, meaning that all identical sequences are reduced to a single sequence. Dereplicated sequences are clustered into operational taxonomic units (OTUs) using the UPARSE algorithm implemented in USEARCH [18]. The clustering involves a de novo chimera removal step. Afterwards, a reference based chimera removal is performed with UCHIME [19]. Taxonomy is subsequently assigned to each OTU by UBLAST alignment against a reference data set. Finally, the initial sequences are mapped on OTU sequences and the result of the mapping is converted to an OTU table.

1. Join all processed sequences.
   cat *_merged_filtered.fasta>AllSamples.fasta

2. Dereplicate all sequences.
   usearch -derep_fulllength AllSamples.fasta -fastaout /
   AllSamples_uniques.fasta -sizeout

3. Cluster sequences in operational taxonomic units.
   usearch -cluster_otus AllSamples_uniques.fasta -otus /
   AllSamples_otus.fasta -relabel OTU_ -sizein

4. Remove chimeras using UCHIME (*see* **Note 6**).
   usearch -uchime_ref AllSamples_otus.fasta –db /
   <PATH_TO_REFERENCE_DATA>-strand plus /
   -nonchimeras AllSamples_otus_uchime.fasta

5. Classify sequences suing UBLAST (*see* **Note 7**).
   usearch -usearch_local AllSamples_otus_uchime.fasta /

```
-db<PATH TO REFERENCE DATA>-id 0.9 -blast6out /
AllSamples_otus_uchime.taxonomy -top_hit_only -strand plus
```

6. Remap all preprocessed sequences on OTU sequences.
   usearch -usearch_global AllSamples.fasta -db /
   AllSamples_otus_uchime.fasta -strand plus /
   -id 0.97 -otutabout AllSamples_otu_table.txt

7. Add taxonomy to obtained OTU table using R.
   ```
   #Reading the generated OTU table
   OTU_TABLE=read.delim("AllSamples_otu_table.txt")
   #Reading the taxonomy file supplied with reference datasets
   FULL_TAX=read.delim("<PATH        TO        TAXONOMY
   DATA>", h=F)
   names(FULL_TAX)=c("Accession", "taxonomy")
   #Reading the first two columns of the local tax file generated /
   by UBLAST alignment against reference data
   UBLAST_TAX=read.delim("AllSamples_otus_uchime.taxon-
   omy", /
   h=F)[,1:2]
   names(LOCAL_TAX)=c("OTU ID", "Accession")
   #Merging local and full Taxonomy Files but deleting the first
   /
   column of the merged file
   JOINED_TAX=merge(LOCAL_TAX,              FULL_TAX,
   by="Accession")[,-1]
   # Merging the generated taxonomy table with the otu table
   TABLE_TAX=merge(TABLE, JOINED_TAX, by.x="X.OTU.
   ID", /
   by.y="OTU ID")
   # Writing output to new file
   write.table(TABLE_TAX, "AllSamples_otu_table_tax.txt", /
   sep="\t", quote=F, dec=".")
   #Generating a biom table for use in QIIME
   write("#OTU table generated with USEARCH", /
   "AllSamples_otu_table_tax_qiime.txt", sep="\t")
   names(TABLE_TAX)[1]="#OTU ID"
   write.table(TABLE_TAX,   "AllSamples_otu_table_tax_qiime.
   txt", /
   sep="\t", quote=F, dec=".", append=T)
   ```

4 Notes

1. Non-fungal ITS sequences are common contaminations. To suppress co-amplification of these sequences, the full region between the 18S rRNA and the 23S rRNA is amplified using oligonucleotides highly specific for fungi. The ITS2 region is subsequently amplified in a nested PCR

approach due to the limited read length of 2× 300 bp of the MiSeq sequencer. Increasing sequencing length might obviate the nested PCR.

2. Add MiSeq sequencing adaptors and/or barcode sequences to primer sequences used in the second PCR.

3. Plant-derived 16S rRNA data sets are usually contaminated with plastid-derived or mitochondrial sequences. The amount of sequence contamination is reduced by application of oligonucleotides suppressing co-amplification of plastid-derived sequences.

4. PCR amplification results in the formation of two PCR products: a mitochondrial product of approximately 1100 bp and a bacterial product of approximately 735 bp.

5. The 32-bit version of USEARCH is usually sufficient for studies with smaller sampling size and the corresponding data sets. However, two steps are usually problematic in terms of memory usage: the dereplication of all sequences and OTU classification. Sample-wise dereplication (*see* Subheading 3.5.2, **step 1**) prior to full-dereplication can bypass the first problem. For the second problem, we recommend to use the 'search_pcr' function implemented in USEARCH in combination with the primer sequences of the second PCR reaction to remove unnecessary sequence flanks.

6. It is usually recommended to use a well-curated 16S rRNA data set, e.g., the latest 16S rRNA training set of the RDP classifier, as reference database for chimera removal. Larger data sets such as SILVA or Greengenes contain many low-quality reads which degrade detection accuracy.

7. It is important that the reference data set used for classification contains sequences of known contaminations as the protocol described here only reduces the contamination rate. Obtained data might still contain non-bacterial and non-fungal sequences, respectively. These have to be removed prior to further sequence analysis.

8. For further sequence analysis, we recommend to use R and the vegan package. This, for example, allows data visualization via ordination analysis (PCA, CCA, NMDS) and calculation of alpha diversity indices.

References

1. Hardoim PR, van Overbeek LS, Berg G, Pirttila AM, Compant S, Campisano A et al (2015) The hidden world within plants, ecological and evolutionary considerations for defining functioning of microbial endophytes. Microbiol Mol Biol Rev 79:293–320

2. Lodewyckx C, Vangronsveld J, Porteous F, Moore ERB, Taghavi S, Mezgeay M et al (2002) Endophytic bacteria and their potential applications. Crit Rev Plant Sci 21:583–606

3. Bulgarelli D, Garrido-Oter R, Münch PC, Weiman A, Dröge J, Pan Y et al (2015)

Structure and function of the bacterial root microbiota in wild and domesticated barley. Cell Host Microbe 17:392–403

4. Gottel NR, Castro HF, Kerley M, Yang Z, Pelletier DA, Podar M et al (2011) Distinct microbial communities within the endosphere and rhizosphere of *Populus deltoides* roots across contrasting soil types. Appl Environ Microbiol 77:5934–5944

5. Wemheuer F, Wemheuer B, Kretzschmar D, Pfeiffer B, Herzog S, Daniel R et al (2016) Impact of grassland management regimes on bacterial endophyte diversity differs with grass species. Lett Appl Microbiol 62:323. doi:10.1111/lam.12551

6. Robinson RJ, Fraaije BA, Clark IM, Jackson RW, Hirsch PR, Mauchline TH (2016) Endophytic bacterial community composition in wheat (*Triticum aestivum*) is determined by plant tissue type, developmental stage and soil nutrient availability. Plant Soil 405:381

7. Toju H, Tanabe AS, Yamamoto S, Sato H (2012) High-coverage ITS primers for the DNA-based identification of ascomycetes and basidiomycetes in environmental samples. PLoS One 7:e40863

8. White TJ, Bruns T, Lee S, Taylor J (1990) Amplification and direct sequencing of fungal ribosomal RNA genes for phylogenetics. PCR Protoc 18:315–322

9. Chelius MK, Triplett EW (2001) The diversity of Archaea and Bacteria in association with the roots of *Zea mays* L. Microb Ecol 41:252–263

10. Lane DJ (1991) 16s/23s rRNA sequencing. In: Stackebrandt E, Goodfellow M (eds) Nucleic acid techniques in bacterial systematics. John Wiley & Sons, New York, NY, pp 115–175

11. Nübel U, Engelen B, Felske A, Snaidr J, Wieshuber A, Amann RI et al (1996) Sequence heterogeneities of genes encoding 16S rRNAs in *Paenibacillus polymyxa* detected by temperature gradient gel electrophoresis. J Bacteriol 178:5636–5643

12. Edgar RC (2010) Search and clustering orders of magnitude faster than BLAST. Bioinformatics 26:2460–2461

13. Abarenkov K, Henrik Nilsson R, Larsson K-H, Alexander IJ, Eberhardt U, Erland S et al (2010) The UNITE database for molecular identification of fungi – recent updates and future perspectives. New Phytol 186:281–285

14. Cole JR, Wang Q, Cardenas E, Fish J, Chai B, Farris RJ et al (2009) The Ribosomal Database Project, improved alignments and new tools for rRNA analysis. Nucleic Acids Res 37:D141–D145

15. Quast C, Pruesse E, Yilmaz P, Gerken J, Schweer T, Yarza P et al (2013) The SILVA ribosomal RNA gene database project, improved data processing and web-based tools. Nucleic Acids Res 41:D590–D596

16. R Core Team (2014) R, a language and environment for statistical computing. Vienna, R Foundation for Statistical Computing. Available at: http://www.R-project.org/

17. Araujo WL, Marcon J, Maccheroni W Jr, Van Elsas JD, Van Vuurde JW, Azevedo JL (2002) Diversity of endophytic bacterial populations and their interaction with *Xylella fastidiosa* in citrus plants. Appl Environ Microbiol 68:4906–4914

18. Edgar RC (2013) UPARSE: highly accurate OTU sequences from microbial amplicon reads. Nat Methods 10:996–998

19. Edgar RC, Haas BJ, Clemente JC, Quince C, Knight R (2011) UCHIME improves sensitivity and speed of chimera detection. Bioinformatics 27:2194–2200

Chapter 7

Shotgun Metagenomic Sequencing Analysis of Soft-Rot *Enterobacteriaceae* in Polymicrobial Communities

James Doonan, Sandra Denman, James E. McDonald, and Peter N. Golyshin

Abstract

Shotgun metagenomic sequencing of bacterial communities in necrotic plant lesions allows insights of host–pathogen molecular interactions. Soft-rot *Enterobacteriaceae* are significant crop pathogens with a wide host range. Reconstructed polymicrobial community DNA from soft-rot affected crops provides details of species relative abundance and functional potential, enabling significant insights into their lifestyle. Here, we describe a workflow for DNA recovery, metagenomic shotgun sequencing and in particular, an in silico analysis of bacterial isolates from affected plant tissue.

Key words Shotgun metagenomics, Host–pathogen molecular interactions, Soft-rot *Enterobacteriaceae*, Polymicrobial, In silico

1 Introduction

1.1 Soft-Rot Enterobacteriaceae

The soft-rot *Enterobacteriaceae* (SRE) are a family of lytic bacterial plant pathogens which include members of the former soft-rot *Erwiniae*, primarily belonging to the *Pectobacterium* and *Dickeya* genera [1]. These bacteria are responsible for substantial commercial loss on arable and horticultural crops and are both represented in the top ten bacterial plant pathogens [2]. SRE are necrotrophic or brute force pathogens which break down plant tissue and establish infection primarily through pathogenicity components known as Plant Cell Wall Degrading Enzymes (PCWDE). Unlike the lipid based structures of mammalian cell walls, plant cell walls are composed of polysaccharides (pectate and cellulose). PCWDE must be armed with the capability to target these particular polysaccharides in order for the pathogen to be virulent [1]. Animal pathogenic *Enterobacteriaceae* also produce PCWDE, but at much lower levels, and have a reduced capacity to macerate plant tissue [3]. SRE discharge specific enzymes which destroy plant cell wall polysaccharides (soft-rot disease) and release nutrients for bacterial

Wolfgang R. Streit and Rolf Daniel (eds.), *Metagenomics: Methods and Protocols*, Methods in Molecular Biology, vol. 1539, DOI 10.1007/978-1-4939-6691-2_7, © Springer Science+Business Media LLC 2017

growth [4]. These species depolymerise host tissues through the release of exoenzymes, including cellulases, proteases, and multiple isoforms of pectinase [5]. Each isoform may be specific to a particular host, the combined capability of these multiple isoforms allows the pathogen to attack various substrates. Cellulases degrade the primary and secondary plant cell walls, but along with proteases, are minor virulence factors in these pathogens. Pectinases are major pathogenicity factors, which break down the middle lamella and plant cell walls, resulting in tissue collapse, cell damage, and leakage [6]. Resultant degraded products are transported across the bacterial cell membrane and catabolized [7]. Catabolism of host tissue is a targeted process reliant on global regulators which dictate translocation of PCWDE at appropriate moments to maximize destruction [8].

1.2 Secretion Systems

To enable macromolecules such as PCWDE to cross bacterial membranes, proteinaceous nanomachines known as secretion systems are employed to facilitate the process. Secretion systems are critical to the study of bacterial virulence, as they enable delivery of many toxins and effectors to recipient cells. Secretion systems are key virulence determinants amongst the *Enterobacteriaceae* [1, 2]. Pathogenicity determinants (including PCWDE) require secretion system mediated transport into the extracellular surroundings or directly into host cells. The basic secretion apparatus consists of "core components"—which are necessary for secretion, and identification of these in silico is typically a strong indicator of functionality [9]. However, it should be noted that in silico validation is not evidence of gene expression as a large number of vestigial secretion system genes may be present without being functional [10].

1.3 Horizontal Gene Transfer

The SRE have a battery of established virulence factors. Their reproductive success in wide ranging hosts is in part due to their proclivity for gene loss and horizontal gene transfer (HGT). This presents a method of virulence gene uptake "*en bloc*," as opposed to the slow evolutionary process of selective point mutations [11]. Additionally, this propensity to exchange genes allows rapid adaptation to novel environments and can ultimately lead to speciation due to the diversifying power of HGT. Virulence genes found within a metagenome can be readily acquired by *Enterobacteriaceae* in the polymicrobial environment and retained if they present an evolutionary advantage, as opposed to nonbeneficial genes which are rapidly lost in the dynamics of genome fluctuation [12]. This gene gain/loss model perpetuates the view of the microbiome as a community genome whose genes are not only the preserve of a single bacterium, but as the property of a collective dynamic entity [13]. To understand community functionality a holistic approach is required to gain a broader view of inter-bacterial relationships acting synergistically and antagonistically. This can be explored through sequenced-based environmental genomics [14].

1.4 Metagenomics

Environmental genomics or metagenomics of diseased plant tissue allows identification of the taxonomic and functional diversity of the polymicrobial community. Metagenomics provides a cultivation-independent approach to align the key organisms and enzymes which are drivers of disease in the ecosystem. A wealth of information can be revealed from metagenomic analyses of microbial communities, including phylogenetic composition, known and novel functional types, adaptation to specific environments and the distribution of gene families across ecosystems [15]. Sequencing methods commonly use Next Generation Sequencing technologies, and many excellent reviews describe these, e.g., [16]. This chapter presents an overview of microbiome analysis of taxonomic and functional diversity. This allows two key questions to be addressed:

1. What is in the community?

2. What functional potential do they have?

2   Materials

2.1 DNA Extraction Chemicals

1. Qiagen (Manchester, UK) Gentra Puregene Yeast/Bact. kit.

2.2 DNA Enrichment Chemicals

1. Qiagen (Manchester, UK) QIAamp DNA microbiome kit.

2.3 DNA Library Preparation Kit

1. Illumina (Illumina UK, Little Chesterford, UK) Nextera DNA library preparation kit.

2.4 Laboratory Equipment

1. Mallet and chisel.

2. Pestle and mortar.

3. Illumina HiSeq 2500 sequencing platform.

4. Qubit Fluorometer v3.0 (Thermo Fisher).

2.5 Software

1. FastQC [17]—initial analysis of metagenomic sequence data.

2. Cutadapt [18]—removes adapters from the sequence data.

3. Trim Galore! [19]—removes adapters and can be used if adapter sequence is unknown.

4. Sickle [20]—removes low quality sequence data.

5. Ray-Meta [21]—assembles metagenomic sequence data.

6. MEGAN [22]—clusters related sequence data into bins.

7. Prokka [23]—general metagenomic taxonomic and functional analysis tool.

8. HUMAnN2 [24]—general metagenomic taxonomic and functional analysis tool.

9. LefSe [25]—statistical package for analysis differences between datasets.

10. GraPhlAn [26]—visualization aid.

11. bCAN [27]—specific annotation tool for CAZymes.

12. T346Hunter [28]—specific annotation tool for Type III, IV, and VI secretion systems.

3   Methods

3.1   Shotgun Metagenomic Sequencing Strategy

1. Random shotgun metagenome sequencing enables the study of entire communities of microorganisms without cultivation. First, total DNA is extracted from the samples prior to pooling in equimolar quantities (if required), shearing, library preparation, and sequencing of the resultant nucleic acid library.

2. Sequencing strategies should be designed to address research questions, if for example extensive coverage of a microbial community is required, then short fragment assemblies are the best option, whereas for more accurate contiguous sequences a combination of short and long fragment sequencing may be more appropriate [29]. This hybrid approach will likely consist of paired-end fragment sequencing, producing sequences of around 150 base pairs (bp) (using the Illumina HiSeq 2500) and a mate pair library with large fragments of between 800 and 1000 bp (using the Roche 454 sequencer), or far longer, highly accurate fragments using the Pacific Biosciences RSII sequencing platform [30]. Clearly, these combined methods increase time and project costs, and they require a far higher concentration of starting material. Currently, there are few studies where complete genomes have been generated from deep sequencing of a metagenome, with notable exceptions such as the near complete reconstruction of the verrucomicrobial class *Spartobacteria* genome from the Baltic Sea using only 454 mate pair, large fragment libraries, but with a sample known to have a high concentration of the bacterium [31]. Through initially sorting cells with a Fluorescence Activated Cell Sorter (FACS) before using shotgun sequencing, 201 uncultivated bacterial and archaeal cells from nine diverse habitats were assembled into finished genomes [32]. However, this "single-cell" genomics method combined with shotgun sequencing is constrained by limitations in throughput, potential for contamination, increased expense and time considerations [33]. For most metagenomic studies, extensive paired end fragment libraries are the most appropriate method, as this will

generate the greatest depth of coverage and allow research questions relating to the composition and functionality of the community to be addressed. Therefore, we focus on the Illumina HiSeq 2500 sequencing platform (Illumina UK, Little Chesterford, UK), which currently produces the highest coverage, is relatively inexpensive and is generally considered to be the most appropriate metagenomic sequencing platform available.

3. Short fragment sequencing platforms produce a large volume of sequences containing nonrandom errors. There are technical difficulties resulting from this approach, the first originates from the sequencing platform, but continues to the assembly process where error strewn sequences are merged into contiguous genomes, producing mis-assemblies as an integral part of the output, of which collapsed repeats, sequence rearrangements and inversions are the classic signatures [34]. The second issue is the nature of microbial communities, which vary greatly in terms of species abundance. Assembly outputs allow relative abundance measurements; however, in a species rich sample, many individuals could be missed due to the finite number of sequence fragments. Therefore prior knowledge of community structure will guide estimations of required assembly depth [29]. This may be practically difficult, especially for novel communities, and therefore, good practice would allow for broad shallow sequencing pilot studies prior to deep sequencing. Overall, it is thought that in large datasets less abundant taxa will be missed; however, dominant clades are expected to play the most significant functional roles under normal conditions [15]. Furthermore, metagenome taxonomic abundance and functional profiles often reflect metatranscriptome expression data [35].

3.2 Experimental Design and Sampling

1. For a statistically robust analysis of biological variation in a community an appropriate number of technical and biological replicates must be sampled, for guidance *see* [36].

3.2.1 Plant Tissue Homogenization

1. The optimal method of host tissue homogenization for bacterial DNA extraction, will vary between samples. For plant roots a ribolyzer (Thermo Savant FastPrep 120 Cell Disrupter System) may be the most appropriate, e.g., [37]. For leaves a bead beater (BeadBeater, Thistle Scientific) may be the most appropriate, e.g., [38]. For homogenization of woody tissue, use a mallet and chisel to remove the lesion, then place the material into an appropriate container and transfer to liquid nitrogen storage. Successful homogenization can be measured by recovery of bacterial DNA; however, for each sample the best method will vary. For all disruption methods, prepare a

container (for example, polystyrene) to contain a volume of liquid nitrogen, and which is able to hold a mortar. Polystyrene is surprisingly adept at holding liquid nitrogen; a polystyrene box works well. Place mortar in container and pour in the liquid nitrogen, also add a small amount into the mortar. Remove sample from the liquid nitrogen storage and transfer to mortar. Using the pestle, homogenize tissue into a fine powder (*see* **Note 1**).

3.2.2   DNA Extraction

1. The Qiagen (Manchester, UK) Gentra Puregene Yeast/Bact. Kit, produces a high total volume of DNA and has successfully isolated bacterial DNA from necrotic plant lesions, e.g., [39] [for alternatives *see* **Note 2**].

3.2.3   Bacterial DNA Enrichment

1. A barrier to maximizing sequencing coverage is the amount of host DNA within the microbiome. Sequencing of diseased plant tissue can result in an overwhelming amount of DNA from the far larger host genome, greatly undermining a true representation of the microbiome [40]. This anomaly can be overcome by selectively enriching microbial DNA. The Qiagen QIAamp DNA microbiome kit takes advantage of the robust morphology of bacterial cells by lysing the more labile eukaryotic cells and enzymatically degrading their DNA, thus depleting the sample of host DNA [for alternatives *see* **Note 3**].

3.2.4   Library Preparation

1. DNA is prepared for sequencing using platform specific library preparation kits. Each sequencing platform, e.g., Pacific Biosciences RSII, Oxford Nanopore MinION or Illumina HiSeq has tailored kits, with a specific workflow. For the Illumina HiSeq, there are three kits available for shotgun metagenomic sequencing, these are; the TruSeq DNA PCR free kit, TruSeq Nano DNA kit and the Nextera DNA kit. The TruSeq kits differ in the amount of input DNA required, with low input volume for the Nano kit (25–75 ng DNA) and high input volume for the PCR free methods (1–2 μg). Due to its enzymatic fragmentation method the Nextera kit offers larger output sequences (300–1500 bp), low input volume (50 ng) and shorter preparation time, compared to the mechanical fragmentation and lower output sequence length (350 or 550 bp) of the TruSeq methods.

3.3   Pre-assembly Data Optimization

The Illumina HiSeq produces sequence data in Fastq format. These are typically left and right or 5′ and 3′, paired end sequences, in large compressed files.

3.3.1   Sequencing Output Data and Quality Control

1. For a rapid check of sequence data quality, the Java based, NGS quality check program FastQC [17] offers an intuitive graphical display of sequence data quality. Fastq files can be directly loaded into the program.

3.3.2 Removing Adapters and Low Quality Sequences

1. Attached sequence adapters should be removed prior to assembly. The Unix based program Cutadapt [18], removes adapters, if the adapter sequence is known, or Trim Galore! [19], a wrapper tool for Cutadapt, can automatically detect and remove adapter sequences.

2. Removing low quality sequence data will improve the accuracy of resultant assemblies, the Unix based NGS tool Sickle [20] trims and discards poor quality data. Resultant trimmed high quality sequence data in Fastq format is now ready for downstream applications.

3.4 Taxonomic Diversity

Metagenome assembly, typically employs de novo methods, based on de Bruijn graph algorithms, where collinear overlapping sequences are merged into contiguous sequences or contigs, in Fasta format.

1. Metagenome assemblers include MetaVelvet [41] and Ray-Meta [21]. Assembly accuracy can be measured using ALE [42]. Assembled genomes can be explored using downstream applications, such as Prokka [23] which uses assembled contigs to predict coding domains and for subsequent function based homology searches.

2. An alternative method is to cluster or bin sequences into either taxonomic groups (this can be order, family, genus, etc.) or distinguishing features such as GC content or sequence similarity to a database. Possibly the most well-known of these tools is MEGAN [22], which uses sequence similarity searches against a database to separate sequences into bins.

3. Assembly and binning can be used in combination, as individual bins can be assembled, allowing greater accuracy [40].

These methods allow for an understanding of the taxonomic diversity of the community (*see* **Note 4**), allowing the first question of metagenomics (i.e., what is there?) to be answered (Fig. 1).

3.5 Taxonomic and Functional Annotation

1. MG-RAST is an open source interactive metagenomic annotation pipeline which provides an excellent starting point for annotation of assembled data and contextualization of results [44]. It requires assembled contigs or unassembled Fastq files (N.B. these take considerably longer for processing) to be uploaded to the server. Data can then be explored and analyzed, with excellent graphical comparison tools to visualize differences in both taxonomic composition and functional abundance between datasets. These images along with a variety of data file formats can be downloaded for use in downstream analysis or as an endpoint.

2. An alternative general annotation method, particularly for those with sensitive data (such as clinical data), is the locally

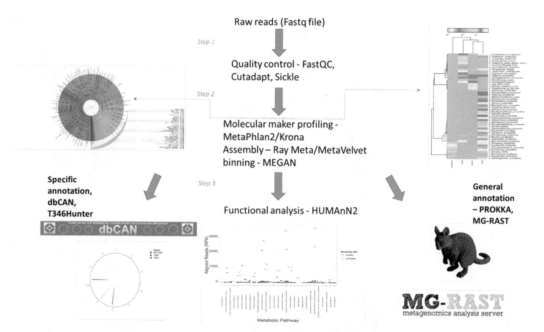

Fig. 1 Flowchart beginning with metagenomic sequencing data. Step 1—Data QC. Step 2—Measure relative species abundance, depicted here using MetaPhlan2 (as part of the HUMAnN software package) and illustrated with a heatmap of the top 100 species present at the genus and species level from healthy and unhealthy plant microbiomes, and a Krona plot [43] of all taxonomic levels. Step 3—Functional analysis, illustrated with output from HUMAnN2, with sample sequences from healthy and unhealthy plant microbiomes aligned against the MetaCyc database. General annotation is helpful for taxonomic and functional data overview illustrated here with PROKKA and MG-RAST. Specific annotation provides a closer examination of community function examining genes/pathways of interest such as PCWDE using the CAZy database, here through dbCAN, and secretion systems using T346Hunter, illustrated within a genome

installable genomic and metagenomic annotation pipeline, Prokka [23]. This customizable Unix based annotation program can incorporate private genomes without adding them to a public database. It requires assembled metagenome Fasta files as input and provides extensively annotated data files in various formats for use in downstream applications such as the genome browser Artemis [45]. Furthermore, tabulated output data can be easily converted for visualization in the genome aesthetic program Circos [46]. Circos can display an array of coordinate dependent data such as metagenomic contigs with aligned annotations or metagenome annotations aligned to individual genomes (Fig. 2).

3. Using standalone BLAST (Basic Local Alignment Search Tool) [47], to query an assembled, structurally annotated metagenome dataset against a locally installed database, remains one of the best methods to understand the relative abundance and functional profile of individual bacteria within a metagenome. This method allows manageable, fine scale analysis of annotated

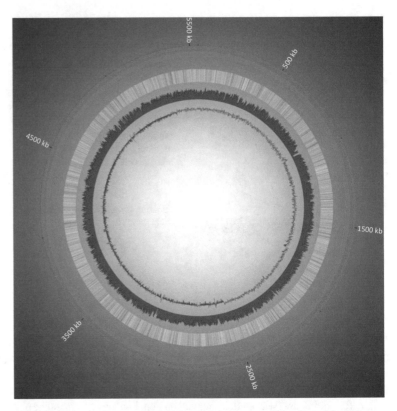

Fig. 2 Circos plot of an annotated bacterial genome with aligned homologous metagenome coding domains. From outer ring; bacterial chromosome, annotated genes, metagenome annotations from several libraries (libraries distinguished by specific color), GC content, GC skew

genes of interest, which can be an important consideration when dealing with prodigious datasets. A compiled database of bacterial proteins (or genes) of interest, queried (using stringent cut-offs) by metagenomic proteins will retrieve homologs between the metagenome and the bacteria, allowing an understanding of the relationship of one or a small number of bacteria to the relative abundance and functional profile of the metagenome. This method is demonstrated using a Circos plot, where a metagenome has been queried against a bacterium (Fig. 2).

4. The Human Microbiome Project Unified Metabolic Analysis Network (HUMAnN) is a functional and taxonomic prediction program, originally developed for the human microbiome project by the Huttenhower lab as part of the bioBakery suite of microbiome tools [24]. HUMAnN2 is an updated extension of this program which can be applied to any sequenced bacterial community. HUMAnN2 first measures relative abundance through MetaPhlan2, then reconstructs the metabolic potential of bacterial communities, based on a large collection

of experimentally verified pathways. It answers the two questions of metagenomic sequencing mentioned above, i.e., (1) What is present? (2) What are they capable of doing?

5. HUMAnN2 takes Fastq files as input data. Sequences are characterized individually, therefore paired end sequences must be concatenated before use. There are three main output files, in tsv format, which provide information on functional gene abundance and their taxonomic origin (genefamilies), metabolic potential of the community (pathabundance) and presence/absence of a metabolic pathway in the community (pathcoverage). The pathabundance data file contains sequences which have aligned to the MetaCyc database and profiles the abundance of sequences per metabolic pathway (Fig. 1). The pathabundance file can be passed to the bioBakery tool LEfSe [25], which uses prior knowledge of the metagenome to create a robust statistical class comparison of taxonomic and metabolic relationships across metagenome phylogenies using biomarkers specific to each metagenome [48]. Resultant differences between taxonomic and functional hierarchies can be visualized using the metagenome phylogeny tool GraPhlAn [26].

3.6 Specific Annotation Tools

1. Biological databases often lack oversight and contain many erroneously identified products. The manually curated CAZy database is an exemplary resource which identifies closely related carbohydrate active enzymes (CAZymes) and actively updates nomenclature in keeping with taxonomic appraisals [49]. CAZymes are enzymes involved in the assembly (glycosyltransferases) and breakdown (glycoside hydrolases, polysaccharide lyases, and carbohydrate esterases) of complex carbohydrates.

2. A simple method to explore annotation data in the CAZy database is through the online server dbCAN [27]. Using hidden Markov models dbCAN searches for CAZyme signature domain regions to identify CAZymes and transfer annotation from the protein database if the CAZyme family is known. Additionally, dbCAN has links to GenBank [50] and Pfam [51] domain-based searches to further explore annotated CAZymes. Submission of data to dbCAN requires a translated protein file. Prokka faa output files can be uploaded directly to dbCAN.

3. Extracting secretion system coding domains from general annotation databases can be laborious and confusing as various nomenclature schemes are used. Using hidden Markov models, the Type 3, 4 and 6 secretion system Hunter (T346Hunter) [28], provides a web-based tool for the prediction of secretion system clusters and unifies the nomenclature. This annotation tool was designed for bacterial genomes, but multi-contig metagenome Fasta files can be uploaded to the server and a

detailed analysis will be provided. Unfortunately, SRE translocate PCWDE across the cell membrane using the Type II secretion system [1], which is not included in the pipeline, and therefore, manual detection of these genes (usually clustered in operons) is required.

4 Notes

1. When homogenizing plant tissue in Subheading 3.2.1, maintain a low level of liquid nitrogen in the polystyrene container and mortar, topping up when necessary.

2. Aside from the DNA extraction method described in Subheading 3.2.2, there are many easy to use alternative methods such as the alkali method [52], which has been used successfully in many plant associated microbial DNA extractions, e.g., [53].

3. The New England BioLabs NEBnext microbiome DNA enrichment kit offers an alternative host DNA removal method, to that described in Subheading 3.2.3, it targets the CpG-methylated DNA of eukaryotes, relying on the rarity of CpG-methylated DNA in bacteria to deplete the sample of eukaryotic DNA.

4. There are a number of metagenomic analysis software packages beyond those described in Subheading 3.4, a further program of note is OneCodex, a recently developed taxonomic abundance measurement package, which offers a user friendly GUI, excellent graphics, and a simple drag-and-drop upload facility [54].

5 Conclusions

Shotgun metagenomic sequencing allows the taxonomic and functional characterization of polymicrobial communities. Here we describe contemporary analysis methods of SRE DNA recovered from affected plant tissue. There are numerous methods to generate and analyze resultant data beyond those described here; however, it is important to choose the most appropriate methods to answer the key questions of metagenomics: (1) What is there? (2) What are they doing?

References

1. Toth IK, Pritchard L, Birch PR (2006) Comparative genomics reveals what makes an enterobacterial plant pathogen. Annu Rev Phytopathol 44:305–336

2. Mansfield J, Genin S, Magori S, Citovsky V, Sriariyanum M, Ronald P et al (2012) Top 10 plant pathogenic bacteria in molecular plant pathology. Mol Plant Pathol 13:614–629

3. Manulis S, Kobayashi DY, Keen NT (1988) Molecular cloning and sequencing of a pectate lyase gene from *Yersinia pseudotuberculosis*. J Bacteriol 170:1825–1830

4. Toth IK, Bell KS, Holeva MC, Birch PR (2003) Soft rot erwiniae: from genes to genomes. Mol Plant Pathol 4:17–30

5. Beaulieu C, Boccara M, Vangijsegem F (1993) Pathogenic behavior of pectinase-defective *Erwinia chrysanthemi* mutants on different plants. Mol Plant Microb Interact 6:197–202

6. Barras F, van Gijsegem F, Chatterjee AK (1994) Extracellular enzymes and pathogenesis of soft-rot erwinia. Annu Rev Phytopathol 32:201–234

7. Nasser W, Reverchon S, Robert-Baudouy J (1992) Purification and functional characterization of the KdgR protein, a major repressor of pectinolysis genes of *Erwinia chrysanthemi*. Mol Microbiol 6:257–265

8. Nykyri J, Niemi O, Koskinen P, Nokso-Koivisto J, Pasanen M, Broberg M et al (2012) Revised phylogeny and novel horizontally acquired virulence determinants of the model soft rot phytopathogen *Pectobacterium wasabiae* SCC3193. PLoS Pathog 8, e1003013

9. Murdoch SL, Trunk K, English G, Fritsch MJ, Pourkarimi E, Coulthurst SJ (2011) The opportunistic pathogen *Serratia marcescens* utilizes type VI secretion to target bacterial competitors. J Bacteriol 193:6057–6069

10. Ochman H, Davalos LM (2006) The nature and dynamics of bacterial genomes. Science 311:1730–1733

11. Dobrindt U, Hochhut B, Hentschel U, Hacker J (2004) Genomic islands in pathogenic and environmental microorganisms. Nat Rev Microbiol 2:414–424

12. Nowell RW, Green S, Laue BE, Sharp PM (2014) The extent of genome flux and its role in the differentiation of bacterial lineages. Genome Biol Evol 6:1514–1529

13. Goldenfeld N, Woese C (2007) Biology's next revolution. Nature 445:369

14. Marchi G, Sisto A, Cimmino A, Andolfi A, Cipriani MG, Evidente A, Surico G (2006) Interaction between *Pseudomonas savastanoi* pv. *savastanoi* and *Pantoea agglomerans* in olive knots. Plant Pathol 55:614–624

15. Knight R, Jansson J, Field D, Fierer N, Desai N, Fuhrman JA et al (2012) Unlocking the potential of metagenomics through replicated experimental design. Nat Biotechnol 30:513–520

16. Loman NJ, Pallen MJ (2015) Twenty years of bacterial genome sequencing. Nat Rev Microbiol 13:787–794

17. Andrews S (2010) FastQC: a quality control tool for high throughput sequence data. Available at: http://www.bioinformatics.babraham.ac.uk/projects/fastqc

18. Martin M (2011) Cutadapt removes adapter sequences from high-throughput sequencing reads. EMBnetJ 17(1):10–12

19. Krueger F (2013) Trim Galore!: a wrapper tool around Cutadapt and FastQC to consistently apply quality and adapter trimming to FastQ files.

20. Joshi N and Fass J (2011) Sickle. A sliding-window, adaptive, quality-based trimming tool for FastQ files.

21. Boisvert S, Raymond F, Godzaridis E, Laviolette F, Corbeil J (2012) Ray Meta: scalable *de novo* metagenome assembly and profiling. Genome Biol 13:R122

22. Huson DH, Auch AF, Qi J, Schuster SC (2007) MEGAN analysis of metagenomic data. Genome Res 17:377–386

23. Seemann T (2014) Prokka: rapid prokaryotic genome annotation. Bioinformatics 30:2068–2069

24. Abubucker S, Segata N, Goll J, Schubert AM, Izard J, Cantarel BL et al (2012) Metabolic reconstruction for metagenomic data and its application to the human microbiome. PLoS Comput Biol 8, e1002358

25. Segata N, Izard J, Waldron L, Gevers D, Miropolsky L, Garrett WS, Huttenhower C (2011) Metagenomic biomarker discovery and explanation. Genome Biol 12:R60

26. Asnicar F, Weingart G, Tickle TL, Huttenhower C, Segata N (2015) Compact graphical representation of phylogenetic data and metadata with GraPhlAn. PeerJ 3:e1029

27. Yin Y, Mao X, Yang J, Chen X, Mao F, Xu Y (2012) dbCAN: a web resource for automated carbohydrate-active enzyme annotation. Nucleic Acids Res 40:W445–W451

28. Martinez-Garcia PM, Ramos C, Rodriguez-Palenzuela P (2015) T346Hunter: a novel web-based tool for the prediction of type III, type IV and type VI secretion systems in bacterial genomes. PLoS One 10, e0119317

29. Vieites JM, Guazzaroni ME, Beloqui A, Golyshin PN, Ferrer M (2009) Metagenomics approaches in systems microbiology. FEMS Microbiol Rev 33:236–255

30. Frank JA, Pan Y, Tooming-Klunderud A, Eijsink VGH, McHardy AC, Nederbragt AJ, Pope PB (2015) Improved metagenome assemblies and taxonomic binning using long-read circular consensus sequence data. bioRxiv doi: 10.1101/026922.

31. Herlemann DP, Lundin D, Labrenz M, Jurgens K, Zheng Z, Aspeborg H, Andersson AF (2013) Metagenomic *de novo* assembly of an aquatic representative of the verrucomicrobial class Spartobacteria. MBio 4:e00569–12

32. Rinke C, Schwientek P, Sczyrba A, Ivanova NN, Anderson IJ, Cheng JF et al (2013) Insights into the phylogeny and coding potential of microbial dark matter. Nature 499:431–437

33. Darling AE, Jospin G, Lowe E, Matsen FA, Bik HM, Eisen JA (2014) PhyloSift: phylogenetic analysis of genomes and metagenomes. PeerJ 2:e243

34. Phillippy AM, Schatz MC, Pop M (2008) Genome assembly forensics: finding the elusive mis-assembly. Genome Biol 9:R55

35. Mason OU, Hazen TC, Borglin S, Chain PS, Dubinsky EA, Fortney JL et al (2012) Metagenome, metatranscriptome and single-cell sequencing reveal microbial response to Deepwater Horizon oil spill. ISME J 6:1715–1727

36. Ju F, Zhang T (2015) Experimental design and bioinformatics analysis for the application of metagenomics in environmental sciences and biotechnology. Environ Sci Technol 49:12628–12640

37. Viebahn M, Veenman C, Wernars K, van Loon LC, Smit E, Bakker PA (2005) Assessment of differences in ascomycete communities in the rhizosphere of field-grown wheat and potato. FEMS Microbiol Ecol 53:245–253

38. Cai R, Lewis J, Yan S, Liu H, Clarke CR, Campanile F et al (2011) The plant pathogen *Pseudomonas syringae* pv. tomato is genetically monomorphic and under strong selection to evade tomato immunity. PLoS Pathog 7, e1002130

39. Maes M, Huvenne H, Messens E (2009) *Brenneria salicis*, the bacterium causing watermark disease in willow, resides as an endophyte in wood. Environ Microbiol 11:1453–1462

40. Sharpton TJ (2014) An introduction to the analysis of shotgun metagenomic data. Front Plant Sci 5:209

41. Namiki T, Hachiya T, Tanaka H, Sakakibara Y (2012) MetaVelvet: an extension of Velvet assembler to *de novo* metagenome assembly from short sequence reads. Nucleic Acids Res 40, e155

42. Clark SC, Egan R, Frazier PI, Wang Z (2013) ALE: a generic assembly likelihood evaluation framework for assessing the accuracy of genome and metagenome assemblies. Bioinformatics 29:435–443

43. Ondov BD, Bergman NH, Phillippy AM (2011) Interactive metagenomic visualization in a Web browser. BMC Bioinformatics 12:385

44. Meyer F, Paarmann D, D'Souza M, Olson R, Glass EM, Kubal M et al (2008) The metagenomics RAST server - a public resource for the automatic phylogenetic and functional analysis of metagenomes. BMC Bioinformatics 9:386

45. Carver T, Harris SR, Berriman M, Parkhill J, McQuillan JA (2012) Artemis: an integrated platform for visualization and analysis of high-throughput sequence-based experimental data. Bioinformatics 28:464–469

46. Krzywinski M, Schein J, Birol I, Connors J, Gascoyne R, Horsman D et al (2009) Circos: an information aesthetic for comparative genomics. Genome Res 19:1639–1645

47. Altschul SF, Gish W, Miller W, Myers E, Lipman D, Park U (1990) Basic local alignment search tool. J Mol Biol 215:403–410

48. Segata N, Boernigen D, Tickle TL, Morgan XC, Garrett WS, Huttenhower C (2013) Computational meta'omics for microbial community studies. Mol Syst Biol 9:666

49. Lombard V, Golaconda Ramulu H, Drula E, Coutinho PM, Henrissat B (2014) The carbohydrate-active enzymes database (CAZy) in 2013. Nucleic Acids Res 42:D490–D495

50. Benson DA, Clark K, Karsch-Mizrachi I, Lipman DJ, Ostell J, Sayers EW (2015) GenBank. Nucleic Acids Res 43:D30–D35

51. Finn RD, Mistry J, Tate J, Coggill P, Heger A, Pollington JE et al (2010) The Pfam protein families database. Nucleic Acids Res 38:D211–D222

52. Niemann S, Pühler A, Tichy HV, Simon R, Selbitschka W (1997) Evaluation of the resolving power of three different DNA fingerprinting methods to discriminate among isolates of a natural *Rhizobium meliloti* population. J Appl Microbiol 82:477–484

53. Brady C, Hunter G, Kirk S, Arnold D, Denman S (2014) *Rahnella victoriana* sp. nov., *Rahnella bruchi* sp. nov., *Rahnella woolbedingensis* sp. nov., classification of *Rahnella* genomospecies 2 and 3 as *Rahnella variigena* sp. nov. and *Rahnella inusitata* sp. nov., respectively and emended description of the genus *Rahnella*. Syst Appl Microbiol 37:545–552

54. Minot SS, Krumm N, Greenfield NB (2015) One codex : a sensitive and accurate data platform for genomic microbial identification. bioRxiv.

Chapter 8

Cloning and Expression of Metagenomic DNA in *Streptomyces lividans* and Subsequent Fermentation for Optimized Production

Yuriy Rebets, Jan Kormanec, Andriy Luzhetskyy, Kristel Bernaerts, and Jozef Anné

Abstract

The choice of an expression system for the metagenomic DNA of interest is of vital importance for the detection of any particular gene or gene cluster. Most of the screens to date have used the gram-negative bacterium *Escherichia coli* as a host for metagenomic gene libraries. However, the use of *E. coli* introduces a potential host bias since only 40% of the enzymatic activities may be readily recovered by random cloning in *E. coli*. To recover some of the remaining 60%, alternative cloning hosts such as *Streptomyces* spp. have been used. Streptomycetes are high-GC gram-positive bacteria belonging to the *Actinomycetales* and they have been studied extensively for more than 15 years as an alternative expression system. They are extremely well suited for the expression of DNA from other actinomycetes and genomes of high GC content. Furthermore, due to its high innate, extracellular secretion capacity, *Streptomyces* can be a better system than *E. coli* for the production of many extracellular proteins. In this article an overview is given about the materials and methods for growth and successful expression and secretion of heterologous proteins from diverse origin using *Streptomyces lividans* has a host. More in detail, an overview is given about the protocols of transformation, type of plasmids used and of vectors useful for integration of DNA into the host chromosome, and accompanying cloning strategies. In addition, various control elements for gene expression including synthetic promoters are discussed, and methods to compare their strength are described. Integration of the gene of interest under the control of the promoter of choice into *S. lividans* chromosome via homologous recombination using pAMR4-based system is explained. Finally a basic protocol for benchtop bioreactor experiments which can form the start in the production process optimization and upscaling is provided.

Key words *Streptomyces*, Expression, Cloning, Actinomycetes, Cloning vectors, Integrative vectors, Plasmids, Protein secretion, Fermentation

The original version of this chapter was revised. The erratum to this chapter is available at:
DOI 10.1007/978-1-4939-6691-2_20

Wolfgang R. Streit and Rolf Daniel (eds.), *Metagenomics: Methods and Protocols*, Methods in Molecular Biology, vol. 1539,
DOI 10.1007/978-1-4939-6691-2_8, © Springer Science+Business Media LLC 2017

1 Introduction

Metagenomics offers unprecedented opportunities for enzyme mining and allows the diversion and exploitation of biochemical pathways. Both sequence-based as well as function-based approaches are used. For sequence-based metagenomics, DNA from environmental samples is sequenced and subsequently analyzed in silico to search for genes of interest. Next degenerate primers are designed based on the amino acid sequence of the target protein, cloned in a suitable vector and expressed in the host of choice. For function-based screening microbial DNA is cloned in high capacity vectors to form libraries that are then transferred to an expression host. For the expression of genes of metagenomics DNA, *Escherichia coli* is most often used as host both for the sequence-driven approach and for function-based screening. However, the number of genes that are being expressed from these metagenomics libraries, particularly for function-based screening, and their corresponding functional and assayable proteins being synthesized is often disappointing [1]. Well-known reasons for this are among others: low metagene expression in the library-hosting cell and frequent rediscovery of enzymes with already known functions, the latter mainly when sequence-based screening is used. To overcome this expression problem several approaches have been tested for *E. coli* including the use of different vectors, strong promoters, adapted ribosome binding site, host-specific codon optimized genes, chaperone co-expression, but often without success. For this reason alternative hosts are being tested [2], which may increase the success of functional metagenomics by providing expression machinery suited to genes from diverse organisms [3]. Since it cannot be predicted which host is suitable for the expression of a particular gene, a battery of several hosts might be used including gram-positive bacteria. Moreover, the latter bacteria, in contrast to gram-negative bacteria, have the property that secretory proteins are released into the culture medium potentially allowing proper folding and function.

In recent years much research has been done to evaluate the potential of *Streptomyces lividans* as a host for the production of heterologous proteins [4] including from metagenomics-derived samples. *S. lividans* has been shown to be an interesting expression system for several proteins that are difficult to express in other bacterial host systems such as *E. coli* (reviewed in ref. 5). Several tools for the construction and functional screening of metagenomic libraries in *S. lividans* have been developed already. In addition, very recently the genome of *S. lividans* TK24 has become available [6] allowing to rationally design a more efficient strain optimization strategy. Although a broad range of genes, both prokaryotic and eukaryotic, has been expressed in this host, *S. lividans* is particularly useful for the expression of genes from actinomycetes and genes from other genomes of high GC content. Given the abundance of actinomycetes in soil samples, it comes as no surprise that the first expression of metagenomic DNA in *Streptomyces* was of a soil sample [7] and resulted in the discovery of novel bioactive compounds. More recently, other examples of the successful use of *S. lividans* have been published [8, 9].

The recent development of *E. coli–S. lividans* cosmid shuttle vectors [10] greatly facilitates the expression of entire metagenomics libraries since they allow the construction of the libraries in the standard host, *E. coli*, while the screening can be performed in either *E. coli* or *S. lividans*. In a next step, proteins of interest can easily be produced in *S. lividans* using a wide range of vector and expression systems. Novel enzymes, identified in soil and marine metagenomic screens, have already been produced to high levels in *S. lividans* [11, 12].

In this chapter we discuss all the protocols necessary for researchers to grow *S. lividans* TK24, the preferred host due to the absence of a methylation/restriction system and a low protease activity, to express entire metagenomics libraries and finally to express single genes of interest in this host. We describe the protocols of transformation, discuss *Streptomyces* vectors and their features, highlight gene expression control elements, and how they can be integrated for efficient expression of the gene of interest. Furthermore, small scale shake flask experiments versus large scale bioreactor experiments (lab-scale versus industrial scale) (culturing and processing conditions) are discussed, and how this can be used to maximize the production of proteins isolated from metagenomics resources.

It is important to note that, while this chapter discusses mostly *S. lividans* TK24, most of these protocols are readily applicable to other *Streptomyces* spp. and where differences occur, this is mentioned in Subheading 7.

2 Transformation of *S. lividans*

2.1 Materials

2.1.1 General Growth Media

1. Phage medium: 0.5 g $MgSO_4 \cdot 7H_2O$, 0.74 g $CaCl_2 \cdot 2H_2O$, 10 g glucose, 5 g tryptone (Becton-Dickinson, cat. no. 211705), 5 g yeast extract (Becton-Dickinson, cat. no. 288620), 5 g Lab Lemco powder (Oxoid, cat. no. LP0029B). Bring to 1 L with deionized water (dH_2O). Adjust the pH of the solution to 7.2 with 5 N NaOH and sterilize.

2. Trace element solution: 40 mg $ZnCl_2$, 200 mg $FeCl_3 \cdot 6H_2O$, 10 mg $CuCl_2 \cdot 2H_2O$, 10 mg $MnCl_2 \cdot 4H_2O$, 10 mg $Na_2B_4O_7 \cdot 10H_2O$, 10 mg $(NH_4)_6Mo_7O_{24} \cdot 4H_2O$. Bring to 1 L with dH_2O and filter-sterilize.

3. TES-buffer: 0.25 M TES, adjusted to pH 7.2.

4. R2 medium (modified): Dissolve 103 g sucrose, 0.25 g K_2SO_4, 10.12 g $MgCl_2 \cdot 6H_2O$, 0.1 g casamino acids (Becton-Dickinson, cat. no. 223050), 1 g yeast extract (Becton-

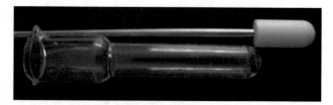

Fig. 1 Potter-Elvehjem cell homogenizer

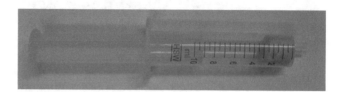

Fig. 2 Syringe with cotton wool, used to filter the spore suspension

Dickinson, cat. no. 288620), 5 g of Lab Lemco powder (Oxoid, cat. no. LP0029B). Add 100 mL TES-buffer, 2 mL of the trace element solution and 10 mL of a KH_2PO_4 (0.5%) solution. Bring to 1 L with dH_2O. Divide the suspension in 4× 250 mL and add 5.5 g of agar to each Erlenmeyer flask. Autoclave for 20 min. Add 1/100 volume of a filter sterilized 3.68% $CaCl_2 \cdot 2H_2O$ and 1/1000 volume of a filter sterilized 2 mM $CuSO_4$ solution (*see* **Notes 1** and **2**) and pour into petri dishes.

5. Glass/Teflon Potter-Elvehjem cell homogenizer (*see* Fig. 1 and **Note 3**).

6. TSB medium: 30 g of Tryptone Soya Broth powder (Oxoid, cat. no. CM129). Bring to 1 L with dH_2O (*see* **Note 4**).

7. Bennet maltose medium [13]: 0.1% Difco Yeast Extract, 0.1% Difco Meat extract, 0.2% Difco Tryptone, 1% maltose, pH 7.2, 1.5% Difco Bacto Agar. Sterilize by autoclaving and pour into petri dishes.

2.1.2 Preparation of S. lividans Spore Suspension

1. 20% glycerol in dH_2O (sterile).

2. 3–4 day old culture of *S. lividans* plated on MS medium.

3. Inoculation loop.

4. Sterilized 10 mL syringes containing nonabsorbent cotton wool (*see* **Note 5** and Fig. 2).

5. 12 mL Falcon tube.

6. 5 mL sterile tip with inserted cotton wool connected with a short silicone tube to 20 mL syringe (see Fig. 3). This instrument can be used for additional filtration of the spore suspension to thoroughly remove traces of the mycelial fragments.

2.1.3 Plasmid Conjugation Between E. coli and S. lividans

1. *E. coli* S17-1 (ATCC #4705) or *E. coli* ET12567[pUZ8002] [14] cells containing the DNA of interest (*see* **Note 6**).

2. Lysogeny (or Luria Bertani) broth (LB): 10 g tryptone (Becton-Dickinson, cat. no. 211705), 5 g yeast extract (Becton-Dickinson, cat. no. 288620), 10 g NaCl. Bring to 1 L with deionized water (dH₂O). Adjust to pH 7.0 with 5 N NaOH and sterilize.

3. 2× YT-medium: 32 g tryptone (Becton-Dickinson, cat. no. 211705), 20 g yeast extract (Becton-Dickinson, cat. no. 288620), 10 g NaCl. Bring to 1 L with dH₂O water and sterilize.

4. Mannitol soya flour (MS) medium. Dissolve 20 g of mannitol in 1 L of tap water. Add 20 g of agar and 20 g of soya flour (*see* **Note 7**) to the solution. Autoclave twice with gentle shaking between both runs. Add 10 mM MgCl₂ and pour into petri dishes.

5. Antibiotic stock solutions (where appropriate): ampicillin (50 mg/mL in dH₂O), apramycin (50 mg/mL in dH₂O), kanamycin (50 mg/mL in dH₂O), nalidixic acid (25 mg/mL in 0.2 N NaOH), thiostrepton (50 mg/mL in DMSO).

2.1.4 Triparental Mating

1. *E. coli* ET12567 [pUB307], BAC of cosmid library in suitable *E. coli* host strain, *S. lividans* lawn-grown culture.

2. Lysogeny broth (LB): *see* above in Subheading 2.1.3.

3. Sterile water.

4. Mannitol soya flour (MS) medium: *see* above in Subheading 2.1.3.

5. Antibiotic stock solutions (where appropriate): ampicillin (50 mg/mL in dH₂O), apramycin (50 mg/mL in dH₂O), kanamycin (50 mg/mL in dH₂O), nalidixic acid (25 mg/mL in 0.2 N NaOH), thiostrepton (50 mg/mL in DMSO), chloramphenicol (25 mg/mL in ethanol).

2.1.5 Preparation of Streptomyces Protoplasts

1. Phage medium (*see* Subheading 2.1.1).

2. 6.5% glucose in dH₂O, filter-sterilized.

3. 20% glycine in dH₂O, autoclaved.

4. S-medium: Dissolve in 800 mL dH₂O: 4 g peptone (Becton-Dickinson, cat. no. 211921), 4 g yeast extract (Becton-Dickinson, cat. no. 288620), 0.5 g MgSO₄·7H₂O, 2 g KH₂PO₄ and 4 g K₂HPO₄. Divide in 3× 266 mL and autoclave for 20 min. Add 50 mL of 6.5% glucose solution and 0.8% glycine (final concentration) to 266 mL medium (*see* **Note 8**).

5. A preculture of *S. lividans* in 5 mL phage medium, grown at 300 rpm for 48 h.

6. A sterile 0.9% NaCl solution.

7. Trace element solution (*see* Subheading 2.1.1).

8. TES-buffer (*see* Subheading 2.1.1).

9. PTC buffer: 103 g sucrose, 0.25 g K_2SO_4, 2.03 g $MgCl_2 \cdot 6H_2O$, 2.94 g $CaCl_2 \cdot 2H_2O$, 80 mL TES-buffer, 2 mL trace element solution. Bring to 1 L with dH_2O and autoclave.

10. Lysozyme (Roche diagnostics, cat. no. 10837059001).

2.1.6 Protoplast Transformation

1. PTC buffer (*see* Subheading 2.1.5).

2. Filter-sterilized solution of 35 % PEG6000 (NBS Biologicals, cat. no. 14808-C) (*see* **Note 9**) in PTC buffer.

3. R2 medium (*see* Subheading 2.1.1).

4. Stock solutions of the appropriate antibiotics.

2.2 Methods

2.2.1 Growth of S. lividans

S. lividans, and *Streptomyces* spp. in general, are relatively easy to grow. However, *S. lividans* grows much slower than *E. coli*: a 5 mL culture can take 48 h to grow to a sufficient density for further experiments. Contrary to *E. coli*, *S. lividans* does not show fully dispersed growth but tends to grow as pellets of mycelium. These pellets can be troublesome to work with, especially when using one culture to inoculate a second one. Mechanical homogenization, or the addition of dispersants or 2 mm glass beads to the medium can greatly reduce this pelleted growth. Here we describe a basic work-flow to grow *Streptomyces* spp. starting from a colony obtained as a spore suspension or glycerol stock and leading to a 50 mL flask culture.

1. Pour 20 mL of R2 medium into a standard petri dish and spread 100 µL of the spore suspension or glycerol stock on the agar using a glass spreader (*see* **Note 10**).

2. After 2–3 days, use an inoculation loop to pick up a single colony and suspend this colony in 5 mL phage medium. This culture can be used as a starter for the 50 mL flask culture (*see* **Note 11**).

3. Incubate at 27 °C at 300 rpm for 48–60 h.

4. Pour the culture into a glass cell homogenizer and move the Teflon piston up and down in the culture to homogenize the mycelium pellets (*see* **Note 12**).

5. Pipette 1 mL of this homogenized culture suspension into an Erlenmeyer flask containing 50 mL of TSB medium and incubate this culture at 27 °C at 300 rpm. After 24–48 h of growth, this culture can be used for further analysis (e.g., enzymatic activity, secondary metabolites).

2.2.2 Preparation of S. lividans Spore Suspension

Streptomyces spore suspensions are a very useful tool. They are easier to work with than with standard glycerol stocks (20 % final glycerol concentration) and inoculation with spore suspension usually results in cultures that faster reach the required density for further

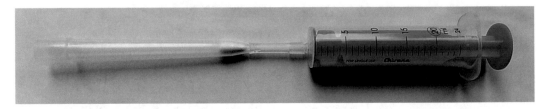

Fig. 3 5 mL sterile tip with inserted cotton wool connected with a short silicone tube to a 20 mL syringe used for additional filtration of the spore suspension

experiments (DNA/RNA isolation, enzyme assays, ...). Furthermore, conjugation to spores is more efficient than conjugation to mycelial fragments. Therefore spore suspensions are essential when conjugating a metagenomic DNA library from *E. coli* to *S. lividans*.

1. Pour 4 MS plates, adding any necessary antibiotics to the plate.

2. Spread 1 mL of an overnight culture of *S. lividans* grown in phage-medium on each plate.

3. Incubate the plates for 4–5 days at 30 °C (*see* **Note 13**).

4. Add 9 mL of sterile dH₂O to the plate.

5. Use an inoculation loop or sterile cotton bud to harvest the spores by gently scraping the surface of the culture. Gradually increase the pressure on the surface and scrape more vigorously, without damaging the agar layer.

6. Pipette or pour the spore suspension into a 12 mL Falcon tube and vortex the suspension at maximum setting to break the spore chains.

7. Filter the suspension through a sterile syringe containing non-absorbent cotton wool (*see* **Note 5** and Fig. 2) and collect in a 12 mL Falcon tube.

8. To remove traces of mycelial fragments thoroughly, filter this spore suspension through the 5 mL sterile tip with inserted cotton wool connected with a short silicone tube to a 20 mL syringe (*see* Fig. 3).

9. Spin the Falcon tube at $5000 \times g$ for 5 min and immediately pour off the supernatant.

10. Resuspend the spores in 1–2 mL of sterile 20% glycerol and vortex briefly. Freeze at −20 °C.

11. It is often desirable to have a rough idea of the amount of spores. Therefore, take 1 µL of the spore suspension and use this to make tenfold dilutions (down to 10^{-9}) in dH₂O. Plate these dilutions on MS medium and incubate at 27–30 °C for 2–3 days after which a CFU count can be made. For this counting, it is better to use transparent Bennet medium.

Depending on the type of vector used introducing DNA into *S. lividans* can be done either by protoplast transformation or by conjugation. The latter has several advantages, the main one being that the vectors can replicate in *E. coli*, greatly facilitating the production of the required constructs. Furthermore, protoplast transformation is very inefficient when large DNA fragments such as cosmids are introduced, while having very little influence on the conjugation efficiency.

Different *Streptomyces* vectors and their features are described in heading 3. *E. coli*–*S. lividans* cosmid shuttle vectors allow the construction of libraries using the standard host *E. coli*, but the subsequent screening can be performed employing *E. coli* or *S. lividans* as hosts. Here we describe a standard protocol to perform the conjugation of these or other cosmids from *E. coli* to *S. lividans*.

1. Transform competent *E. coli* S17-1 (ATCC #4705) or *E. coli* ET12567 [pUZ8002] cells containing the DNA of interest with the *oriT* containing cosmid (*see* **Note 6**).

2. Inoculate the cells of a colony into 5 mL of LB medium, supplemented with the appropriate antibiotic(s) to select for the *oriT* containing plasmid and grow overnight at 30 °C (*see* **Note 14**).

3. Dilute the overnight culture 1:100 in fresh LB medium and grow at 37 °C to an OD_{600} of 0.4–0.5.

4. Centrifuge the cells at $5000 \times g$ for 5 min.

5. Decant the supernatant and resuspend the cell pellet in an equal volume of ice cold LB.

6. Repeat **steps 4–5–4** in this order

7. Finally, resuspend the cell pellet in 0.1 volume of ice cold LB and place the suspension on ice.

8. While washing the *E. coli* cells, add 10^8 *S. lividans* spores to 0.5 mL of 2× YT medium.

9. Centrifuge the spores at $13,000 \times g$ for 1 min

10. Decant the supernatant and resuspend the spores in 0.5 mL of 2× YT medium.

11. Repeat **steps 9–10–9–10** in this order

12. Use a heat block to incubate the spore mix at 59 °C for 10 min, then allow the mixture to cool to room temperature.

13. Add 500 μL of the *E. coli* cells to the spore mixture. Vortex and spin briefly.

14. Pour off the supernatant and resuspend the pellet in the remaining fluid.

15. Plate on MS agar [15] supplemented with 10 mM $MgCl_2$ (*see* **Note 15**) and incubate the plates at 27–30 °C for 16–20 h.

16. Overlay the plate with 1 mL dH$_2$O containing 0.5 mg nalidixic acid and the appropriate antibiotic to select for proper exconjugants (*see* **Note 16**).

17. Spread the antibiotic solution evenly (*see* **Note 17**).

18. Continue incubation at 27–30 °C for 3–4 more days.

19. Pick off potential exconjugants to selective media containing (25 μg/ml) and proper antibiotic for plasmid selection.

2.2.4 Triparental Mating

1. Inoculate cells of a colony of *E. coli* ET12567 (pUB307) into 5 mL of LB medium, supplemented with chloramphenicol (25 μg/mL) and kanamycin (25 μg/mL), grow overnight at 37 °C (but not more than 16 h).

2. Inoculate *E. coli* carrying the BAC or cosmid library based on *oriT* containing vector from a glycerol stock into 5 mL of LB medium supplemented with the appropriate antibiotic. Grow overnight at 37 °C.

3. Centrifuge the cells at 5000×*g* for 5 min.

4. Decant the supernatant, wash the cells with 5 mL of LB to remove antibiotics. Centrifuge the cells at 5000×*g* for 5 min.

5. Resuspend the cell pellet in 0.5 mL of LB and place the suspension on ice.

6. While washing the *E. coli* cells prepare *S. lividans* spore suspension in sterile water or TSB medium. Transfer the spores into 1.5 mL microcentrifuge tubes.

7. Centrifuge the spores at 13,000×*g* for 1 min.

8. Decant the supernatant and resuspend the spores in the remaining liquid.

9. Incubate the spores at 42–45 °C for 10 min, then allow cooling to room temperature (We have found that lowering the temperature for spore heat shock increases the efficiency of plasmid transfer).

10. Add 100 μL of the *E. coli* helper and donor cells to the spore mixture. Vortex.

11. Plate on MS agar [15] supplemented with 10 mM MgCl$_2$ (*see* **Note 15**) and incubate the plates at 27–30 °C for 12 h.

12. Overlay the plate with 1 mL dH$_2$O containing 0.5 mg nalidixic acid and the appropriate antibiotic (for apramycin 1 mg should be used) to select for successful exconjugants (*see* **Note 16**).

13. Spread the antibiotic solution evenly (*see* **Note 17**).

14. Continue incubation at 27–30 °C for 3–4 more days.

15. Pick off potential exconjugants to selective media containing nalidixic acid (25 μg/mL) and antibiotic for plasmid selection.

2.2.5 Preparation of Streptomyces Protoplasts

Once an enzymatic activity (or a bioactive compound) of interest has been identified in an *S. lividans* library, it might be desirable to express a single gene instead of an entire genome region. Several vector and expression systems are currently available for *S. lividans*, with different advantages and disadvantages [4, 15]. The expression cassette can be constructed either in shuttle vectors which can replicate in both *E. coli* and *S. lividans*, or immediately in an *S. lividans* vector. In the former case, *S. lividans* will have to be transformed with purified plasmid DNA, while in the latter case they have to be transformed with a ligation mixture. Transformation of *S. lividans* cells is done using protoplasts. *S. lividans* protoplasts can be readily transformed by plasmid DNA at very high frequency in the presence of PEG. In the two following paragraphs, the protocol for the preparation and transformation of protoplasts is discussed.

1. Preculture *S. lividans* in 5 mL phage-medium for 48 h. If necessary, add the appropriate antibiotic.

2. Homogenize culture (as described in Subheading 2.2.1) and inoculate 50 mL S-medium with 2 mL preculture. Incubate this culture at 27–30 °C at 280 rpm for 20–24 h.

3. Harvest the culture by centrifugation at $5000 \times g$ for 5 min

4. Decant the supernatant and resuspend the cells in 0.9 % NaCl.

5. Centrifuge the cells at $5000 \times g$ for 5 min

6. Carefully decant the supernatant and resuspend the cells in 15 mL PTC-buffer.

7. Centrifuge the cells at $5000 \times g$ for 5 min

8. During this centrifugation step, prepare, per sample, 5.5 mL of PTC-buffer containing 10 mg/mL of lysozyme and filter-sterilize this solution.

9. Resuspend the cell pellet in 5 mL of the lysozyme solution and incubate the cell suspension at 27–30 °C on a shaker (120 rpm) for 15–30 min (*see* **Note 18**).

10. Check the formation of protoplasts using a microscope (*see* **Note 19**).

11. When enough protoplasts are formed, continue to **step 12**, otherwise prolong the incubation in the lysozyme solution.

12. Add 10 mL PTC buffer, gently pipette the suspension up and down and centrifuge the suspension at 800 rpm. This will leave the protoplasts in suspension while the mycelium fragments will form a pellet.

13. Gently transfer the protoplast containing supernatant to another tube.

14. Centrifuge the suspension at $5000 \times g$ for 5 min.

15. Decant the supernatant and resuspend the protoplasts in 10 mL of PTC buffer.

16. Centrifuge the suspension at $5000 \times g$ for 5 min.

17. Decant the supernatant and resuspend the protoplasts in PTC buffer to an OD_{600} of ~1.0.

18. Divide the protoplast suspension in aliquots of 0.4–1.4 mL (0.2 mL needed for a transformation) and put them in the freezer ($-80\ °C$).

2.2.6 Protoplast Transformation

1. Take the protoplasts suspension out of the freezer and thaw it quickly (*see* **Note 20**) without too much heating.

2. Put 200 µL of the thawed protoplast suspension in an Eppendorf tube.

3. Add the DNA (or ligation mixture) to the protoplast suspension and mix gently by pipetting up and down.

4. *Immediately* add 500 µL of the 35 % PEG6000 solution and mix by gently pipetting up and down.

5. Leave the mixture at room temperature for 5 min.

6. Plate the mixture on R2 plates (*see* **Note 21**) and incubate the plates at 27–30 °C for 16–20 h allowing the protoplasts to regenerate.

7. Overlay the plate with 1 mL dH_2O containing the appropriate antibiotic (*see* **Note 16**).

8. Spread the antibiotic solution evenly (*see* **Note 17**).

---

3   *Streptomyces* Vectors and Their Features

Efficient library generation is a necessary prerequisite for the successful screening of metagenomic samples for desired features. The use of *S. lividans* as a host requires dedicated vectors for library generation, screening and expression of genes of interest. Dependent on the desired size of the insert, the plasmid, cosmid, or BAC vectors are available. The majority of the current vectors can be maintained in *E. coli* and *Streptomyces*.

The plasmid-based vectors allow cloning of small inserts up to 15 kb thus increasing the number of clones in the library required for sufficient coverage. This subsequently increases the number of clones to be screened. The plasmid vectors are not suitable for cloning pathways that are encoded by large operons or gene clusters. On the other hand, cloning in plasmid vectors is technically simple and set lower requirements to the DNA samples quality. A relatively high copy number of plasmids allow detection of weakly expressed genes. Lastly, the plasmid vectors can be easily reacquired from *S. lividans*.

Several cosmids and BAC shuttle vectors for *Streptomyces* are also available. The inserts up to 300 kb (with average inserts size of around 150 kb) can be cloned and efficiently introduced into *S. lividans* using these vectors. Most of the *Streptomyces* cosmid and BAC vectors are integrative but several low copy number replicatives exist. These vectors are suitable for cloning large operons or gene clusters. The large insert size decreases the size of the library and thus screening efforts. Otherwise construction of library requires high quality DNA samples especially in terms of fragment size. The recovery of cosmid or BAC clones from the *Streptomyces* host is more difficult or impossible. The cosmid and BAC based libraries are mostly used for screening in *E. coli* followed by expression of selected clones in the *Streptomyces* host.

The general features of *Streptomyces* vectors are described in Table 1. Protocols for plasmid and genomic DNA preparation as well as several key *Streptomyces* promoters used for gene expression and their characteristics will be discussed. Protocols for cloning the target gene under control of promoter as well as modification of large insert cosmid or BAC clone are described.

Three types of vectors can be propagated in *Streptomyces*: (1) replicative vectors containing autonomous replication origins. (2) Integrative vectors inserted into *Streptomyces* chromosomes by site-specific integration. (3) Vectors which are able to integrate DNA via homologous recombination between cloned DNA and the *Streptomyces* chromosome.

1. Replicative plasmid vectors

   Most of the replicative vectors for *Streptomyces* are built around replicons originating from natural plasmids. The replicon of the high copy number plasmid pIJ101 isolated from *S. lividans* ISP5434 is used in many vectors [34]. It provides up to 300 copies per chromosome. pSG5 is a natural temperature-sensitive plasmid isolated from *S. ghanaensis* [35]. This plasmid has a moderate copy number of up to 50 copies per chromosome and is used in vectors, mainly for gene inactivation, but also for gene cloning and expression. SCP2 is a large conjugative plasmid isolated from *S. coelicolor* A3(2) [36]. The high fertility variant SCP2* was studied in detail and its replicon was used for construction of cloning vectors [37, 38]. SCP2* is a low copy number plasmids (1–5 copies per chromosome). SCP2* based vectors are highly stable and suitable for cloning inserts of large size. The specific partition function is required to ensure the stable inheritance of large constructs. Some of the SCP2* based vectors lack it and should be maintained under antibiotic pressure. A high copy number variant of SCP2* replicon (from 10 to up to 1000 copies per chromosome) lacking 45 bp (SCP2α) was described [39]. However, these plasmids are unstable and found limited use [40]. Several other natural plasmids are used to construct *Streptomyces*

Table 1
Overview of plasmid, cosmid, and BAC vectors for use in *S. lividans*

Vector name	Size, kb	E. coli		Streptomyces		Features	Ref.
		Replicon	Marker	Replicon	Marker		
Plasmid and phage vectors							
pL97	7.4	pUC18	*aac(3)IV*	pIJ101	*aac(3)IV*	*ermEp*; oriT RK2	[16]
pL98	7.4	pUC18	*aac(3)IV*	pIJ101	*aac(3)IV*	*ssrAp*; oriT RK2	[16]
pL99	7.6	pUC18	*aac(3)IV*	pIJ101	*aac(3)IV*	*nitAp, nitR*; oriT RK2	[16]
pHZ1271	~9	pUC18	*bla*	pIJ101	*neo, tsr*	*tipAp*	[17]
pHZ1272	~9	pUC18	*bla*	pIJ101	*neo, tsr*	*tipAp*; N-terminal 6× His-tag	[17]
pTONA5		pUC18	*neoS* (*Km*)	pIJ101	*neoS, tsr*	metalloendopeptidase (*SSMP*) promoter; oriT RK2	[18]
pWHM3/pWHM4	7.2	pUC18	*bla*	pIJ101	*tsr*	*lacZ*	[19]
pSOK101	7.1	ColE1	*aac(3)IV*	pIJ101	*aac(3)IV*	oriT RK2	[20]
pUWLoriT		pUC18	*bla*	pIJ101	*tsr*	*ermEp*; oriT RK2	[21]
pUCS75	13.9	pUC18	*bla, aacCI*	pIJ303	*aacCI, tsr*	*lacZ*; pIJ101 replicon with *ssi* site (copy number up to 400)	[22]
pKC1139	6.5	p15A	*aac(3)IV*	pSG5	*aac(3)IV*	*lacZ*; oriT RK2	[23]
pAL1		pUC18	*aac(3)IV*	pSG5	*tsr, bph*	*tipAp*; oriT RK2	[21]
pKC1218	5.8	p15A	*aac(3)IV*	SCP2*	*aac(3)IV*	*lacZ*; oriT RK2	[23]

(continued)

Table 1
(continued)

Vector name	E. coli		Streptomyces		Features	Ref.
	Size, kb	Replicon	Marker	Replicon	Marker	
pSET152	5.5	pUC	*aac(3)IV*	int∅C31	*aac(3)IV*	*lacZ*; oriT RK2	[23]
pTES	5.9	pUC	*aac(3)IV*	int∅C31	*aac(3)IV*	pSET152 derivative; *attP* flanked by *loxP* sites; *ermEp*; *t*fd terminator	[24]
pKC824	5.3	pUC	*aac(3)IV*	int pSAM2	*aac(3)IV*	*lacZ*	[25]
pKTO2	6.0	pUC	*bla*	intVWB	*tsr*		[26]
pSOK804	5.3	ColE1	*aac(3)IV*	intVWB	*aac(3)IV*	oriT RK2	[27]
pTOS	5.4	ColE1	*aac(3)IV*	intVWB	*aac(3)IV*	pSOK804 derivative; *attP* flanked by *rox* sites; oriT RK2	[24]
Cosmid vectors							
pOJ446	10.4	p15A	*aac(3)IV*	SCP2*	*aac(3)IV*	(cos)3λ; oriT RK2	[23]
pKC505	18.7	ColE1	*aac(3)IV*	SCP2* replicon and *tra* genes	*aac(3)IV*	(cos)3λ	[28]
pOJ436	10.4	pUC	*aac(3)IV*	int∅C31	*aac(3)IV*	(cos)3λ; oriT RK2	[23]
pMM436	10.4	pUC	*aac(3)IV*	int∅C31	*aac(3)IV*	(cos)3λ; derivative of pOJ436 with *attP* and *int* gene flanked with the *PacI* restriction site.	[8]
pKC767	8.7	pUC	*aac(3)IV*	int pSAM2	*aac(3)IV*	(cos)3λ	[25]

Name	Size	Replicon (E. coli)	Selection (E. coli)	int	Selection (Streptomyces)	Comments	Ref.
pOS700I	not stated	ColEI	*bla*, *byg*	int pSAM2	*byg*	(cos)3λ; pWED1 derivative	[10]
BAC and PAC vectors							
pSMART BAC-S	~10.5	*F1 single copy, oriV* inducible	*cat*, *aac(3)IV*	intøC31	*aac(3)IV*	pSMART BAC v2.0 (BAC vector) derivative; average insert size 110 kb; *cosN*; oriT RK2	Lucigen
pPAC-S1	22.5	P1	*kan*	intøC31	*tsr*	pCYPAC2 (PAC vector) derivative; up to 300 kb, with average 140 kb	[29]
pESAC13	23.3	P1	*kan*	intøC31	*tsr*	Derivative of pPAC-S1; average insert size 75 kb oriT RK2	[30]
pSTREPTOBAC V	16	F1	*aac(3)IV*	intøC31	*aac(3)IV*	pBACe3.6 derivative; oriT RK2	[31]
pSBAC	12.0	F1	*aac(3)IV*	intøBT1	*aac(3)IV*	pCC1BAC derivative; oriT RK2	[32]
pAMR4	10.5	pUC	*aac3(IV)*	no	*aac3(IV)*	*oriT RK2, bpsA*	[33]

vectors. Among them pJV1, with the replicon similar to pIJ101, but with lower copy number (up to 150 copies per chromosome). Low copy number (1–10 copies per chromosome) *S. coelicolor* episome SLP1.2 is used in several vectors strictly dedicated to *S. lividans*, since it integrates into the chromosome of other strains.

2. Integrative plasmid and phage vectors

The vectors based both on bacteriophage and plasmids integration systems are found in a wide array of applications in *Streptomyces* genetics due to the stable inheritance in absence of selective pressure. Despite the obvious advantages of integrative vectors the main drawback for their utilization in metagenomics libraries construction is the difficulty in recovering the construct of interest from the selected clone. Due to this, metagenomics libraries based on integrative BACs or cosmids are usually prescreened in *E. coli* and selected clones are then functionally tested in *Streptomyces*. Recently, the cosmid vector pMM436, derivative of the commonly used pOJ436, was published [8]. The introduction of the rare *Pac*I recognition sites flanking the integration system of the vector allows retrieving the entire construct from the selected positive *S. lividans* clone.

The integrase gene (*int*) and *attP* site of the wide host range actinophage φC31 are used in the majority of integrative vectors for streptomycetes. The phage φC31 lysogenizes its host by site-specific recombination between the *attP* site and chromosomal *attB* site [41]. The small size of the integrase gene and *attP* locus makes construction of small integrative vectors based on φC31 system possible. The majority of the investigated *Streptomycetes* has one *attB* site for φC31 in the chromosome, however some species might carry one or more pseudo *attB* sites resulting in integration of two copies of the vector [42, 43].

As alternative to the φC31 system *S. venezuelae* ETH14630 VWB actinophage *int-att* locus is used for integrative vectors construction [44]. The VWB system has a broad host specificity and can be used not only in *S. venezuelae* and *S. lividans* but in many other streptomycetes [26]. Several other phage systems were applied for vectors construction including φBT1 phage from *S. coelicolor* J1929 [45], *SV1* from *S. venezuelae* [46], and *TG1* from *S. avermitilis* [47].

pSAM2 episomal plasmid found in *S. ambofaciens* JI3212 was shown to exist both as ccc-plasmid and integrated into a tRNA^{pro} gene [48, 49]. It integrates into the chromosome by site-specific recombination. The *int* and *xis* genes with *attP* site and *rep* operon of pSAM2 were used for integrative vector constructions [50].

3. Vectors integrating DNA into *Streptomyces* chromosome via homologous recombination

Homologous recombination is a highly conserved process present in all forms of life, from bacteria to eukaryotes [51]. Several vectors based on this process (e.g., pKC1132; [23]) have been developed in *Streptomyces* spp., mainly for disruption or deletion of genes. Such deletion in streptomycetes generally involves the use of a non-replicative vector carrying targeted DNA, with selection for antibiotic resistance resulting in integration of the construct into the *Streptomyces* genome by homologous recombination, yielding the first crossover recombinant. The resulting strain is then screened for loss of the resistance marker encoded in the vector to identify the required second crossover recombination. However, it can be a very laborious and time-consuming process requiring screening hundreds of colonies. Thus the main obstacle for these vectors is positive selection for double crossover. Recently, we have overcome this problem by creation of pAMR4 plasmid vector with positive selection of a double crossover event [33]. This non-replicative plasmid contains the apramycin resistance gene with the conjugational *oriT* flanked by two polylinkers with several single sites for the rare restriction enzymes used in streptomycetes. In addition, it contains a kanamycin resistance gene which also directs the expression of the downstream *bpsA* gene encoding the biosynthetic enzyme for blue pigment indigoidine. The double crossover recombinants can be easily recognized as non-colored colonies (Fig. 4).

In addition to its use for deletion of genes in *Streptomyces*, pAMR4 can be used also for efficient and stable integration of foreign DNA into the *Streptomyces* chromosome. This foreign DNA could contain genes under the control of various promoters, or cluster of genes for biosynthesis of the metabolite of interest. In comparison with the integrative plasmids, this vector system has several advantages. It is more stable and can integrate foreign DNA to any position in the chromosome. Moreover, it can be used for any *Streptomyces* spp.

Other Features of Streptomyces Plasmids

1. Antibiotics resistance selection markers

Streptomycetes are resistant to a large number of antibiotics used as selection marker. *S. lividans* is resistant to tetracycline, erythromycin, chloramphenicol and β-lactams, limiting the choice of selective markers. Most of the current *Streptomyces* vectors harbor *aac(3)IV* apramycin resistance and *tsr* thiostrepton resistance genes (Tables 1 and 2) [53, 54]. *aac(3)IV* is used in many vectors due to its extremely low frequency of resistant mutations, its bifunctionality (it is active in both

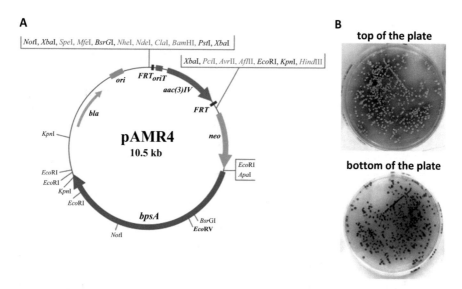

Fig. 4 (**a**) Restriction map of the plasmid pAMR4. It contains the promoterless *bpsA* gene, the kanamycin resistance gene from Tn*5* (*neo*), and the apramycin resistance gene *aac3*(*IV*) with *oriT* and FRT regions from the plasmid pIJ773 [52] in the backbone of the *E. coli* plasmid pBluescript II SK+. Unique restriction sites are colored *red*. (**b**) Example of colonies of TK24 after conjugation of the plasmid pAct1LL to delete the actinorhodin cluster [33] to distinguish between single crossover (*blue* colonies) and double crossover (*white* colonies)

Table 2
Antibiotic resistance selective markers for use in *Streptomyces*

Gene	Function	Resistance	S^a (µg/mL)	E^b (µg/mL)	Origin
aac(3)IV	apramycin acetyltransferase	apramycin	100	50	*Klebsiella pneumoniae*
aacC1	gentamicin acetyltransferase	gentamicin	20	10	*E. coli* Tn1696
aadA	spectinomycin adenyltransferase	spectinomycin/ streptomycin	100/50	50/25	*Pseudomonas* plasmid R100.1
hyg	hygromycin phosphotransferase	hygromycin	50	50–100	*S. hygroscopicus*
neo/aphII	aminoglycoside phosphotransferase	neomycin/ kanamycin	100/100	–	*E. coli* Tn5
tsr	23S rRNA methylase	thiostrepton	50	–	*S. azureus*
vph	viomycin phosphotransferase	viomycin	50	50	*S. vinaceus*
ermE	23S rRNA dimethylase	erythromycin	20	–	*Saccharopolyspora erythraea*

[a]*S*—concentration to be used for selection in *Streptomyces* strains
[b]*E*—concentration to be used for selection in *E. coli*

E. coli and *Streptomyces*) and it is a non-expensive drug. The *tsr* marker cannot be used in *E. coli* as a consequence of natural resistance. Vectors carrying the *tsr* gene also have an additional marker mainly *bla* for selection in *E. coli*. Care should be taken when growing the strains with *tsr* gene on MS medium since higher thiostrepton concentration might be required due to background growth. *aadA* spectinomycin/streptomycin and *hyg* hygromycin resistance genes are also used in some vectors as alternative to *aac(3)IV* and *tsr*. Both genes are active in *E. coli* and *Streptomyces*. The hygromycin selection in *E. coli* strongly depends on the salt concentration in the medium. Media with higher sodium chloride concentrations require higher concentration of the antibiotic.

2. The transfer function for intergeneric *E. coli–Streptomyces* conjugation

    Most of the current *E. coli–Streptomyces* shuttle vectors carry the *oriT* fragment of the broad host range plasmid RK2 (RP4) for DNA transfer by conjugation [55]. The use of methylation-deficient *E. coli* as plasmid donor helps to overcome the restriction systems present in most of *Streptomyces* strains [56, 57]. Also, triparental conjugation is often used in the case of metagenomics libraries to avoid DNA purification step. Attention should be paid to the *E. coli* strain used in the triparental conjugation. Strains with integrated *tra* genes (*E. coli* S17-1) or *tra* genes on a plasmid lacking the *oriT* (*E. coli* ET12567/pUZ8002) cannot be used as a helper. Strains with plasmids carrying transfer function and *oriT* site like pRK2013 or pUB307 are the most efficient in this procedure.

3.1 Materials

3.1.1 Isolation of pDNA by Alkaline Lysis with Potassium Acetate Precipitation

1. 2 and 1.5 mL microcentrifuge tubes, microcentrifuge with at least $15,000 \times g$, water bath 37 °C, ice bath.

2. Small 2–4-day-old culture (TSB, YEME or Phage medium) of *S. lividans* strain harboring the plasmid of interest. Yeast extract-malt extract medium (YEME): yeast extract—3 g/L, Bacto peptone—5 g/L, oxoid malt extract 3 g/L; glucose 10 g/L, sucrose 340 g/L. Mix all ingredients and dissolve in 1 L of distilled water. After autoclaving add 2 mL/L of 2.5 M $MgCl_2 \cdot 6H_2O$ solution (final concentration 5 mM). For TSB and Phage medium (*see* Subheading 2.1.1).

3. STE Buffer: 75 mM NaCl, 25 mM EDTA, 20 mM Tris–HCl (pH 8.0).

4. Lysozyme solution 50 mg/mL in STE buffer. RNase A solution 1 mg/mL.

5. SDS/NaOH buffer—1% SDS, 0.2 N NaOH. Prepare fresh. Mix 2 mL of 1 N NaOH, 1 mL of 10% SDS and 7 mL of distilled water.

6. 3 M potassium acetate, pH 4.8. Mix 60 mL of 5 M potassium acetate, 11.5 mL of glacial acetic acid and 28.5 mL of distilled water.

7. Isopropanol, 70 % ethanol, 5 M potassium acetate, 5 M sodium chloride.

8. TE buffer. 1 mM EDTA, 10 mM Tris–HCl (pH 8.0).

3.1.2 Isolation of Low-Copy Number Plasmids from S. lividans Using the QIAGEN Plasmid Midi Kit

1. 50 mL conical centrifuge tubes, centrifuge for 50 mL tubes with at least $15,000 \times g$, water bath 37 °C, freezer −20 °C, ice bath, glass microscopy slide, QIAGEN Plasmid Midi kit with QIAGEN-tip 100.

2. 50–100 mL 2–4 days old culture of *S. lividans* strain harboring the plasmid in TSB, YEME or Phage medium.

3. 10.3 % sucrose solution, sterilized by autoclaving.

4. Lysozyme. Weight 50 mg of lysozyme into 50 mL tube. Dissolve the enzyme in 10 mL of P1 buffer. Store on ice before use.

5. P1 (resuspension) buffer: 50 mM Tris–HCl (pH 8.0), 10 mM EDTA, RNase A 100 µg/mL (RNase is optional, already supplemented in QIAGEN Plasmid Midi kit). P2 (lysis buffer): 200 mM NaOH, 1 % SDS (v/v). P3 (neutralization) buffer: 3 M potassium acetate (pH 5.5). QBT (equilibration) buffer: 750 mM NaCl, 50 mM MOPS (pH 7.0), 15 % isopropanol (v/v), 0.15 % Triton X-100 (v/v). QC (washing) buffer: 1.0 M NaCl, 50 mM MOPS (pH 7.0), 15 % isopropanol (v/v). QF (elution) buffer: 1.25 M NaCl, 50 mM Tris–HCl (pH 8.5), 15 % isopropanol (v/v).

6. RNase A solution 10 mg/mL, 10 % SDS solution, Isopropanol, 70 % ethanol, TE buffer, pH 8.0.

3.1.3 Miniprep Isolation of Total DNA with Potassium Acetate Precipitation

1. 2 and 1.5 mL microcentrifuge tubes, microcentrifuge with at least $16,000–18,000 \times g$ speed, water bath 37 and 65 °C, ice bath.

2. STE25 buffer, 75 mM NaCl, 25 mM EDTA, 25 mM Tris–HCl (pH 8.0).

3. RNase A solution, 10 mg/mL.

4. Lysozyme. Weight 50 mg of lysozyme in 50 mL tube. Dissolve the enzyme in 10 mL of STE25 buffer. Store on ice before use.

5. 5 M sodium chloride, 10 % SDS, 5 M potassium acetate, isopropanol, 70 % ethanol.

3.1.4 Salting Out Protocol for Isolation of Genomic DNA

1. 50 mL conical centrifuge tubes, 2 mL microcentrifuge tube, centrifuge for 50 mL tubes with at least $5000 \times g$, water bath 37 and 55 °C, ice bath, microscopy slide.

2. STE25 buffer, 75 mM NaCl, 25 mM EDTA, 25 mM Tris–HCl (pH 8.0).

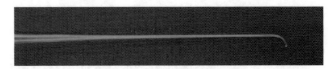

Fig. 5 Sealed Pasteur pipette for spooling the total DNA from solution

3. Proteinase K solution: dissolve 20 mg of proteinase K in 1 mL of buffer containing 20 mM Tris–HCl (pH 8.0), 3 mM CaCl and 40% glycerol. Store at −20 °C.

4. 10% SDS, 5 M sodium chloride, chloroform, isopropanol, 70% ethanol, TE buffer.

5. Pasteur pipette. Seal the end of the glass pipette by keeping it in the flame for a few seconds. The tip could be bent to form a hook (Fig. 5).

3.2 Methods

3.2.1 Plasmid DNA Purification

Several protocols for plasmid DNA purification from *Streptomyces* cells were successfully adapted. In all cases the efficiency of plasmid purification depends on the replicon used in the vector, age of the culture, size of the plasmid. The small replicative shuttle plasmids with pIJ101 or pSG5 replicon can be easily purified from recombinant *S. lividans* using the protocol described below. Generated pDNA is suitable for further manipulations like for PCR, *E. coli* transformation, and restriction endonucleases mapping. The DNA is not suitable for sequencing. For large constructs with low copy number and for sequencing purposes, an alternative protocol is described using the QIAGEN pDNA isolation kit.

Isolation of pDNA by Alkaline Lysis with Potassium Acetate Precipitation

1. Transfer 0.5–1 mL of 2–4 days old culture of *S. lividans* containing the pDNA into 2 mL tube. Harvest cells by centrifugation at 5,000×*g* for 5 min. Decant the supernatant (*see* **Note 22**).

2. Wash cells with 1 mL of STE buffer (*see* **Note 23**).

3. Resuspend cells in 180 μL of STE buffer; add 20 μL lysozyme solution to a final concentration of 5 mg/mL. Add 4 μL of RNase A solution (final concentration 20 μg/mL). Incubate 30 min at 37 °C.

4. Add 400 μL of SDS/NaOH buffer, mix by inverting several times (do not shake or vortex). Incubate at RT for 10–15 min.

5. Add 300 μL of 3 M potassium acetate pH 4.8. Mix by inverting. Place on ice for 10 min.

6. Centrifuge for 10 min at 16,000–18,000×*g*. Transfer supernatant into new 1.5 mL tube.

7. Add 540 μL of room temperature isopropanol. Mix by inverting. Centrifuge for 10 min at 16,000–18,000×*g*. Decant supernatant.

8. *Optional.* Spin down tube for a few seconds. Remove all liquid, dry at room temperature and subsequently dissolve in 500 μL of TE buffer. Add 30 μL of 5 M potassium acetate (unbuffered), 30 μL of 5 M sodium chloride, and 920 μL of ethanol. Mix by inverting. Centrifuge for 10 min at 16,000–18,000×g. Decant supernatant (*see* **Note 24**).

9. Add 700 μL of 70 % ethanol. Centrifuge for 5 min at 16,000–18,000×g. Decant supernatant. Spin down for a few seconds and remove all liquid. Dry the DNA at RT.

10. Dissolve the DNA in 30–50 μL of TE buffer.

Isolation of Low-Copy Number Plasmids from *S. lividans* Using the QIAGEN Plasmid Midi Kit

This protocol is suitable for large size low copy number plasmid and cosmid constructs. The yield and purity of DNA is sufficient for enzymatic digestion and sequencing.

1. Harvest the bacterial cells by centrifugation at 5000×g for 10 min at 4 °C. *S. lividans* TSB grown culture from 50 to 100 mL of media is sufficient for this protocol. Collect biomass in one sterile 50 mL centrifuge tube.

2. Wash the pellet in 20–30 mL 10.3 % sucrose. Centrifuge at 3000×g for 10 min. Freeze at −20 °C.

3. Add 8 mL Buffer P1 containing 5 mg/mL of lysozyme. Resuspend the cells. Incubate 30–60 min at 37 °C, mix by inversion every 15 min. Control the lysis by mixing 10 μL of cell suspension with 1 μL of 10 % SDS on a microscope slide.

4. Add 8 mL of Buffer P2, mix gently inverting 4–6 times, incubate at room temperature for 5–15 min (*see* **Note 25**).

5. Add 8 mL of chilled Buffer P3, mix immediately by inverting 4–6 times, and incubate on ice for 30–60 min.

6. Centrifuge at 15,000–20,000×g for 30 min at 4 °C. Gently transfer supernatant containing DNA into new tube.

7. Centrifuge for another 10 min at 15,000–20,000×g.

8. During centrifugation equilibrate a QIAGEN-tip 100 by applying 4 mL Buffer QBT. Allow the column to empty by gravity flow (2 min) (*see* **Note 26**).

9. Apply the supernatant immediately after centrifugation to the QIAGEN-tip 100 and allow it to flow through the resin by gravity flow (5 min) (*see* **Note 27**).

10. Wash the QIAGEN-tip 100 with 2× 10 mL Buffer QC.

11. Elute the DNA with 5 mL Buffer QF (*see* **Note 28**).

12. Combine the eluted DNA solution in one tube. Add 7 mL room temperature isopropanol. Mix by inverting.

13. Centrifuge at 15,000×g for 30 min at 4 °C.

14. Wash the DNA pellet twice with 1 mL ice-cold 70% ethanol, centrifuge at $15,000 \times g$ for 10 min, and carefully decant the supernatant without disturbing the pellet. Spin down for a few seconds and remove all liquid.

15. Air-dry the pellet for 5 min and dissolve the DNA in 50–100 μL TE by incubation at 4 °C overnight.

3.2.2 Total DNA Isolation from S. lividans

In many cases the plasmid DNA cannot be directly obtained from *S. lividans* culture due to large size, low copy number, integration into chromosome. In such cases the construct can be recovered by isolation of the total DNA. The replicative constructs can then be used to transform *E. coli* and subsequently be purified. Here we describe two protocols for isolation of total DNA from *S. lividans* and other actinobacteria.

Quick Isolation of Total DNA with Potassium Acetate Precipitation

This procedure is simple and a fast way to purify total DNA from *Streptomyces* strains. The entire protocol takes around 2 h. The DNA might still contain contaminating proteins and polysaccharides, but is suitable for downstream applications like enzymatic digestion, DNA hybridization, and PCR.

1. Transfer 1 mL of 2–3 days old culture of *S. lividans* into 2 mL centrifuge tube. Harvest biomass by centrifugation for 1 min at $5,000 \times g$. Decant supernatant.

2. Wash cells with 1 mL of STE25 buffer.

3. Resuspend cells in 450 μL of STE25 buffer containing RNase A (20 μg/mL final concentration) and lysozyme 5 mg/mL. Incubate at 37 °C for 30–60 min. Mix cells by inverting every 15 min.

4. Preheat the water bath to 65 °C.

5. Add 50 μL of 5 M NaCl to the lysate. Immediately mix by inverting 2–3 times.

6. Add 120 μL of 10% SDS. Immediately mix by inverting 2–3 times.

7. Incubate the tube at 65 °C for 15–20 min. The lysate should become clear.

8. Chill the lysate at room temperature for 2 min. Add 240 μL of prechilled 5 M potassium acetate (unbuffered). Mix by inverting. Incubate on ice for 30 min.

9. Centrifuge at $16,000–18,000 \times g$ or 15 min at 4 °C. Move the supernatant containing DNA into fresh 1.5 mL centrifuge tube.

10. Add 500 mL of isopropanol. Mix gently by inverting. Incubate at RT for 5 min. Centrifuge at $16,000–18,000 \times g$ for 15 min. Remove supernatant.

11. Add 700 μL of 70% ethanol. Centrifuge for 5 min at 16,000–18,000×*g*. Decant supernatant. Spin for a few seconds and remove all liquid. Dry the DNA at room temperature (Never dry samples completely because DNA will become insoluble).

12. Dissolve the DNA in 50 μL of TE buffer (*see* **Note 29**).

3.2.3 High Quality Genomic DNA Isolation

This protocol is more time consuming but provides a high quality and high yield of genomic DNA. The DNA is suitable for any downstream manipulations including library construction, genome sequencing, PCR, enzymatic digestion.

1. Transfer 30 mL of 2–3 days old culture of *S. lividans* into 50 mL centrifuge tube. Harvest biomass by centrifugation for 10 min at 5000×*g*. Decant supernatant.

2. Wash cells with 30 mL of STE25 buffer. Resuspend cells in 5 mL of STE25 buffer containing RNase A (20 μg/mL) and lysozyme 5 mg/mL. Incubate at 37 °C for 30–60 min. Mix cells by inverting every 15 min. Control the lysis by mixing 10 μL of cells with 1 μL of 10% SDS on glass microscopy slide.

3. Add 140 μL of Proteinase K solution, mix by inverting several times. Add 600 μL of 10% SDS, mix by inverting. Incubate 55 °C for 2 h. Mix occasionally.

4. Add 2 mL of 5 M sodium chloride solution, mix thoroughly by inverting.

5. Add 5 mL of chloroform. Mix by inverting for 10 min at room temperature (*see* **Note 30**). Centrifuge for 5 min at 3000×*g* at 20 °C. Transfer aqueous (upper) phase to a fresh 50 mL tube.

6. Repeat **step 5**.

7. Transfer aqueous (upper) phase to a fresh 50 mL tube. Add 100 μL of RNase A. Incubate at 37 °C for 30 min.

8. Add 5 mL of isopropanol. Gently mix by inverting. DNA will appear as white hank of filaments. Spool DNA onto sealed Pasteur pipette, transfer into 2 mL tube with 1.5 mL of 70% ethanol. Centrifuge for 3 min 15,000×*g*. Wash DNA with 2 mL of 70% ethanol. Dry and dissolve in 1–2 mL of TE at 55 °C.

4   Gene Expression Control Elements for Use in *Streptomyces*

Genes originated from streptomycetes are usually expressed in *S. lividans* from their own promoters. However, often when genes from other bacteria are cloned into *S. lividans* the transcriptional and translational control elements should be provided to insure proper expression. Features of some of the widely used *Streptomyces* promoters are summarized in Table 3.

Table 3
Streptomyces **promoters used in expression vectors**

Promoter	Description	Reference
ermEp	Strong, constitutive promoter from erythromycin resistance gene, partially inducible in *S. erythreae*.	[58]
ermEp*	Modification of *ermEp* with increased activity. Strong, constitutive.	[59]
actIp	Promoter of major actinorhodin biosynthesis operon of *S. coelicolor*. Strong, temporally controlled. Activity of *actIp* requires actII-ORF4 gene product.	[60]
vsi	Promoter of the highly secreted subtilisin inhibitor (VSI) of *S. venezuelae* CBS762.70, strong, constitutive.	[61]
hrdBp	Promoter of RNA polymerase principal sigma factor gene from *S. coelicolor*. Strong, constitutive.	[62]
kasOp*	Modified promoter of *cpkO* (*kasO*) gene from *S. coelicolor* coelimycin P1 gene cluster. Strong, constitutive. Shown to be more active than *ermEp** and *SF14p*.	[63]
A1p-D4p	Library of synthetic promoters with consensus −10 and −35 sequences recognized by HrdB sigma polymerase. Constitutive promoters of different strengths are available. Activity of the strongest variant does not exceed the activity of *ermEp**.	[64]
P21p	Library of synthetic promoters based on −10 and −35 sequences of *ermEp1*. Constitutive promoters of different strengths are available. Activity of the strongest variant P21 exceeds the activity of *ermEp** by 1.6-fold.	[65]
tipAp	Strong, thiostrepton inducible promoter from *S. coelicolor*. Induction range up to 200-fold. Requires TipA protein for activation. Leaky.	[66]
tcp830p	Strong, tetracycline inducible promoters combining *ermEp1* sequence and *tet* operators from *E. coli* Tn5. Induction range up to 270-fold in the case of *tcp830p*. Requires TipA protein for activation. Leaky.	[67]
T7p	T7p/T7 RNA polymerase system adopted from *E. coli*. Strong, thiostrepton inducible. Large range of induction, suitable for transcription of long DNA fragments. Tightly controlled, not leaky. Strain construction required.	[68]
nitAp	Nitrilase gene promoter from *Rhodococcus rhodochrous*. Strong, inducible with ε-caprolactam. Requires repressor gene *nitR*. Tightly controlled and expression level strictly depends on inducer concentration.	[69]
P21pCymO	Strong inducible promoter system. Inducer cumate. Tightly controlled and expression level strictly depends on inducer concentration.	[70]
P21RolO	Strong inducible promoter system. Inducer resorcinol. Tightly controlled and expression level strictly depends on inducer concentration.	[70]
gylP	Glycerol-inducible promoter from *S. coelicolor*. Requires *gylR* regulator for activity.	[71]
TREp	Temperature-induced promoter from *S. nigrifaciens* plasmid pSN22. Requires *traR* gene for activity. Induced by incubation at 37 °C.	[72]

The promoter of the erythromycin resistance gene from
S. erythreae is one of the most studied and used in *Streptomyces*
genetics [58]. The original *ermEp* region contains two different
promoters, *ermEp1* and *ermEp2* [59]. Deletion of TGG in the −35
region of the *ermEp1* resulted in a higher initiation rate. This new
upregulated variant was named *ermEp** and has been used in numerous applications including construction of expression vectors.

The use of housekeeping gene promoters from the host bacteria may improve expression of the target gene since many of them
(e.g., those encoding ribosomal proteins, RNA polymerase, etc.)
are usually transcribed at very high level. A panel of housekeeping
gene promoters were characterized for *S. albus* and *S. lividans*
expanding the choice of promoters to be used for gene expression
[73, 74]. However, activity of these promoters may be susceptible
to changes in growth conditions and other internal and external
factors. As an alternative to native streptomycete promoters, synthetic promoters could be used. In such case transcription of the
target gene is less dependent on the host factors. Several reports of
generating synthetic *Streptomyces* promoters have been published
[63, 75]. Virolle et al. generated a set of 38 synthetic promoters of
different strength by randomizing the spacer region between the
−10 and −35 consensus sequences of *Streptomyces* promoters recognized by the major vegetative sigma factor HrdB [64]. A similar
approach was used in our laboratory to generate a library of
Streptomyces synthetic promoters based on the −10 and −35 sequences of *ermEp1* [65]. The library of 56 synthetic promoters has
activity ranging from 2 to 319% compared to parental *ermEp1*.
The great advantage of both these libraries is the small size of
promoters (up to 45 bp). This allows inserting the promoter of
choice into the primer for target gene amplification.

Several inducible promoter systems are also used in *Streptomyces*
genetic manipulations. The *tipAp* promoter is able to boost transcription of *tipA* gene in the presence of thiostrepton [76]. *tipAp*
is a strong promoter activated up to 200-fold in *S. lividans* following addition of thiostrepton to the culture medium [66, 77]. This
promoter has, however, several drawbacks: the thiostrepton resistance gene is necessary in many cases to protect host cells against
toxicity from the inducer compound; *tipAp* is a leaky promoter
that cannot be fully repressed due to the nature of its regulation
[78]. Despite these disadvantages *tipAp* remains the most used
inducible promoter in *Streptomyces* genetics.

Several other inducible systems are available for gene expression in *Streptomyces*. A set of synthetic inducible promoters based
on *ermEp1* and *tetO1/O2* TetR operators from the *E. coli* transposon Tn*10* were reported to be tightly regulated [67]. Similarly, an
E. coli T7-polymerase based expression system was adapted for use
in streptomycetes [68]. However, this system requires construction
and is currently available only in *S. lividans*. The *nitAp* promoter

of the nitrilase gene and the corresponding regulator NitR of actinomycetes *Rhodococcus rhodochrous* are also adopted for gene expression in streptomycetes [69]. Expression from *nitAp* is induced by ε-caprolactam and is highly dose-dependent. *nitAp/ nitR* based vectors are often used for protein production in *S. lividans*. Similar systems were adapted from *Pseudomonas putida* and *Corynebacterium glutamicum* [70]. They are based on cumate and resorcinol dependent transcriptional repressors CymR and RolR and their operator sequences. Used inducer compounds are non-toxic, inexpensive, water-soluble and they easily penetrate cells. Both systems showed dose-dependent induction profiles that allow the modulation of gene expression by varying the concentration of inducer. Unfortunately, the cloning into existing vectors carrying these inducible expression systems is somewhat limited.

In summary, a set of vectors with well-characterized promoters of different strengths for gene expression in streptomycetes are available. If strong and constitutive expression is required promoters of major housekeeping genes or well-studied promoters from secondary metabolism genes would be a preferable choice. However, if inducible gene expression or tuned expression of genes or operons is desired several natural and artificial inducible promoter systems are available.

The correct termination of transcripts influences their stability. The use of terminators in cloning vectors ensures controlled expression of the target gene from the desired promoter and prevents their expression from promoters of vector components. Several *rho*-independent terminators have been characterized and used in streptomycetes. Cloning of the *S. fradiae aph* gene terminator downstream of the human interferon gene significantly improved production of this protein in *S. lividans* presumably by preventing generation of long unstable transcripts [79]. This terminator was found to provide 90% termination efficiency. Most used terminators in *Streptomyces* genetics originate from *E. coli* bacteriophages fd (t_{fd}) [80] and λ (t_0) [81].

4.1   Materials

4.1.1   Cloning of Target Gene Under Control of Synthetic Promoter of Choice

1. Primers designed as described in the Methods section (*see* Subheading 4.2).

2. Phusion® high fidelity DNA polymerase or any other thermostable DNA polymerase with proofreading activity.

3. The cloning vector of choice and appropriate restriction endonuclease enzymes to perform the cloning.

4.1.2   Modification of Large Clones by Insertion of Promoter Cassettes

Amplification of Activation Cassette

1. Primers designed as described in the procedure section.

2. The plasmid carrying promoter cassette of choice (accession numbers: *hyg*: strong promoter: KP234256; moderate promoter KP234259; weak promoter: KP234261; *aadA*: strong promoter KP234258; moderate promoter KP234260; and *aac(3)IV*: strong promoter KP234257).

3. Phusion, *Taq* or any other thermostable DNA polymerase. *Bam*HI and *Hin*dIII endonuclease enzymes, thermocycler.

4. Agarose gel system, power supply, TAE buffer, gel DNA purification kit (for example QIAquick Gel Extraction Kit but any other commercial kits can be used).

Recombination Procedure

1. *E. coli* BW25113/pIJ790, BAC or cosmid to be modified, PCR product from previous procedure.

2. Electroporator, 0.2 cm electroporation cuvettes, microcentrifuge, shaker incubator for 37 °C, incubator for 37 °C, ice bath, 15 mL culture tube, 1.5 and 2 sterile microcentrifuge tubes.

3. LB and LB agar media, chloramphenicol and antibiotics for selection of BAC and promoter cassette of choice (hygromycin, apramycin or spectinomycin), sterile distilled water, sterile 10 % glycerol solution, sterile 10 % arabinose solution (filter sterilized).

4. Primers for verification of activation cassette integration, Taq DNA polymerase, thermocycler.

Marker Removal

1. *E. coli* ET12567 (pUB307 or pUZ8002) harboring pUWLint31 plasmid with φC31 integrase gene [82].

2. Liquid TSB media, MS agar plates, LB agar, thiostrepton, antibiotics for promoter cassette selection and vector selection.

3. Verification primers, Taq DNA polymerase and thermocycler.

4.2 Methods

4.2.1 Cloning of Target Gene Under Control of Synthetic Promoter of Choice

Below we will describe the procedure for cloning of the target gene for functional expression in *S. lividans*. In many cases the vectors provide the promoter for gene expression. However, the choice of restriction nucleases that can be used is limited by the vector Multiple Cloning Site. In addition, the choice of promoters is limited. Majority of *Streptomyces* expression vectors are built around *ermEp* and *tipAp*. In most cases these promoters will be sufficient for functional expression of the target gene. However, if a specific tuning of gene expression or particular vector is required the promoter sequence can be introduced into the construct by PCR. The promoters of different strength can be obtained from the synthetic library [65]. The procedure for cloning of desired gene into pSOK101 vector under control of synthetic promoter is described below. The same procedure can be used for other *Streptomyces* vectors.

1. *Primers design*. The forward primer for cloning of the target gene should be designed in the following way: TATGG ATCC<u>TGTGCG</u>**GGCTC**TAACACGTCCTAGTATGG**TAG GAT**GAGCAA(NNNNNN**AAAGGAGG**NNNNN)**A/C**T**G** *NNNNNNNNNNNNNNNNNNNNN* GGATCC—*Bam*HI cloning site.

P21 promoter sequence is underlined. −10 and −35 promoter regions shown in bold.

If needed the RBS sequence can be included in the primer (in scopes). If gene of interest will be cloned with its own RBS the additional RBS in the primers is not needed.

N indicates the region annealing to the target gene (italic).

2. Reverse primer should include *Eco*RI or *Kpn*I site. If needed the terminator sequence can be included into reverse primer similar to promoter sequence in the forward primer.

t_{fd} TTAAAGGCTCCTTTTGGAGCCTTTTTTTTT

3. PCR and cloning procedure are performed according standard protocols (*see* **Note 31**).

4.2.2 Modification of Large Clones by Insertion of Promoter Cassettes

In case the library is built on cosmid or BAC vectors a different approach can be used to reprogram the transcriptional regulation of the target gene or operon. For this purpose the promoter can be introduced as a cassette containing resistance marker by means of Red/ET recombination technique (Dr. Myronovskyi, unpublished data). Several such cassettes are built including strong, moderate, and weak promoters and *aac(3)IV*, *hyg*, or *aadA* resistance genes (Fig. 6) (accession numbers: KP234256, KP234259; KP234261; KP234258; KP234260 and KP234257). The resistance markers are flanked by the modified φC31 integrase recognition sites allowing simple removal of the marker from the cassette in *S. lividans* [82].

Amplification of Activation Cassette

1. Primers have to be designed as follow:
   Forward: NNNNNNNNNNNNNNNNNNNNNNNNNNNNNN NNNNNNNNNNNNNGTCGACCCTCTAGGGTA CCCT
   Reverse: NNNNNNNNNNNNNNNNNNNNNNNNNNNNNNN NNNNNNNNNNNNNNGTGTAGGCTGGAGCTGCTTC
   N—40 bp sequence flanking the region where the promoter cassette will be inserted (Fig. 6b). We recommend replacing the native gene promoter.

2. Digest 5–10 μg of plasmid DNA with *Bam*HI and *Hin*dIII for 1 h at 37 °C. Run the digested DNA on gel and purify the band that corresponds to 1.3 kb fragment (promoter cassette with *hyg* marker) from gel.

3. Amplify the cassette using long primers from **step 1**. The annealing temperature for amplification with Taq polymerase should be 52 and 62 °C for Phusion polymerase.

4. Purify the PCR product from gel. Elute DNA from column with 10–20 μL of distilled water to gain a concentration of DNA of appr. 100–200 ng/μL.

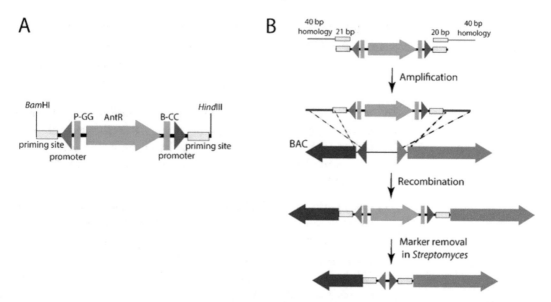

Fig. 6 (**a**) The structure of promoter cassette. AntR—antibiotic resistance gene; P-GG and B-CC recombination sites for antibiotic resistance marker removal [82]. (**b**) Scheme of promoter replacement and antibiotic resistance gene removal

Recombination Procedure

1. Red/ET recombination. Transform *E. coli* BW25113/pIJ790 strain with the cosmid or BAC clone to be modified. Plate on LB agar plates containing 30 μg/mL of chloramphenicol for pIJ790 selection and appropriate antibiotic for selection of BAC. Grow overnight at 30 °C (*see* **Note 32**).

2. Pick one fresh colony of the *E. coli* BW25113/pIJ790 carrying the BAC clone and inoculate into 15 mL tube with 1 mL of fresh LB media supplemented with 30 μg/mL of chloramphenicol. Grow at 30 °C till OD_{600} 0.2 (approx. 2–3 h).

3. Add 30 μL of sterile 10% arabinose solution to induce expression of recombinase genes. Grow at 30 °C till OD_{600} 0.4–0.5 (approx. 2 h).

4. Transfer cells into sterile 1.5 mL tube. Spin down at $10,000 \times g$ for 30 sec.

5. Wash cells with 1 mL of sterile distilled water three times.

6. Wash cells with 1 mL of sterile 10% glycerol. Resuspend the cell pellet in the remaining 10% glycerol.

7. Mix 50 μL cell suspension with ~100 ng (1–2 μL) of PCR product. For electroporation use 0.2 cm ice-chilled electroporation cuvettes. Parameter: 200 Ω, 25 μF, and 2.5 kV. Immediately add 1 mL of ice-cold LB and incubate with shaking for 1 h at 37 °C.

8. Plate cell onto LB containing antibiotics for selection of BAC and promoter cassette. Incubate overnight at 37 °C.

9. Verify the correct integration of cassette by colony PCR or restriction endonuclease mapping (*see* **Note 33**).

Removal of the Marker

In case the marker in the promoter cassette should be reused, it can be removed by expression of φC31 integrase in the recombinant *S. lividans* strain. If the used vector is based on φC31 integration system the marker will be removed during conjugation (efficiency of removal 50–95 % after one passage).

1. Conjugate the pUWLint plasmid into strain harboring the constructed cosmid or BAC clone with the promoter cassette. Select exconjugants on thiostrepton-containing medium.

2. Plate one colony on MS media containing thiostrepton (30 μg/mL) to obtain lawn growth. After 4–5 days scrape spores and prepare the spore suspension.

3. Plate serial dilutions of spore suspension in TSB on MS plates without antibiotics.

4. Pick 20 colonies from dilutions plating and transfer on LB agar plates with antibiotic for selection of promoter cassette and LB agar plates with antibiotic for vector selection. Select the colonies that are not growing in presence of the first antibiotic.

5. Verify the removal of antibiotic resistance marker by PCR with the same primers that were used for verifying the integration of promoter cassette.

5 Integration of the Gene of Interest Under the Control of the Promoter of Choice into *S. lividans* Chromosome via Homologous Recombination Using pAMR4-Based System

Here we describe the procedure for the insertion of the gene of interest under the control of a selected promoter into the *S. lividans* TK24 chromosome via homologous recombination using pAMR4-based vector system. The strategy is described in Fig. 7.

5.1 Materials

1. Primers designed as described in the Methods section (see above).

2. *Pfu* DNA polymerase or other proof reading DNA polymerase.

3. The cloning plasmid pAMR4, appropriate restriction enzymes, T4 DNA ligase.

4. Competent cells from appropriate *E. coli* cloning host strain (e.g., *E. coli* DH5α).

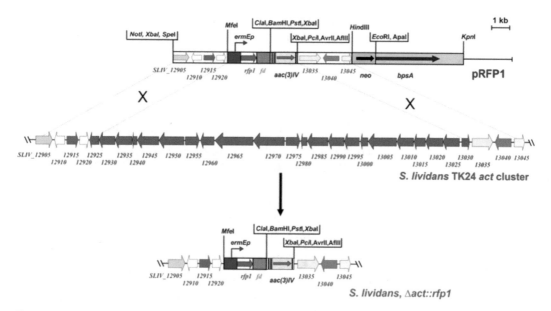

Fig. 7 Scheme of the *act* cluster replacement in *S. lividans* TK24 by the *rfp1* gene for *red* fluorescent protein under the control of the *ermEp* promoter using the plasmid pRFP1. This plasmid contains 3 kb DNA regions upstream and downstream of the *act* cluster cloned in pAMR4, followed by cloning of the *rfp1* gene controlled by *ermEp* and terminated by the *fd* terminator. *Thick arrows* denote the direction and size of genes. *Bent arrow* indicates the position of the *ermEp* promoter. Gene labeling is based on the genomic sequence of *S. lividans* TK24 (GenBank Acc. No. CP009124)

5. Agarose gel system, power supply, TAE buffer [83], gel DNA purification kit (e.g., commercial QIAquick Gel extraction kit, Qiagen).

6. Solid LB agar medium [83] with apramycin (50 mg/mL).

7. Solid MS agar medium [15] and solid Bennet medium [13] apramycin (50μg/mL) or kanamycin (50μg/mL).

5.2 Methods

1. Amplify 3 kb DNA fragment by PCR using the *S. lividans* TK24 chromosomal DNA as a template and a pair of primers containing 24 bp homologous regions from the 3 kb region upstream the *S. lividans* TK24 actinorhodin gene cluster (containing genes *SLIV_12905* to *SLIV_12920*; Fig. 7) flanked at the 5′ end with the sequence containing *Spe*I and *Mfe*I recognition sites (5′-CCCCCACTAGT and 5′-CCCCCAATTG), preferentially using *Pfu* proofreading DNA polymerase.

2. Extract the mixture by phenol/chloroform and chloroform, add 5 μg of glycogen (Roche), and precipitate with ethanol. Dissolve in water, digest with *Spe*I and *Mfe*I, and purify the DNA fragment after preparative agarose electrophoresis by some commercial kit (Qiaprep etc.). Clone the fragment into pAMR4 digested by *Spe*I and *Mfe*I by standard protocol [83].

3. Similarly amplify and clone downstream region of the actinorhodin cluster (containing genes *SLIV_13035* to

SLIV_13045; Fig. 4) between AflII and HindIII sites in the previous resulting recombinant plasmid.

4. Clone the gene of interest or cluster of genes (in the example case containing rfp1 gene under the control of the ermEp promoter and followed by the strong fd terminator, Fig. 7) in the previous resulting recombinant between MfeI and ClaI sites, resulting in the final pRFP1 recombinant plasmid (Fig. 7).

5. Transfer the plasmid by conjugation into S. lividans TK24 with selection to apramycin resistance (as already described in this chapter).

6. Pick up spores from one blue colony into 100 μL of sterile water and spread them to a plate with solid Bennet medium and grow for 7 days at 28 °C to complete grey sporulation.

7. Repeat the procedure of non-selective sporulation.

8. Perform several dilutions of the spores and spread them on a plate with solid Bennet medium and grow for 7 days at 28 °C to complete sporulation.

9. Pick up several white colonies and prepare spore stocks (as already described in this chapter).

10. Test the kanamycin sensitive phenotype after spreading to Bennet medium with kanamycin.

11. Verify the correct integration by Southern blot hybridization or by PCR as described in ref. 83.

6   Fermentations with Recombinant S. lividans

After construction of a recombinant S. lividans with the heterologous gene or gene cluster of interest, culturing conditions should be optimized in a bioreactor and upscaling needs to be conducted. Medium optimization is required to determine a culture medium that ensures good biomass growth as well as high product yield, and preferably also high productivity. Sufficient biomass needs to be formed since the final product yield will be proportional to the amount of cells in the reactor. Sufficient biomass needs to be formed since the final product yield will be proportional to the final amount of cells in the reactor, but growth and product formation are not always occurring simultaneously. D'Huys and coauthors [84] observed a distinct difference in protein yield (in this case, for mTNF-α) during exponential growth and the stationary phase, where the protein yield in the stationary phase was the highest. This might not be so surprising since active biomass formation imposes competition for building blocks (amino acids), energy (ATP, GTP), and reductive power (NADPH). In case of protein production, protease activity can occur during the stationary phase and typically when pH rises [11]. Hence, the optimal fermentation time for production needs to be determined.

This section provides a basic protocol for benchtop bioreactor experiments which can form the start in the production process optimization and upscaling. Whereas many screenings are commonly performed in shake flasks, which are time- and cost-effective experiments, bioreactors have the great advantage of process control. On the one hand, process parameters can be kept constant at optimal values, e.g., dissolved oxygen, pH, temperature. On the other hand, process operation can be adjusted from batch to fed-batch or even to continuous modus. A controlled substrate feeding during a fed-batch process can in some cases increase biomass formation and potentially heterologous product secretion by avoiding by-product formation related to overflow metabolism (e.g., [85, 86]). Operational parameters (e.g., stirrer speed, aeration rate) as well as medium requirements (e.g., composition, C/N ratio), which need optimization, are mentioned.

6.1   Materials

6.1.1   Fermentation Media

For general growth media and media for inoculum preparation: *see* Subheading 2.1. Two basic media for fermentation studies are the following:

1. Minimal medium (MM; adjusted from [87]): Per liter, use 1.8 g NaH_2PO_4 (Sigma—S0751), 2.6 g K_2HPO_4 (Chem-Lab—CL00.1156), 0.6 g $MgSO_4 \cdot 7H_2O$ (Chem-Lab—CL00.1324), 3 g $(NH_4)_2SO_4$ (Chem-Lab—CL00.0148), 10 g glucose (Fisher—G/0500/60), 25 mL trace elements solution (*see* **Note 34**).

2. Trace element solution (40× concentrated): dissolve 40 mg $ZnSO_4 \cdot 7H_2O$ (Chem-Lab—CL00.2629), 40 mg $FeSO_4 \cdot 7H_2O$ (Fluka—44970), 40 mg $MnCl_2 \cdot 4H_2O$ (Acros—205895000), 40 mg $CaCl_2$ (Sigma—21074) in 1 L deionized water. Filter-sterilize (0.2 μm) and store at 4 °C away from the light (*see* **Note 35**).

3. Modified minimal liquid medium (NMMP): minimal medium supplemented with 5 g/L Casamino acids (Bacto DB) (*see* **Note 36**).

6.1.2   Bioreactor

1. Any commercial bioreactor for microbial fermentations can be used. Rushton turbines are suitable for *Streptomyces* fermentation.

2. For pH control, prepare a 1 M KOH and a 1 M H_2SO_4 solution. Autoclave solutions in the addition flask with addition tubes attached (*see* **Note 37**).

3. For foam prevention, acquire an antifoaming agent such as Antifoam Y-30 (Sigma, A5758). Autoclave and add desired amounts to the medium during the fermentation to avoid excessive foam formation (*see* **Note 38**).

6.2   Methods

6.2.1   Inoculum Preparation

Standardization for reproducible culturing of *S. lividans* in physiological and fermentation studies is important and starts with a suitable inoculum preparation. Precultures can be started from (1) a mycelium stock prepared in a complex rich medium (e.g., phage medium) with 20% glycerol frozen at −80 °C, (2) a spore suspension in water with 20% glycerol frozen at −20 °C (*see* Subheading 2.2.2), or (3) a fully developed culture (i.e., aerial mycelium showing grey spores) formed on a mannitol soya (MS) agar plate (which is less than 3 weeks old). Precultures are preferably subcultured twice to avoid history effects of storage and to obtain sufficient biomass. Prior to inoculation, the preculture is washed to remove spent medium from the preculture. The cells are washed with a saline solution and resuspended in fresh bioreactor medium, i.e., the medium that will be used in the bioreactor experiment.

A basic preculturing method:

1. Scrape aerial mycelium and spores from the MS agar plate with a loop needle and bring the cell material in 5 mL Phage medium in a test tube (repeat three times).

2. Incubate the test tubes shaken at 250–300 rpm for 48–60 h at 27–30 °C.

3. Collect the preculture in an Elvehjem homogenizer and homogenize.

4. Transfer 1 mL in 50 mL Phage medium in a 250 mL baffled shake flask (*see* **Note 39**).

5. Incubate on an orbital shaker at 250–300 rpm for 24–48 h at 30 °C.

6. Collect culture broth in a centrifuge tube.

7. Centrifuge for 10 min at 3200–4000 × g and discard the supernatant (gently such that the pellet stays intact; if necessary use a pipette to remove spent medium).

8. Resuspend the pellet in a small aliquot (few mL) of 0.9% w/v sterile saline solution, vortex and repeat **step 6**.

9. Resuspend the pellet in a small aliquot (few milliliters) of fresh bioreactor medium.

10. Inoculate the bioreactor (*see* **Note 14**).

6.2.2   Medium Selection

Media for research purposes focusing on in-depth characterization of understanding, e.g., metabolic flux analysis, require a minimal medium containing a single carbon and nitrogen source (e.g., MM). A richer medium is more suitable for preliminary testing of expression, e.g., NMMP.

Media for production can be very diverse and are typically undefined complex media, e.g., NMMP, TSB, NB. Amino acids are typically supplied from a protein hydrolysate, e.g., casamino acids results from a casein hydrolysate, or result from the degradation of proteins by proteolytic enzymes secreted by the streptomycetes. Soya flour is one of the most commonly used protein sources in streptomycetes fermentation media. Pharmaceutical applications may, however, require a defined medium composition in which the amino acid composition can be optimized, e.g., [88]. Finally, addition of precursors for secondary metabolites can also reside in higher product yields, e.g., [89]. NMMP is a basic medium applicable for starting screening of heterologous expression in *S. lividans* TK24.

6.2.3 Small-Scale Batch Fermentations

The following protocol describes a batch fermentation in a standard 5 L benchtop bioreactor.

1. Fill the reactor with medium and autoclave (*see* **Notes 36** and **40**).

2. Add sterile trace element solution to obtain the desired final medium composition.

3. Set process operation conditions (*see* **Note 41**).

    (a) Temperature: 30 °C.

    (b) pH: 6.8 (control by automatic addition of 1 M KOH and 1 M H_2SO_4).

    (c) Agitation speed: 400 rpm (*see* **Note 42**).

    (d) Aeration: 2 L/min compressed air (*see* **Note 43**).

    (e) DO control: – (*see* **Note 44**).

4. Add 500 μL/L of Y-30 antifoaming agent (*see* **Note 45**).

5. Inoculate the bioreactor with the desired amount of washed preculture (*see* **Note 46**).

   The fermentation for *S. lividans* wild-type strain takes typically 48–72 h. The duration is determined by the doubling time during exponential growth and thus by the nutritional properties of the medium as well as the metabolic burden imposed by metagene expression. Since secretion is often observed in the (early) stationary phase, the culture is typically maintained for a determined period in this condition. Proteolytic activity may cause degradation of secreted heterologous proteins and determines the final fermentation time.

6.2.4 Biomass Determination

Quantification of product yield as well as evaluation of the growth dynamics in the bioreactor requires the determination of the biomass concentration (or amount) in the bioreactor. A suitable, common way for quantification of the biomass dry weight reads as follows.

1. Dry at 105 °C and pre-weigh a micropore filter (0.22 μm, PES, ⌀ 45 mm).

2. Put filter on bottle-top vacuum filter system and apply vacuum (pump).

3. Pipette carefully 5 mL of well-mixed culture on the filter (*see* **Note 47**).

4. Wash the biomass on the filter with deionized water (*see* **Note 48**).

5. Put filter with cells in oven at 105 °C and dry overnight (12–24 h) until constant weight.

6. Calculate the biomass dry weight concentration in the bioreactor (g_{DW}/L).

Product analysis is dedicated and dependent on the type of secreted product (e.g., ELISA, enzymatic essays, chromatography, mass spectrometry). Nowadays, physiological studies include metabolomics analysis on the basis of chromatographic techniques. Protocols for endo- and exo-metabolome analysis can be found in, e.g., [84] and [90].

6.2.5 Upscaling Strategies

Medium and process conditions optimization start with lab-scale fermentations in 1–10 L bioreactors. The final and challenging phase includes production process upscaling to 5,000–10,000 L for high-added value products like biopharmaceuticals, up to more than 100,000 L for industrial enzymes. Biological, chemical and physical factors impact upscaling and should be carefully evaluated, and if possible accounted for beforehand, e.g., [91].

The number of generations (cell divisions) in a large scale production will be much higher than in the small bioreactor and a seed train (i.e., cells are grown to a particular volume and density through a series of increasingly sized fermenters) is set up to inoculate the large reactor tank. Consequently, recombinant production strains must be stable (e.g., no loss of the plasmid with heterologous gene) during the seed train and production process. Mixing is no longer homogeneous in large-scale bioreactors and local substrate gradients will affect the metabolic capacity of the production strain and the observed overall production yield. Increasing stirrer speed avoids heterogeneity but is limited by cell damage or lysis due to shear stress and by foaming problems which are especially pronounced with filamentous microorganisms grown in nutritionally rich media. Besides mixing, transfer of oxygen to the liquid phase is slow and critical in large-scale aerobic bioreactors. Oxygen availability is important to maintain desired product yields in streptomycetes fermentations.

Empirical relations between geometric, physical and process operation parameters (e.g., stirrer speed, tank diameter, impeller type, viscosity) and mixing and mass transfer efficiency in large-scale bioreactors can be guiding tools in process upscaling and are described in many handbooks on bioreactor engineering, e.g., [86,

92, 93]. Selection of tank diameter and impeller rotation number fix many of these parameters and important tuning parameters in large bioreactors. Notwithstanding advancing opportunities for computer-based modeling of large reactors at the level of mass transfer and metabolic activity, the use of rules of thumb is common practice. Scale-up strategies can be based on geometric similarity, constant impeller tip speed, constant gassed power per unit volume or constant mixing time. For filamentous microorganisms, it is recommended to keep the impeller tip speed constant. Whereas upscaling for single cell growing microorganisms is preferably based on a constant DO strategy [94].

7   Notes

1. Addition of $CaCl_2 \cdot 2H_2O$ and $CuSO_4$ to the medium before autoclaving will result in precipitation.

2. When using salt-sensitive antibiotics (e.g., kanamycin, apramycin), Ca^{2+} and Cu^{2+} can hinder antibiotic activity. It is therefore sometimes desirable to omit these components from the medium. This is possible, but will result in slower growth of the *S. lividans* colonies.

3. *S. lividans*, and many other *Streptomyces* spp., grow in pellets. The Potter cell homogenizer (also known as tissue grinder), consisting of a glass tube and a Teflon piston, is used to homogenize the pellets in the precultures.

4. TSB is used routinely as standard rich medium. However, a variety of other rich media are possible for the growth of *Streptomyces* spp. [15].

5. The syringe, containing nonabsorbent cotton wool will be used as a filter to separate the spores from mycelium fragments.

6. *E. coli* S17-1 cells are methylation proficient and can be used for the conjugational transfer of DNA to *S. lividans*. For other species, it might be necessary to use the methylation deficient ET12567 strain.

7. Using cheap, regular soya flour from any supermarket yields the same result as using the expensive flour from specialized growth media suppliers.

8. For *S. lividans*, 0.8% of glycine is added to the culture. This concentration can vary from 0.5 to 1% for other *Streptomyces* spp.

9. While PEG 6000 can be obtained from different suppliers, it should be noted that testing PEG from different origin results in large differences in protoplast transformation efficiency.

10. Spore suspensions can also be inoculated directly into 5 mL phage medium (~10^6 spores) and the same holds true for glycerol stocks (50–100 µL). This is a more logical step if there is no later need for colonies on plate since it allows researchers to skip growing *S. lividans* on plate which takes 2–3 days.

11. This culture can also be used for preliminary tests (e.g., enzymatic activity), but it is important to note that the Phage medium is mostly geared towards biomass formation and that other media (such as TSB) are better suited for enzyme/secondary metabolite production.

12. In general, the pelleted growth of *S. lividans* does not interfere with later experiment. Should there be a problem after all, it is possible to reduce the pellet formation by using flasks containing baffles. A simple baffle can be obtained by inserting a stainless steel spring (30 cm length, 1.3 cm diameter, 19sw gauge) into an Erlenmeyer flask. Alternatively, 2 mm glass beads can be used. If this still does not sufficiently solve the problem, addition of 34% sucrose, which *S. lividans* cannot catabolize, can further reduce pellet formation. Finally, it is also possible to achieve a more dispersed growth by use of other media, containing PEG or Junlon, both of which favor dispersed growth (*see* [15]).

13. Incubate the plates until the entire culture lawn shows the dark-grey color of *Streptomyces* spores. A white or light grey color indicates the presence of non-sporulating aerial mycelium which will result in a lower final yield.

14. When starting from a glycerol stock, inoculate into 3 mL LB-medium + antibiotic and grow for 5–6 h. Dilute this preculture for the overnight incubation described above.

15. Drying the MS plates for 1 h in a laminar flow hood before plating greatly helps absorbing the 1 mL suspension added in the following step.

16. Apramycin and/or kanamycin resistance are the most often used selection markers; for these, add 1 mg per plate. For thiostrepton, add 750 µg per plate. When using apramycin, add the nalidixic acid first to the suspension.

17. Spreading the solution can be done either with a spreader, very lightly, barely touching the plate, or manually, gently shaking the plate in a rotating movement.

18. The time needed for lysozyme treatment to form sufficient protoplasts varies greatly between strains. For *S. lividans*, we find that 15–20 min is usually enough while other strains (e.g., *S. coelicolor*) may require up to 60 min. It should also be noted that *S. lividans* will not lyse when incubated for longer periods (up to 1 h), but the same does not hold true for other *Streptomyces* spp.

19. Protoplasts will be visible under the microscope as spheres among the mycelial clumps of *S. lividans*. The protoplasts should fill the majority of the microscopic field. If there are few protoplasts visible, a prolonged incubation is advised since otherwise the final yield will generally be poor.

20. Thawing the protoplast suspension is best done in either a warm water bath (40–45 °C) or by gentle shaking of the frozen tube under running warm water.

21. For ligation mixtures, we routinely plate one mixture on four R2 plates (4× 150 μL). In the case of transformation with pure DNA, it might be desirable to make tenfold dilutions in PTC and then plate the protoplasts.

22. Grow the culture in presence of glass bead (5–10 mm diameter, 10–20 beads per 50 mL flask) or stainless-steel spring with the ends hooked to form a circle. This will result in more disperse growth of mycelia allowing better lysis. Use 2–5 times lower antibiotics concentration than in solid media (apramycin 20 μg/mL, thiostrepton 10 μg/mL). Use 0.2–0.3 g of wet biomass for each tube. Too much of biomass will lead to viscous lysate and thus in poor precipitation of proteins, too few will lead to low yield of pDNA.

23. Washing will remove the extracellular nucleases, proteinases and polysaccharides.

24. This step is optional. It will remove the traces of SDS and salts.

25. Incubating for 15 min will increase the plasmid yield.

26. The buffer should drain completely.

27. The QIAGEN-tip 100 can accommodate up to 12 mL of lysate. Store the remaining 12 mL of lysate on ice. Repeat **steps 7–11** with the same tip and remaining lysate.

28. For large construct over 50 kb pre-warming the QF buffer to 65 °C might increase the yield.

29. Incubation of tubes at 55 °C will accelerate DNA dissolving. Do not pipette, this will shear the DNA.

30. This step is crucial for DNA isolation. Intensive mixing will result in shearing the DNA and it's loss. Not enough mixing will result in protein contamination of samples. We do not recommend using shaker.

31. Calculate the primers melting temperature only for the region that will anneal to the target gene.

32. pIJ790 will be lost at 37 °C.

33. For PCR verification, primers annealing approximately 100 bp outside of the cassette integration site will usually produce both modified size fragment and wild-type fragment. The latter results from the remaining wild-type DNA that will be lost during re-transformation.

34. Some modifications are made as compared to the minimal medium by [87]. The concentration of $(NH_4)_2SO_4$ is increased 1.5 times such that growth becomes carbon-limited. PEG 6000 (polyethylene glycol) is removed to avoid foam formation in the bioreactor and avoid interference with offline measurements, e.g., dry weight, chromatographic analyses.

35. Prior to use, the solution needs to be well mixed to obtain a homogeneous solution. The required volume is added to the medium in the bioreactor or shake flask which has been autoclaved.

36. If possible, prepare and autoclave the glucose solution separately from the other compounds to avoid Maillard reaction (brown color formation) between glucose and amino acids or peptides in the medium during autoclaving. Glucose solutions are poured into the bioreactor using a sterile funnel or pipetted into a shake flask.

37. Use more concentrated base and acid solutions (from 1 to 4 M) when pH changes during the fermentation are considerable as base/acid addition alters the medium volume too drastically.

38. Y-30 is an aqueous-silicone emulsion. Mix (shake) the antifoaming agent well before pipetting to remove phase separation. Other antifoaming agents can also be suitable.

39. Other medium volumes may be used in the second preculturing step but a typical volume ratio of 1/50 is applied for inoculation, and a shake flask should not contain too much medium to allow sufficient oxygen transfer from the head space.

40. Follow instructions from the manufacturer. Calibrate pH electrode prior to autoclaving the reactor with medium. Calibrate the dissolved oxygen probe after autoclaving at the operational parameters of temperature, stirring speed and aeration flow.

41. Process operation parameters can be altered depending on the strain and medium. Temperature is typically set at 28 or 30 °C. pH is typically chosen around neutrality (pH 6.8–7.3).

42. Too high stirrer speeds induce excessive foam formation and fragmentation of the biomass which can negatively affect expression. Streptomycetes are known to be sensitive to shear stress.

43. To keep the dissolved oxygen concentration high enough during the fermentation, oxygen enriched air (up to 40%) can be used for sparging, in case of high-value products.

44. Streptomyces grows aerobically. To prevent the dissolved oxygen in the medium to drop drastically, the DO control of the bioreactor can be used to keep a set-point of 30%. Aeration (flow rate of compressed air) and agitation (rotation per minute)

are automatically increased by a master–slave controller action to keep the DO constant. Maximum aeration speed and agitation speed should be selected such that excessive shear stress and foam formation are avoided.

45. Foam formation becomes a huge problem in rich media with a lot of soy meal and when working at high cell densities requiring high aeration rates to keep the culture aerobic. Add more antifoaming agent when excessive foam formation is observed.

46. The bioreactor is typically inoculated at 5–10% v/v (preculture/medium volume), e.g., a bioreactor with 3 L medium is inoculated with 4× 50 mL preculture.

47. Heterogeneous pipetting and loss of cell pellets can greatly affect the measurement. Vortex before each pipetting action.

48. This wash step removes salts remaining on the filter and causing an overestimation of the dry weight. In many studies and literature sources, this rinsing step is not included and the dry weight is overestimated.

Acknowledgment

The research leading to these results has received funding from the European Commission's Seventh Framework Program (FP7/2007–2013) under the grant agreement STREPSYNTH (Project No. 613877). In addition, Jan Kormanec was also supported by the Slovak Research and Development Agency under the contracts APVV-15-0410 and DO7RP-0037-12, and by the VEGA grant 2/0002/16 from Slovak Academy of Sciences.

References

1. Gabor EM, Alkema WB, Janssen DB (2004) Quantifying the accessibility of the metagenome by random expression cloning techniques. Environ Microbiol 6:879–886

2. Liebl W, Angelov A, Juergensen J, Chow J, Loeschcke A, Drepper T et al (2014) Alternative hosts for functional (meta)genome analysis. Appl Microbiol Biotechnol 98:8099–8109

3. Rondon MR, August PR, Bettermann AD, Brady SF, Grossman TH, Liles MR et al (2000) Cloning the soil metagenome: a strategy for accessing the genetic and functional diversity of uncultured microorganisms. Appl Environ Microbiol 66:2541–2547

4. Vrancken K, Anné J (2009) Secretory production of recombinant proteins by *Streptomyces*. Future Microbiol 4:181–188

5. Anné J, Vrancken K, Van Mellaert L, Van Impe J, Bernaerts K (2014) Protein secretion biotechnology in Gram-positive bacteria with special emphasis on *Streptomyces lividans*. Biochim Biophys Acta 1843:1750–1761

6. Rückert C, Albersmeier A, Busche T, Jaenicke S, Winkler A, Friethjonsson OH et al (2015) Complete genome sequence of *Streptomyces lividans* TK24. J Biotechnol 199:21–22

7. Wang GY, Graziani E, Waters B, Pan W, Li X, McDermott J et al (2000) Novel natural products from soil DNA libraries in a streptomycete host. Org Lett 2:2401–2404

8. McMahon MD, Guan C, Handelsman J, Thomas MG (2012) Metagenomic analysis of *Streptomyces lividans* reveals host-dependent functional expression. Appl Environ Microbiol 78:3622–3629

9. Kang HS, Brady SF (2014) Mining soil metagenomes to better understand the evolution of natural product structural diversity: pentangular polyphenols as a case study. J Am Chem Soc 136:18111–18119

10. Courtois S, Cappellano CM, Ball M, Francou FX, Normand P, Helynck G et al (2003) Recombinant environmental libraries provide access to microbial diversity for drug discovery from natural products. Appl Environ Microbiol 69:49–55

11. Sianidis G, Pozidis C, Becker F, Vrancken K, Sjoeholm C, Karamanou S et al (2006) Functional large-scale production of a novel *Jonesia sp.* xyloglucanase by heterologous secretion from *Streptomyces lividans.* J Biotechnol 121:498–507

12. Meilleur C, Hupe JF, Juteau P, Shareck F (2009) Isolation and characterization of a new alkali-thermostable lipase cloned from a metagenomic library. J Ind Microbiol Biotechnol 36:853–861

13. Horinouchi S, Hara O, Beppu T (1983) Cloning of a pleiotropic gene that positively controls biosynthesis of A-factor, actinorhodin, and prodigiosin in *Streptomyces coelicolor* A3(2) and *Streptomyces lividans.* J Bacteriol 155: 1238–1248

14. Macneil DJ, Gewain KM, Ruby CL, Dezeny G, Gibbons PH, Macneil T (1992) Analysis of *Streptomyces avermitilis* genes required for avermectin biosynthesis utilizing a novel integration vector. Gene 111:61–68

15. Kieser T, Bibb MJ, Buttner MJ, Charter KF, Hopwood D (2000) Practical *Streptomyces* genetics. John Innes Foundation, Norwich

16. Sun N, Wang ZB, Wu HP, Mao XM, Li YQ (2012) Construction of over-expression shuttle vectors in *Streptomyces.* Ann Microbiol 62:1541–1546

17. Yang R, Hu Z, Deng Z, Li J (1998) Construction of *Escherichia coli-Streptomyces* shuttle expression vectors for gene expression in *Streptomyces.* Chin J Biotechnol 14:1–8

18. Hatanaka T, Onaka H, Arima J, Uraji M, Uesugi Y, Usuki H et al (2008) pTONA5: a hyperexpression vector in Streptomycetes. Protein Expr Purif 62:244–248

19. Vara J, Lewandowskaskarbek M, Wang YG, Donadio S, Hutchinson CR (1989) Cloning of genes governing the deoxysugar portion of the erythromycin biosynthesis pathway in *Saccharopolyspora erythraea* (*Streptomyces erythreus*). J Bacteriol 171:5872–5881

20. Zotchev S, Haugan K, Sekurova O, Sletta H, Ellingsen TE, Valla S (2000) Identification of a gene cluster for antibacterial polyketide-derived antibiotic biosynthesis in the nystatin producer *Streptomyces noursei* ATCC 11455. Microbiology 146(Pt 3):611–619

21. Fedoryshyn M, Petzke L, Welle E, Bechthold A, Luzhetskyy A (2008) Marker removal from actinomycetes genome using Flp recombinase. Gene 419:43–47

22. Dyson PJ, Evans M (1996) pUCS75, a stable high-copy-number *Streptomyces Escherichia coli* shuttle vector which facilitates subcloning from pUC plasmid and M13 phage vectors. Gene 171:71–73

23. Bierman M, Logan R, Obrien K, Seno ET, Rao RN, Schoner BE (1992) Plasmid cloning vectors for the conjugal transfer of DNA from *Escherichia coli* to *Streptomyces spp.* Gene 116: 43–49

24. Herrmann S, Siegl T, Luzhetska M, Petzke L, Jilg C, Welle E et al (2012) Site-specific recombination strategies for engineering actinomycete genomes. Appl Environ Microbiol 78: 1804–1812

25. Kuhstoss S, Richardson MA, Rao RN (1991) Plasmid cloning vectors that integrate site-specifically in *Streptomyces* spp. Gene 97: 143–146

26. Van Mellaert L, Mei LJ, Lammertyn E, Schacht S, Anné J (1998) Site-specific integration of bacteriophage VWB genome into *Streptomyces venezuelae* and construction of a VWB-based integrative vector. Microbiology 144: 3351–3358

27. Sekurova ON, Brautaset T, Sletta H, Borgos SEF, Jakobsen OM, Ellingsen TE et al (2004) In vivo analysis of the regulatory genes in the nystatin biosynthetic gene cluster of *Streptomyces noursei* ATCC 11455 reveals their differential control over antibiotic biosynthesis. J Bacteriol 186:1345–1354

28. Richardson MA, Kuhstoss S, Solenberg P, Schaus NA, Rao RN (1987) A new shuttle cosmid vector, pKS505, for streptomycetes—its use in the cloning of 3 different spiramycin-resistance genes from a *Streptomyces ambofaciens* library. Gene 61:231–241

29. Sosio M, Giusino F, Cappellano C, Bossi E, Puglia AM, Donadio S (2000) Artificial chromosomes for antibiotic-producing actinomycetes. Nat Biotechnol 18:343–345

30. Jones AC, Gust B, Kulik A, Heide L, Buttner MJ, Bibb MJ (2013) Phage P1-derived artificial chromosomes facilitate heterologous expression of the FK506 gene cluster. PLoS One 8:e69319

31. Miao V, Coeffet-LeGal MF, Brian P, Brost R, Penn J, Whiting A et al (2005) Daptomycin biosynthesis in *Streptomyces roseosporus*: cloning

and analysis of the gene cluster and revision of peptide stereochemistry. Microbiology 151: 1507–1523

32. Liu H, Jiang H, Haltli B, Kulowski K, Muszynska E, Feng XD et al (2009) Rapid cloning and heterologous expression of the meridamycin biosynthetic gene cluster using a versatile *Escherichia coli-Streptomyces* artificial chromosome vector, pSBAC. J Nat Prod 72: 389–395

33. Knirschova R, Novakova R, Mingyar E, Bekeova C, Homerova D, Kormanec J (2015) Utilization of a reporter system based on the blue pigment indigoidine biosynthetic gene *bpsA* for detection of promoter activity and deletion of genes in *Streptomyces*. J Microbiol Methods 113:1–3

34. Kieser T, Hopwood DA, Wright HM, Thompson CJ (1982) pIJ101, a multi-copy broad host-range *Streptomyces* plasmid: functional analysis and development of DNA cloning vectors. Mol Gen Genet 185:223–238

35. Muth G, Wohlleben W, Pühler A (1988) The minimal replicon of the *Streptomyces ghanaensis* plasmid pSG5 identified by subcloning and Tn5 mutagenesis. Mol Gen Genet 211: 424–429

36. Schrempf H, Goebel W (1977) Characterization of a plasmid from *Streptomyces coelicolor* A3(2). J Bacteriol 131:251–258

37. Lydiate DJ, Malpartida F, Hopwood DA (1985) The *Streptomyces* plasmid SCP2star - its functional analysis and development into useful cloning vectors. Gene 35:223–235

38. Bibb MJ, Hopwood DA (1981) Genetic studies of the fertility plasmid Scp2 and its Scp2 star variants in *Streptomyces coelicolor* A3(2). J Gen Microbiol 126:427–442

39. Hu ZH, Hopwood DA, Hutchinson CR (2003) Enhanced heterologous polyketide production in *Streptomyces* by exploiting plasmid co-integration. J Ind Microbiol Biotechnol 30:516–522

40. Fong R, Vroom JA, Hu ZH, Hutchinson CR, Huang JQ, Cohen SN, Kao CM (2007) Characterization of a large, stable, high-copy-number *Streptomyces* plasmid that requires stability and transfer functions for heterologous polyketide overproduction. Appl Environ Microbiol 73:4094

41. Kuhstoss S, Rao RN (1991) Analysis of the integration function of the streptomycete bacteriophage Phi C31. J Mol Biol 222:897–908

42. Combes P, Till R, Bee S, Smith MCM (2002) The *Streptomyces* genome contains multiple pseudo-attB sites for the phi C31-encoded site-specific recombination system. J Bacteriol 184:5746–5752

43. Bilyk B, Luzhetskyy A (2014) Unusual site-specific DNA integration into the highly active pseudo-attB of the *Streptomyces albus* J1074 genome. Appl Microbiol Biotechnol 98: 5095–5104

44. Anné J, Wohlleben W, Burkardt HJ, Springer R, Pühler A (1984) Morphological and molecular characterization of several actinophages isolated from soil which lyse *Streptomyces cattleya* or *Streptomyces venezuelae*. J Gen Microbiol 130:2639–2649

45. Gregory MA, Till R, Smith MCM (2003) Integration site for streptomyces phage phi BT1 and development of site-specific integrating vectors. J Bacteriol 185:5320–5323

46. Fayed B, Younger E, Taylor G, Smith MCM (2014) A novel *Streptomyces spp.* integration vector derived from the *S. venezuelae* phage, SV1. BMC Biotechnol 14:51

47. Morita K, Yamamoto T, Fusada N, Komatsu M, Ikeda H, Hirano N, Takahashi H (2009) The site-specific recombination system of actinophage TG1. FEMS Microbiol Lett 297: 234–240

48. Pernodet JL, Simonet JM, Guerineau M (1984) Plasmids in different strains of *Streptomyces ambofaciens* - free and integrated form of plasmid pSAM2. Mol Gen Genet 198:35–41

49. Boccard F, Pernodet JL, Friedmann A, Guerineau M (1988) Site-specific integration of plasmid Psam2 in *Streptomyces lividans* and *Streptomyces ambofaciens*. Mol Gen Genet 212:432–439

50. Smokvina T, Mazodier P, Boccard F, Thompson CJ, Guerineau M (1990) Construction of a series of pSAM2-based integrative vectors for use in actinomycetes. Gene 94:53–59

51. West SC (2003) Molecular views of recombination proteins and their control. Nat Rev Mol Cell Biol 4:435–445

52. Gust B, Challis GL, Fowler K, Kieser T, Chater KF (2003) PCR-targeted *Streptomyces* gene replacement identifies a protein domain needed for biosynthesis of the sesquiterpene soil odor geosmin. Proc Natl Acad Sci U S A 100: 1541–1546

53. Cundliffe E (1978) Mechanism of resistance to thiostrepton in the producing-organism *Streptomyces azureus*. Nature 272:792–795

54. Stanzak R, Matsushima P, Baltz RH, Rao RN (1986) Cloning and expression in *Streptomyces lividans* of clustered erythromycin biosynthesis genes from *Streptomyces erythreus*. Nat Biotechnol 4:229–232

55. Labigneroussel A, Harel J, Tompkins L (1987) Gene transfer from *Escherichia coli* to *Campylobacter* species - development of shuttle

vectors for genetic analysis of *Campylobacter jejuni*. J Bacteriol 169:5320–5323

56. Mazodier P, Petter R, Thompson C (1989) Intergeneric conjugation between *Escherichia coli* and *Streptomyces* species. J Bacteriol 171:3583–3585

57. Flett F, Mersinias V, Smith CP (1997) High efficiency intergeneric conjugal transfer of plasmid DNA from *Escherichia coli* to methyl DNA-restricting streptomycetes. FEMS Microbiol Lett 155:223–229

58. Bibb MJ, Janssen GR, Ward JM (1985) Cloning and analysis of the promoter region of the erythromycin resistance gene (ErmE) of *Streptomyces erythraeus*. Gene 38:215–226

59. Bibb MJ, White J, Ward JM, Janssen GR (1994) The mRNA for the 23S rRNA methylase encoded by the ermE gene of *Saccharopolyspora erythraea* is translated in the absence of a conventional ribosome-binding site. Mol Microbiol 14:533–545

60. McDaniel R, Ebertkhosla S, Hopwood DA, Khosla C (1993) Engineered biosynthesis of novel polyketides. Science 262:1546–1550

61. Van Mellaert L, Lammertyn E, Schacht S, Proost P, Van Damme J, Wroblowski B et al (1998) Molecular characterization of a novel subtilisin inhibitor protein produced by *Streptomyces venezuelae* CBS762.70. DNA Seq 9:19–30

62. Du D, Zhu Y, Wei JH, Tian YQ, Niu G, Tan HR (2013) Improvement of gougerotin and nikkomycin production by engineering their biosynthetic gene clusters. Appl Microbiol Biotechnol 97:6383–6396

63. Wang WS, Li X, Wang J, Xiang SH, Feng XZ, Yang KQ (2013) An engineered strong promoter for streptomycetes. Appl Environ Microbiol 79:4484–4492

64. Seghezzi N, Amar P, Koebmann B, Jensen PR, Virolle MJ (2011) The construction of a library of synthetic promoters revealed some specific features of strong *Streptomyces* promoters. Appl Microbiol Biotechnol 90:615–623

65. Siegl T, Tokovenko B, Myronovskyi M, Luzhetskyy A (2013) Design, construction and characterisation of a synthetic promoter library for fine-tuned gene expression in actinomycetes. Metab Eng 19:98–106

66. Kuhstoss S, Rao RN (1991) A thiostrepton-inducible expression vector for use in *Streptomyces* spp. Gene 103:97–99

67. Rodriguez-Garcia A, Combes P, Perez-Redondo R, Smith MCA, Smith MCM (2005) Natural and synthetic tetracycline-inducible promoters for use in the antibiotic-producing bacteria *Streptomyces*. Nucleic Acids Res 33

68. Lussier FX, Denis F, Shareck F (2010) Adaptation of the highly productive T7 expression system to *Streptomyces lividans*. Appl Environ Microbiol 76:967–970

69. Herai S, Hashimoto Y, Higashibata H, Maseda H, Ikeda H, Omura S, Kobayashi M (2004) Hyper-inducible expression system for streptomycetes. Proc Natl Acad Sci U S A 101: 14031–14035

70. Horbal L, Fedorenko V, Luzhetskyy A (2014) Novel and tightly regulated resorcinol and cumate-inducible expression systems for *Streptomyces* and other actinobacteria. Appl Microbiol Biotechnol 98:8641–8655

71. Hindle Z, Smith CP (1994) Substrate induction and catabolite repression of the *Streptomyces coelicolor* glycerol operon are mediated through the GylR protein. Mol Microbiol 12:737–745

72. Kataoka M, Tatsuta T, Suzuki I, Kosono S, Seki T, Yoshida T (1996) Development of a temperature-inducible expression system for *Streptomyces spp.* J Bacteriol 178:5540–5542

73. Shao ZY, Rao GD, Li C, Abil Z, Luo YZ, Zhao HM (2013) Refactoring the silent spectinabilin gene cluster using a plug-and-play scaffold. ACS Synth Biol 2:662–669

74. Luo YZ, Zhang L, Barton KW, Zhao HM (2015) Systematic identification of a panel of strong constitutive promoters from *Streptomyces albus*. ACS Synth Biol 4:1001–1010

75. Bai CX, Zhang Y, Zhao XJ, Hu YL, Xiang SH, Miao J et al (2015) Exploiting a precise design of universal synthetic modular regulatory elements to unlock the microbial natural products in *Streptomyces*. Proc Natl Acad Sci U S A 112:12181–12186

76. Murakami T, Holt TG, Thompson CJ (1989) Thiostrepton-induced gene expression in *Streptomyces lividans*. J Bacteriol 171: 1459–1466

77. Schmittjohn T, Engels JW (1992) Promoter constructions for efficient secretion expression in *Streptomyces lividans*. Appl Microbiol Biotechnol 36:493–498

78. Chiu ML, Folcher M, Katoh T, Puglia AM, Vohradsky J, Yun BS et al (1999) Broad spectrum thiopeptide recognition specificity of the *Streptomyces lividans* TipAL protein and its role in regulating gene expression. J Biol Chem 274:20578–20586

79. Pulido D, Jimenez A (1987) Optimization of gene expression in *Streptomyces lividans* by a transcription terminator. Nucleic Acids Res 15:4227–4240

80. Ward JM, Janssen GR, Kieser T, Bibb MJ, Buttner MJ, Bibb MJ (1986) Construction

and characterization of a series of multi-copy promoter-probe plasmid vectors for *Streptomyces* using the aminoglycoside phosphotransferase gene from Tn5 as indicator. Mol Gen Genet 203:468–478

81. Scholtissek S, Grosse F (1987) A cloning cartridge of lambda-to terminator. Nucleic Acids Res 15:3185

82. Myronovskyi M, Rosenkranzer B, Luzhetskyy A (2014) Iterative marker excision system. Appl Microbiol Biotechnol 98:4557–4570

83. Ausubel FM, Brent R, Kingston RE, Moore DO, Seidman JS, Smith JA, Struhl K (1995) Current protocols in molecular biology. Wiley, New York, NY

84. D'Huys PJ, Lule I, Van Hove S, Vercammen D, Wouters C, Bernaerts K et al (2011) Amino acid uptake profiling of wild type and recombinant *Streptomyces lividans* TK24 batch fermentations. J Biotechnol 152:132–143

85. Eiteman MA, Altman E (2006) Overcoming acetate in *Escherichia coli* recombinant protein fermentations. Trends Biotechnol 24:530–536

86. Villadsen J, Nielsen JH, Lidén G (2011) Bioreaction engineering principles. Springer, New York, NY

87. Hodgson DA (1982) Glucose repression of carbon source uptake and metabolism in *Streptomyces coelicolor* A3(2) and its perturbation in mutants resistant to 2-deoxyglucose. J Gen Microbiol 128:2417–2430

88. Nowruzi K, Elkamel A, Scharer JM, Cossar D, Moo-Young M (2008) Development of a minimal defined medium for recombinant human interleukin-3 production by *Streptomyces lividans* 66. Biotechnol Bioeng 99:214–222

89. Gajzlerska W, Kurkowiak J, Turlo J (2015) Use of three-carbon chain compounds as biosynthesis precursors to enhance tacrolimus production in *Streptomyces tsukubaensis*. New Biotechnol 32:32–39

90. Muhamadali H, Xu Y, Ellis DI, Trivedi DK, Rattray NJW, Bernaerts K, Goodacre R (2015) Metabolomics investigation of recombinant mTNF alpha production in *Streptomyces lividans*. Microb Cell Fact 14

91. Takors R (2012) Scale-up of microbial processes: impacts, tools and open questions. J Biotechnol 160:3–9

92. Doran PM (2013) Bioprocess engineering principles. Elsevier, Amsterdam

93. Shuler ML, Kargi F (2002) Bioprocess engineering: basic concepts. Prentice Hall, Upper Saddle River, NJ

94. Garcia-Ochoa F, Gomez E (2009) Bioreactor scale-up and oxygen transfer rate in microbial processes: an overview. Biotechnol Adv 27:153–176

Chapter 9

Degradation Network Reconstruction Guided by Metagenomic Data

Rafael Bargiela and Manuel Ferrer

Abstract

Network reconstruction procedures based on meta-"omics" data are an invaluable tool for inferring total and active set of reactions mediated by different members in a microbial community. Within them, network-based methods for automatic analysis of catabolic capacities in metagenomes are currently limited. Here, we describe the complete workflow, scripts, and commands allowing the automatic reconstruction of biodegradation networks using as an input meta-sequences generated by direct DNA sequencing.

Key words AromaDeg, Aromatics, Biodegradation, Metagenomics, Network reconstruction, Next-generation sequencing, Pathways, Pollutants

1 Introduction

The analysis of microbial communities begins by assessing the structure of the population, which is currently often achieved using partial $16S$ ribosomal RNA (rRNA) gene sequences obtained by non-assembled metagenomic data [1]. The next step consists of characterizing the metabolic capacity of the microbial community, mostly by applying computational methods. Traditional approaches described in the literature typically map data for genes, proteins or metabolites onto well-known pathways or Gene Ontology terms [2]. This enables identifying molecular functions of identified proteins in light of metabolic pathways that are commonly found in many microbial genomes. However, the high connectivity among biological pathways has shifted the focus to networks [3, 4], which allows us to capture more global properties [5]. Molecular networks integrate different pathways and constitute a more general framework for interpreting "omics" data [6]. In particular, a number of approaches have been specifically designed to incorporate gene and protein expression data [7–9] and metabolite and flux levels [10, 11] into metabolic pathways. These approaches (such as the Model SEED) start from the annotated genome of an organism

Wolfgang R. Streit and Rolf Daniel (eds.), *Metagenomics: Methods and Protocols*, Methods in Molecular Biology, vol. 1539, DOI 10.1007/978-1-4939-6691-2_9, © Springer Science+Business Media LLC 2017

[12, 13] or an annotated metagenome and a reference metabolic database as input information to create a meta-network using a graph theoretical approach [14–17].

Reconstruction methods integrating pathways supported by accurately predicted genes may constitute a more general framework for interpreting "omics" data and for deciphering catabolic capacities. These methods may address systematic errors produced by standard methods of protein function prediction. This is particularly noticeable for the functional classification of key genes, particularly those encoding proteins of aromatic compounds' degradation. Recently, the AromaDeg Web-based resource has been created [18]. It contains an up-to-date and manually curated database that includes an associated query system which exploits phylogenomic analysis of the degradation of aromatic compounds. This database addresses systematic errors produced by standard methods of protein function prediction by improving the accuracy of functional classification of key genes encoding proteins of aromatic compounds' degradation. In brief, each query sequence from a genome or metagenome that matches a given protein family of AromaDeg is associated with an experimentally validated catabolic enzyme performing an aromatic compound degradation reaction. Here, an automatic meta-network graphical approach is described, which directly leads to a network that includes catabolic reactions associated to genes encoding enzymes annotated in the genomes of the community organisms. The approach focuses on the usage of the Web-based AromaDeg resource [18] and the usage of meta-genomic data. The method herein reported has been successfully applied to draft the catabolic networks of different meta-sequences generated by direct sequencing from crude oil-contaminated marine sediments and enrichment microcosms set up with those [19, 20].

2   Materials

All computations can be performed on a 64-bit Limux UBUNTU machine, Intel Core 8 at 2.4 GHz and 24 GB of RAM. The inputs are predicted meta-sequences (>50 amino acid length) generated by extensive high-throughput Next-Generation Sequencing.

1. AromaDeg [18].

2. Whole genome or metagenome shotgun sequences (for examples *see* refs. 19 and 20).

3   Methods

Here, we present a procedure for catabolic network reconstruction using meta-genomic data. Briefly, sequences encoding catabolic enzymes, identified by using the Web-based AromaDeg resource [18], are used to create a nodes table on the basis of which an automatic reconstruction of a degradation network is developed under *R* language, as described below.

3.1 Identification of Catabolic Genes in the Meta-Sequences

The Web-based AromaDeg resource [18] is used for catabolic network reconstruction. AromaDeg is a Web-based resource with an up-to-date and manually curated database that includes an associated query system which exploits phylogenomic analysis of the degradation of aromatic compounds. Each query sequence from a genome or metagenome that matches a given protein family of AromaDeg is associated with an experimentally validated catabolic enzyme performing an aromatic compound degradation reaction.

1. AromaDeg Web-based resource (*see* **Note 1**) is used to filter predicted open reading frames in the metagenomic DNA sequences (*see* **Note 2**) by alignment length (>50 amino acids) and minimum percentage of homology (>50 %).

2. After a manual check, a final list of gene sequences encoding enzymes potentially involved in degradation is prepared.

3.2 Creating a Degradation Node Table

1. Each connection in the network represents a step in the degradation pathway (a degradation reaction), connecting a product with its substrate (nodes), which is assigned to a gene encoding a catabolic enzyme (for examples *see* Table 1). Thus, degradation pathways are represented from the initial substrate to the main common intermediaries and the final steps until the tricarboxylic acid (TCA) substrates. A table connecting pollutant products, intermediates, and final degradation products to catabolic enzymes of interest should be prepared before a network is reconstructed (*see* **Note 3**). An example of the naphthalene-to-catechol-to TCA pathways is summarized in Fig. 1.

2. Relative abundance (*see* **Note 4**) for each type of gene encoding catabolic enzymes found for each metagenomes (according to the list of detected gene sequences encoding enzymes potentially involved in degradation) is used to set up the nodes table, resulting in a list of weights that specifies the size of the connections in each step of the network for each sample, as exemplified in Table 1.

3.3 Setting Up the Nodes of the Network

1. Network structure is set up under the programming language *R*, using the functions provided by the package *igraph* and the information given in the nodes Table 1. The process starts calling the functions of the package, opening the table under the *R* environment and creating a new graph object with the substrates/products of the table like nodes:

```
> library(igraph)
> edgelist <-read.table("NodesTable.txt",
```

Table 1
Table with nodes and connections for graphical visualization of degradation networks

Substrate	Product	Enzyme	Rel. ab. genes MG1	MG2
Phenylpropionate	2,3-Dihydroxyphenylpropionate	Multiple	0	0
2,3-Dihydroxyphenylpropionate	2-Hydroxy-6-ketonona-2,4-dienedioate	Dpp	0	1
2-Hydroxy-6-ketonona-2,4-dienedioate	TCA	Multiple	0	0
Phenanthrene	1-Hydroxy-2-naphthoate	Multiple	0	0
1-Hydroxy-2-naphthoate	2′-Carboxybenzalpyruvate	Hna	1	2
2′-Carboxybenzalpyruvate	2-Carboxybenzaldehyde	Multiple	0	0
2-Carboxybenzaldehyde	Phthalate	Multiple	0	0
Phthalate	Protocatechuate	Pht	1	0
Protocatechuate	2-Carboxy-*cis,cis*-muconate	Pca	1	0
2-Carboxy-*cis,cis*-muconate	TCA	-	0	0
Quinoline	2-Oxo-1,2-dihydroquinoline	NID	0	0
2-Oxo-1,2-dihydroquinoline	TCA	Odm	2	2
Dibenzofuran	2,2′,3-Trihydroxybiphenyl	NID	0	0
2,2′,3-Trihydroxybiphenyl	Salicylate	Thb	2	0
Salicylate	Catechol	-	0	0
4-Aminobenzenesulfonate	4-Sulfocatechol	Abs	2	0
4-Sulfocatechol	3-Sulfomuconate	Multiple	0	0
3-Sulfomuconate	TCA	Multiple	0	0
Catechol	2-Hydroxymuconate semialdehyde	Cat	14	17
2-Hydroxymuconate semialdehyde	TCA	Multiple	0	0
Naphthalene	1,2-Dihydroxynaphthalene	NaDi	0	0
1,2-Dihydroxynaphthalene	Salicylate	NID	0	0
Salicylate	Gentisate	Multiple	0	0
Gentisate	Maleylpyruvate	Gen	10	1
Maleylpyruvate	TCA	Multiple	0	0
2-Chlorobenzoate	Catechol	2CB	5	3
Benzene	Catechol	Bzn	0	1
p-Cumate	*cis*-2,3-Dihydroxy-2,3-dihydro-*p*-cumate	Cum	2	0

(continued)

Table 1
(continued)

Substrate	Product	Enzyme	Rel. ab. genes MG1	MG2
cis-2,3-Dihydroxy-2,3-dihydro-*p*-cumate	2-Hydroxy-3-carboxy-6-oxo-7-methylocta-2,4-dienoate (HCOMOD)	NID	0	0
HCOMOD	TCA	Multiple	0	0
Biphenyl	2,3-Dihydroxybiphenyl	Bph	1	1
2,3-Dihydroxybiphenyl	2-Hydroxy-6-oxo-6-phenylhexa-2,4-dienoate (HOPD)	Dhb	6	3
HOPD	Benzoate	NID	0	0
Benzoate	Catechol	Bzt	4	1
Homoprotocatechuate	5-Carboxymethyl-2-hydroxy-muconic semialdehyde (CMHMS)	Hpc	0	1
CMHMS	TCA	Multiple	0	0
Ibuprofen	Ibuprofen-CoA	NID	0	0
Ibuprofen-CoA	1,2-*cis*-Diol-2-hydroibuprofen-CoA	Ibu	0	1
1,2-*cis*-Diol-2-hydroibuprofen-CoA	2-hydroxy-5-isobutylhexa-2,4-dienoate	NID	0	0
2-Hydroxy-5-isobutylhexa-2,4-dienoate	TCA	Multiple	0	0
Orcinol	2,3,5-Trihydroxytoluene	Orc	0	2
2,3,5-Trihydroxytoluene	2,4,6-Trioxoheptanoate	NID	0	0
2,4,6-Trioxoheptanoate	TCA	-	0	0
Indole-3-acetic acid	Catechol	Ind	1	1

Association between biodegradation reactions and genes encoding catabolic enzymes is shown. As described in text, each query sequence from a metagenome that matches a given protein family of the AromaDeg [18] is associated to a key catabolic enzyme for an aromatic degradation reaction. Based on bibliographic records, the substrates and intermediates products can be linked to form a biodegradation network. For network reconstruction, each query sequence encoding a catabolic enzyme was assigned to a degradation reaction (with a code assigned by AromaDeg) involving a metabolic substrate and a product, which were further used for the network reconstruction using appropriated scripts and commands described in Subheading 3. The relative abundance (rel. ab.) of genes encoding each of the catabolic enzymes (to avoid artifacts due to differences in sample size) needed to proceed with the network reconstruction, is shown. Gene names as in Fig. 3 legend

NaDi naphthalene dioxygenase, *MG1* metagenome 1, *MG2* metagenome 2 (*see* **Note 5**)

```
+    header=TRUE,dec=",",sep="\t",check.
names=FALSE)
> g <-graph.empty(directed=TRUE)
> u <-unique(c(as.character(edgelist[,2]),
```

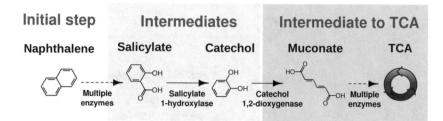

Fig. 1 Description of the general pattern used to draw each degradation pathway. Using the naphthalene degradation pathway as an example, naphthalene is the initial substrate of the pathway, which through several reactions (represented by *dashed lines*) is converted to salicylate (intermediate 1) that is degraded to catechol by a direct reaction (*solid line*). Catechol is further converted into muconate by a direct reaction (*solid line*). Finally, muconate is addressed to the TCA pathway

```
+                        as.character(edgelist[,3])))
>   g<-add.vertices(g,length(u),name=u,
+                        size=size,degree=degre
e,dist=dist)
```

2. After creating a new graph with *graph.empty*, all the substrate/ product names are listed in a value with *unique* and added as nodes of the new graph with *add.vertices*, where some attributes like the size of the node or the position for the labels can be set up using values like *size*, *degree*, or *dist*.

3.4 Adding the Connections Between Nodes to the Network

1. There are two different types of connections for the network. Those with 0 abundance of the gene of interest in all samples (empty connections) and the connections with at least one sample with an abundance >0 (positive connections). We make this difference in order to set up independently the drawing attributes of both types of connections, like the type and curve of the line in the arrows. *See* Fig. 2.

2. Empty connections are added first. A loop checking the data is needed:
```
> for(i in 1:nrow(edgelist)){
+     if (sum(edgelist[i,4:ncol(edgeli
st)])==0){
+                g<- add.edges(g,rbind(edgelist
[i,2],edgelist[i,3]),
+                        attr=list(color=
"grey60",curve=0,
+                        name=as.
character(edgelist[i,1])))
+     }
+}
```

3. Connections are introduced in the graph with the function *add.edges*. Calculating the total abundance in each network step (row) from the nodes table (Table 1), it is possible to see

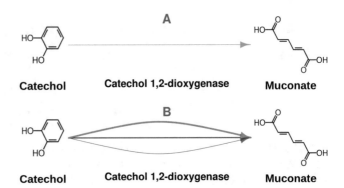

Fig. 2 Description of the two distinct types of connections in the catabolic networks. Multiple connections are used when multiple metagenomes are compared. (**a**) an empty connection with 0 abundance in all the samples, meaning that no genes encoding catabolic enzymes for this reaction was found in the metagenomes. (**b**) a positive connection with abundance >0 in three different metagenomes (arbitrarily represented in *green*, *red*, and *blue* colored-lines), with the size of the line according to the relative abundance value of catabolic gene for each sample

whether the abundance is 0 in all the samples; in this case a simple connection is added to the graph with a grey arrow. Another loop is run to add the positive connections (abundance >0 at least in one sample):

```
> curve<-0
> for(i in 4:ncol(edgelist)){
+           from<-NA
+           to<-NA
+           weights<-NA
+           name<-NA
+           newfrom<-na.omit(from)
+           newto<-na.omit(to)
+           weights<-na.omit(weights)
+           name<-na.omit(name)
+       for(j in 1:nrow(edgelist)){
+           if (edgelist[j,i] > 0){
+             from<-append(from,
+
as.character(edgelist[j,2]),
+
after=length(from))
+                 to<-append(to,
+
as.character(edgelist[j,3]),
+                             after=length(to))
+             weights<-append(weights,
+                             edgelist[j,i],
+
after=length(weights))
```

```
+                 name<-append(name,
+
as.character(edgelist[j,1]),
+
after=length(name))
+                 }
+             }
+     g<- add.edges(g,rbind(from,to),
+
attr=list(weight=weights,
+                              color=color,cu
rve=curve),name=name)
+
+             if (curve%%2==0){
+                 curve<-abs(curve)
+             }
+             else{
+                 curve<- -curve
+             }
+
+             if (curve<0){
+                 curve<-curve
+             }
+             else{
+                 curve<-abs(curve)+0.2
+             }
+
+}
```

4. In the case of abundance >0 (at least in one sample) the loop is more complicated. In the first part, empty vectors for each sample are created to save (using the function *append*) the different attributes of the connections in each case (name, weight, and nodes of the connections). The connections for each sample are added to the graph at the final of the loop again with *add.edges*. The attribute *curve* is configured before running this step and is changed at the end of the loop to set the curve for the next sample.

5. Reason for running two independent loops and checking twice the whole table, is simple. Checking empty connections needs to look over the table row by row, like in the first loop, but checking the positive connections needs to look over the table column by column (sample by sample), like in the second loop.

6. Note that the line for empty connections is drawn in grey color, which means that abundance in this case is 0, and the width of the line is not representing any percentage of gene presence. Also, these connections can represent a single step in the pathway (straight line) or multiple reactions (dashed line).

3.5 Setting Up the Coordinates of the Nodes in the Network

1. Coordinates of the nodes determine the position of each node (substrate/product) in the final draw of the network. These coordinates can be set manually, in order to obtain a customized layout for the network, saved in a file, which is used when needed to draw a new network, without a new manual setup:

```
> p <- tkplot(g)
> Coords <- tkplot.getcoords(p)
> write.table(Coords,"Coords.txt",row.
names=FALSE,col.names=FALSE)
> Coords<- matrix(scan("Coords.
txt"),nc=2,byrow=TRUE)
```

2. Function *tkplot* displays a new interactive screen where one can point each node in the desired position and then save the coordinates in a value with *tkplot.getcoords*. Using *write.table* is possible to print the value with the coordinates in an output file, and read it again using *matrix* and *scan*.

3.6 Drawing the Degradation Network

1. Network can be drawn using the coordinates and the configuration in the prior steps:

```
>   jpeg("Network.jpg",width=5796,height=3561,
+       res=300,quality=100,units="px")
> par(mar=c(0,0,0,0),xpd=TRUE)
>   plot.igraph(g,
+                layout=Coords,
+       vertex.shape=shape,
+       vertex.size=size1,
+       vertex.size2=size2,
+       vertex.size2=size2,
+       vertex.label=labels,
+       vertex.label.dist=V(g)$dist,
+       vertex.label.degree=V(g)$degree,
+       vertex.label.dist=V(g)$dist,
+       vertex.label.degree=V(g)$degree,
+       edge.width=ifelse(E(g)$weight<=0.01,1,
+              ifelse(E(g)$weight>0.10,10,E(g)$
weight*100)),
+       edge.lty=lty
+       )
+ dev.off()
```

2. Functions *jpeg* and *dev.off* are used to save the plot in a *jpeg* file. The main function to draw the network is *plot.igraph*, using the coordinates saved before as layout, and the parameters provided when the vertices were added to the graph object to set up the different options of the function. Other options can be modified using vector objects with values for the different vertices/connections. Abundances for each node in each sample are used as the width of the connections (saved as connection

weight in the **step 2**) but are adapted, with a conditional loop (*ifelse*), to make them fit in the plot. Herein, an abundance of 0.01 is equal 1 in the *edge.width* parameter, so this value will be the abundance multiply by 100 (0.02 is equal to 2, 0.05 is equal to 5). When the *edge.width* value is higher than 10 (for abundances >0.1) the value is set in 10, and if the value is lower than 1 (abundances <0.01) the width is set in 1. For empty connections abundance is set as 0, but in the network will be drawn with a size of 1 as is configured in the parameter *edge.width*. This is because a size >0 must be indicated in the script in order to draw a visible connection; however a grey color is used in these connections to specify the absence of abundance in these reaction/s. Figure 3 provides an example of the degradation capacities of two distinct metagenomes.

4   Notes

1. AromaDeg Web server is available at http://aromadeg.siona.helmholtz-hzi.de/. Parameters used in the Subheading 3.1 for filtering the sequence with the AromaDeg Web resource by minimum homology and alignment length can be set up as needed. Standard settings are used in this case. AromaDeg database contains sequences of key aromatic catabolic gene families (and subfamilies) involved in the degradation of aromatic pollutants [18].

2. Individual query sequences from a genome or metagenome or complete query meta-sequences can be used when searching in AromaDeg Web server.

3. The node tables should be prepared for all pollutants of interest. The Table 1 only provides information for the transformation of a limited number of pollutants. For other pollutants, an appropriate node table should be developed [19, 20].

4. Utilization of values of relative abundance of genes encoding catabolic enzymes is recommended to avoid artifacts due to differences in sample size and metagenome sequence coverage.

5. The meta-sequences of the two metagenomes were taken from the National Center for Biotechnology Information (NCBI). The Whole Genome Shotgun metagenomes are available at NCBI/DDBJ/EMBL/GenBank under the accession numbers PRJNA222663 and AZIK00000000 (for metagenome 1) and PRJNA222664 and AZIH00000000 (for metagenome 2).

6. Not all sequences encoding catabolic enzymes involved in the complete degradation of pollutants can be identified using the Web-based AromaDeg resource [18]. In this case, we added the abbreviation NID in case a reaction (in black color in Fig. 3) is supported by a catabolic enzyme not included in the database.

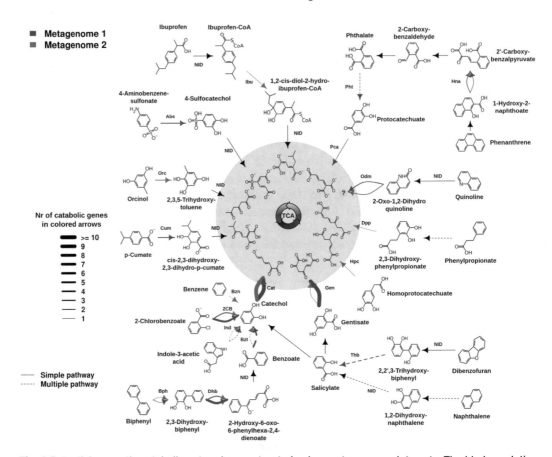

Fig. 3 Potential aromatic catabolic networks constructed using metagenome data sets. The biodegradation network reconstruction was performed as in Subheadings 3.2–3.6, for two arbitrary metagenomes represented by *red* and *blue* color (*see* **Note 5**). Briefly, catabolic genes were identified as described in Subheading 3.1. For network reconstruction, each sequence subsequently was assigned to a metabolic substrate as well as a product (as defined by [18]) with an assigned code. The putative substrates and products processed in the sample were connected, creating a metabolic network using appropriate scripts and commands [19, 20]. The number of each catabolic gene assigned to degradation reactions, is represented by the thickness of the lines in the figure and the complete list of substrates possibly degraded by the communities are summarized. Common and sample-specific initial pollutants or intermediates for which presumptive degradation signatures are identified are specifically indicated in the figure. Solid lines represent single step reactions while dotted lines represent degradation steps where multiple reactions are involved [19, 20]. Gene names or codes (*see* **Note 6**) as follows: *Abs* 4-aminobenzenesulfonate 3,4-dioxygenase, *Bph* biphenyl dioxygenase, *Bzn* benzene dioxygenase, *Bzt* benzoate dioxygenase, *Cat* catechol 2,3-dioxygenase, *2CB* 2-chlorobenzoate dioxygenase, *Cum* *p*-cumate dioxygenase, *Dhb* 2,3-Dihydroxybiphenyl dioxygenase, *Dpp* 2,3-dihydroxyphenylpropionate dioxygenase, *Gen* gentisate dioxygenase, *Hna* 1-hydroxy-2-naphthoate dioxygenase, *Hpc* homoprotocatechuate 2,3-dioxygenase, *Ibu* ibuprofen-CoA dioxygenase, *Ind* Rieske oxygenase involved in indole acetic acid degradation, *Odm* 2-oxo-1,2-dihydroxyquinoline monooxygenase, *Orc* orcinol hydroxylase, *Pca* protocatechuate 3,4-dioxygenase, *Pht* phthalate 4,5-dioxygenase, *Thb* 2,2′,3-trihydroxybiphenyl dioxygenase

Acknowledgments

The authors gratefully acknowledge the financial support provided by the European Community projects KILL-SPILL (FP7-KBBE-2012-312139), MAGIC-PAH (FP7-KBBE-2009-245226), and ULIXES (FP7-KBBE-2010-266473). This project has received funding from the European Union's Horizon 2020 research and innovation program [Blue Growth: Unlocking the potential of Seas and Oceans] under grant agreement No [634486]. This work was further funded by grants BIO2011-25012, and BIO2014-54494-R from the Spanish Ministry of Economy and Competitiveness. The authors gratefully acknowledge the financial support provided by the European Regional Development Fund (ERDF).

References

1. Röling WF, Ferrer M, Golyshin PN (2010) Systems approaches to microbial communities and their functioning. Curr Opin Biotechnol 21:532–538

2. Yamada T, Letunic I, Okuda S, Kanehisa M, Bork P (2011) iPath2.0: interactive pathway explorer. Nucleic Acids Res 39:W412–W415

3. Letunic I, Yamada T, Kanehisa M, Bork P (2008) iPath: interactive exploration of biochemical pathways and networks. Trends Biochem Sci 33:101–103

4. Palsson B (2009) Metabolic systems biology. FEBS Lett 583:3900–3904

5. McCloskey D, Palsson BO, Feist AM (2013) Basic and applied uses of genome-scale metabolic network reconstructions of *Escherichia coli*. Mol Syst Biol 9:661

6. Bordbar A, Palsson BO (2012) Using the reconstructed genome-scale human metabolic network to study physiology and pathology. J Intern Med 271:131–141

7. Jerby L, Shlomi T, Ruppin E (2010) Computational reconstruction of tissue-specific metabolic models: application to human liver metabolism. Mol Syst Biol 6:401

8. Rezola A, Pey J, de Figueiredo LF, Podhorski A, Schuster S, Rubio A, Planes FJ (2013) Selection of human tissue-specific elementary flux modes using gene expression data. Bioinformatics 29:2009–2016

9. Tobalina L, Bargiela R, Pey J, Herbst FA, Lores I, Rojo D et al (2015) Context-specific metabolic network reconstruction of a naphthalene-degrading bacterial community guided by metaproteomic data. Bioinformatics 31:1771–1779

10. Zamboni N, Kummel A, Heinemann M (2008) anNET: a tool for network-embedded thermodynamic analysis of quantitative metabolome data. BMC Bioinformatics 9:199

11. Pey J, Tobalina L, de Cisneros JP, Planes FJ (2013) A network-based approach for predicting key enzymes explaining metabolite abundance alterations in a disease phenotype. BMC Syst Biol 7:62

12. Bachmann H, Fischlechner M, Rabbers I, Barfa N, Branco dos Santos F, Molenaar D, Teusink B (2013) Availability of public goods shapes the evolution of competing metabolic strategies. Proc Natl Acad Sci U S A 110:14302–14307

13. Zomorrodi AR, Suthers PF, Ranganathan S, Maranas CD (2012) Mathematical optimization applications in metabolic networks. Metab Eng 14:672–686

14. Henry CS, DeJongh M, Best AA, Frybarger PM, Linsay B, Stevens RL (2010) High-throughput generation, optimization and analysis of genome-scale metabolic models. Nat Biotechnol 28:977–982

15. Branco dos Santos F, de Vos WM, Teusink B (2013) Towards metagenome-scale models for industrial applications--the case of Lactic Acid Bacteria. Curr Opin Biotechnol 24:200–206

16. Zomorrodi AR, Maranas CD (2012) OptCom: a multi-level optimization framework for the metabolic modeling and analysis of microbial communities. PLoS Comput Biol 8:e1002363

17. Khandelwal RA, Olivier BG, Roling WF, Teusink B, Bruggeman FJ (2013) Community flux balance analysis for microbial consortia at balanced growth. PLoS One 8:e64567

18. Duarte M, Jauregui R, Vilchez-Vargas R, Junca H, Pieper DH (2014) AromaDeg, a novel database for phylogenomics of aerobic bacterial degradation of aromatics. Database (Oxford) 2014:bau118

19. Bargiela R, Gertler C, Magagnini M, Mapelli F, Chen J, Daffonchio D et al (2015) Degradation network reconstruction in uric acid and ammonium amendments in oil-degrading marine microcosm guides by metagenomic data. Front Microbiol 6:1270

20. Bargiela R, Mapelli F, Rojo D, Chouaia B, Tornes J, Borin S et al (2015) Bacterial population and biodegradation potential in chronically crude oil-contaminated marine sediments are strongly linked to temperature. Sci Rep 5:11651

Chapter 10

Novel Tools for the Functional Expression of Metagenomic DNA

Nadine Katzke, Andreas Knapp, Anita Loeschcke, Thomas Drepper, and Karl-Erich Jaeger

Abstract

Functional expression of genes from metagenomic libraries is limited by various factors including inefficient transcription and/or translation of target genes as well as improper folding and assembly of the corresponding proteins caused by the lack of appropriate chaperones and cofactors. It is now well accepted that the use of different expression hosts of distinct phylogeny and physiology can dramatically increase the rate of success. In the following chapter, we therefore describe tools and protocols allowing for the comparative heterologous expression of genes in five bacterial expression hosts, namely *Escherichia coli*, *Pseudomonas putida*, *Bacillus subtilis*, *Burkholderia glumae*, and *Rhodobacter capsulatus*. Different broad-host-range shuttle vectors are described that allow activity-based screening of metagenomic DNA in these bacteria. Furthermore, we describe the newly developed transfer-and-expression system TREX which comprises genetic elements essential to allow for expression of large clusters of functionally coupled genes in different microbial species.

Key words Metagenomic library, Environmental DNA, Activity-based screening, Functional expression, Multi-host screening, Shuttle vector, *Escherichia coli*, *Pseudomonas putida*, *Bacillus subtilis*, *Rhodobacter capsulatus*, *Burkholderia glumae*, Transposon

1 Introduction

Metagenomics comprise a large number of methods to access genes of microbial communities by culture-independent methods, aiming either at the elucidation of microbial diversity and ecosystem organization [1] or at the discovery of novel biocatalysts and natural products [2]. The selection of the environment for sampling represents an essential step in such endeavors. Sampling sites with a high microbial diversity such as soils or sediments [3, 4] are promising targets for the discovery of a number of highly diverse biocatalysts. On the other hand, habitats harboring lower diversity microbial communities may allow to access smaller numbers of biocatalysts or natural products, albeit with specific properties.

Wolfgang R. Streit and Rolf Daniel (eds.), *Metagenomics: Methods and Protocols*, Methods in Molecular Biology, vol. 1539, DOI 10.1007/978-1-4939-6691-2_10, © Springer Science+Business Media LLC 2017

Such habitats often provide extreme conditions regarding pH, temperature, salt concentration, or pressure [5–9], or they are inherently enriched in target biocatalysts [10, 11]. Enrichment strategies, e.g., by applying selective growth conditions, can further boost the search for new biocatalysts in environmental samples and thus narrow down the natural biodiversity to a subset of microorganisms offering the desired biocatalytic activity [12–14].

Screening approaches for metagenomics libraries can be divided into two different categories, namely sequence-based and activity-based strategies. Sequence-based (genome mining) strategies make use of genome and metagenome databases to identify new candidates of a desired enzyme family, thereby limiting the potential to find completely new enzyme groups [15–17]. Activity-based screenings, on the other hand, employ enzymatic activity assays which allow to identify a specific biocatalytic function in metagenomics libraries. To this end, high-throughput screening methods are usually applied where the desired enzymatic activity is easily detectable, e.g., by a change of color of a given substrate or by halo formation around colonies grown on agar plates. However, the discovery of new biocatalysts is limited here by the availability of appropriate screening systems and by the expression efficiency of the corresponding targeted genes [18–21]. The simultaneous and efficient expression of all genes located on a specific metagenome-derived DNA fragment comprises a peculiar challenge for activity-based screenings. Size, orientation and organization of the contained genes, as well as recognition of promoters or regulatory elements by the expression host are additional common bottlenecks for function-based screenings [18, 19]. Even after correct transcription and translation of environmental genes, yields of active enzymes are often limited by the availability of suitable chaperones and specific cofactors or the capability of the host organism for posttranslational modifications and secretion of target proteins [22, 23].

A common strategy to overcome these limitations is the comparative expression of metagenome-derived genes using different expression hosts. This has led to the development of broad-host-range vectors and synthetic biology tools which allow efficient cloning in *Escherichia coli* and subsequent transfer into specialized screening host strains [24, 25]. In addition, there is an increasing interest to develop and establish new microbes with unique physiological properties for efficient expression [24–28].

In this chapter, we present strategies to employ various bacterial expression hosts for efficient screening of metagenomic libraries and overexpression of candidate genes. In the first section, a method is described for the isolation and purification of metagenomic DNA from bacterial consortia to create metagenomic libraries. Library construction is based on the broad-host-range shuttle vector pEBP18 [29] which can be used for comparative expression in *E. coli*, *P. putida*, and *B. subtilis*. The second section describes the

TREX expression system which allows efficient expression of large native gene clusters (size >20 kb) [30] in *E. coli*, *P. putida*, and *R. capsulatus* [31]. Here, target DNA is integrated into the host genome by transposition using two DNA cassettes, L-TREX and R-TREX, which are integrated upstream and downstream of the targeted gene cluster. Bacteriophage T7 derived promoters included in both cassettes enable the bidirectional transcription of the clustered genes, rendering expression independent of their orientation. In the last two sections, handling of and protein production with the Gram-negative bacteria *B. glumae* and *R. capsulatus* are addressed. *B. glumae* PG1 is a nonhuman pathogenic species of the *Burkholderia* group [32, 33] which is known to efficiently produce and secrete a biotechnologically relevant lipase [34, 35] and is therefore regarded as an interesting alternative to existing bacterial expression hosts. *R. capsulatus* is a phototrophic, facultative anaerobic purple bacterium which forms under phototrophic growth conditions an intracyto-plasmic membrane system capable of accommodating large quantities of heterologous membrane proteins, which are considered difficult-to-express because of the limited membrane space available in commonly used expression hosts like *E. coli* [36]. Table 1 shows an overview of advantageous features of the five different expression hosts described in this chapter.

Table 1
Features of bacterial expression host strains

Expression host	Features
Escherichia coli	• well-established industrial expression host • molecular genetics known • numerous tools for cloning and expression available
Pseudomonas putida	• molecular genetics known [37] • plenty of methods available for cultivation and genetic manipulation [38] • produces numerous cofactors, suitable for expression of oxidoreductases [39, 40] • versatile metabolism with high diversity of enzymes [37] • high tolerance against antibiotics and organic solvents [41, 42]
Bacillus subtilis	• well-established industrial expression host highly efficient secretion systems for heterologous proteins • cost-effective purification of heterologous proteins [43]
Burkholderia glumae	• nonhuman pathogen lacking characteristic virulence factors [33] • methods available for cultivation and genetic manipulation • effective secretion of enantioselective lipase [34, 35]
Rhodobacter capsulatus	• facultative anaerobic bacterium suitable for functional expression of oxygen-sensitive proteins and pathways • intracytoplasmic membrane system to accommodate heterologous membrane proteins and enzymes [44] • produces a variety of different metal-containing cofactors [45, 46] • possesses non-toxic LPS [47]

2 Materials

Chemicals were obtained from Carl Roth GmbH (Karlsruhe, Germany) if not noted otherwise.

1. *E. coli* DH5α (Thermo Fisher Scientific, Waltham, Massachusetts, USA) is used for DNA cloning and *E. coli* S17-1 [48] for conjugational transfer of plasmids to *R. capsulatus* and *B. glumae* PG1 (*see* **Note 1**).

2. *P. putida* KT2440 [37] and *B. subtilis* TEB1030 [43] are used for screening and expression with the pEBP18 and TREX system.

3. *B. glumae* PG1 [32] is used for transformation with plasmids or transposons.

4. *R. capsulatus* B10S is used for expression with plasmids of the pRhok series. Strain B10S-T7 is used for T_7-dependent expression [49].

5. Luria–Bertani (LB) medium [50] contains 10 g/L tryptone (peptone from casein), 5 g/L yeast extract, and 5 g/L NaCl solubilized in deionized water and autoclaved (121 °C, 2 bar, 20 min). 2× LB medium contains the same components at doubled concentration.

6. EM medium is prepared by dissolving 20 g/L tryptone (peptone from casein), 5 g/L yeast extract, and 5 g/L NaCl in deionized water, adjusting pH to 7.2 and autoclaving (121 °C, 2 bar, 20 min). After sterilization and cooling, 5 mL/L of sterile glucose solution (50% (w/v) α-D(+)-glucose monohydrate) is added to obtain a final concentration of 0.5% (w/v).

7. EM1 medium is EM medium containing 1% (w/v) glucose.

8. Minimal Medium E (MME) is prepared as 50× stock solution [51]. 10 g $MgSO_4 \cdot 7H_2O$, 100 g citric acid × $1H_2O$, 500 g K_2HPO_4, and 175 g $NaNH_4HPO_4 \cdot 4H_2O$ are dissolved successively in 670 mL deionized water, resulting in approximately 1 L stock, and autoclaved (121 °C, 2 bar, 20 min). After 50-fold dilution with autoclaved water the resulting medium has a pH of 7.0. For MME agar plates, 1.5% (w/v) agar, dissolved in water, is autoclaved and subsequently supplemented with 0.5% (w/v) glucose, 1/50 volume of MME stock solution and appropriate volumes of antibiotic solutions added after cooling to about 60 °C.

9. RCV minimal medium for cultivation of *R. capsulatus* is prepared according to Table 2. This solution is autoclaved (121 °C, 2 bar, 20 min). After cooling, add 9.6 mL 1 M phosphate buffer (81.3 g KH_2PO_4 and 78.7 g K_2HPO_4 in 500 mL deionized water, pH 6.8), 40 mL of a 10% DL-malate solution (pH 6.8) and 10 mL of a 10% $(NH_4)_2SO_4$ solution (*see* **Note 2**).

Table 2
RCV minimal medium composition (modified from ref. [49])

Basic RCV medium (1 L)				
Solution	[Stock][a]	Sterilization[b]	Storage	Volume
EDTA	1% (w/v)	121 °C	RT	2 mL
MgSO$_4$	20% (w/v)	121 °C	RT	1 mL
Trace element solution[c]	see below	121 °C	RT	1 mL
CaCl$_2$	7.5% (w/v)	121 °C	RT	1 mL
FeSO$_4$[d]	0.5% (w/v)	121 °C	RT	2.4 mL
Thiamine	0.1% (w/v)	121 °C	RT	1 mL
MilliQ water			RT	add 1000 mL
Trace element solution (250 mL)				
Compound	[Concentration]			
MnSO$_4 \cdot 1H_2O$	0.40 g			
H$_3$BO$_3$	0.70 g			
Cu(NO$_3$)$_2 \cdot 3H_2O$	0.01 g			
ZnSO$_4 \cdot 7H_2O$	0.06 g			
Na$_2$MoO$_4 \cdot 2H_2O$	0.02 g			
MilliQ water	Add 250 mL			

RT room temperature
[a]Indicates the concentration of stock solutions
[b]By autoclaving at 121 °C, 2 bar, for 20 min
[c]Compounds of trace element solution will only poorly dissolve; thus, it is important to stir well prior to pipetting
[d]1 mL of 37% HCl is added to the solution prior to sterilization to prevent oxidation of FeSO$_4$

10. PY medium: The complex medium for *R. capsulatus* contains 10 g/L Bacto peptone (BD, Sparks, USA) and 0.5 g/L Bacto yeast extract (BD, Sparks, USA). After autoclaving (121 °C, 2 bar, 20 min), let the medium cool down and add 2 mL/L of each 1 M MgCl$_2$, 1 M CaCl$_2$ and 2.4 mL/L of a 0.5% FeSO$_4$ solution (supplemented with 2 mL/L 37% HCl). For conjugation, prepare this medium without addition of FeSO$_4$ (*see* **Note 3**).

11. Fructose solution: 1.2 M fructose solution is used for induction of T7-dependent expression in strain *R. capsulatus* B10S-T7. After sterilization (121 °C, 2 bar, 20 min) the solution is stored at room temperature.

12. If necessary, antibiotics are added to culture media at concentrations shown in Table 2.

13. Agar plates are prepared by supplementing liquid media with 1.5% (w/v) agar prior to sterilization. For *R. capsulatus*, use Select Agar (Thermo Fisher Scientific, Waltham, Massachusetts, USA); for all other bacteria, agar-agar (Carl Roth GmbH,

Karlsruhe, Germany) can be used. Agar plates for *B. glumae* require additional supplements (*see* **item 8**).

14. Starch plates are LB agar plates containing 1% (w/v) corn starch (Mondamin, distributed by local supermarkets); sterilized by autoclaving (121 °C, 2 bar, 20 min). For coloring of starch plates use iodine solution consisting of 0.5% (w/v) iodine (Fluka, Sigma-Aldrich Chemie GmbH, Munich, Germany) and 1% (w/v) potassium iodine (AppliChem GmbH, Darmstadt, Germany) solubilized in deionized water (note that solubilization needs several days).

15. SP resuspension buffer for washing and mechanical disruption of *R. capsulatus* cells contains 22 mM KH_2PO_4, 40 mM K_2HPO_4 and 150 mM NaCl. When used for cell disruption, buffer is supplemented with protease inhibitor tablets (e.g., Complete, EDTA-free; Roche, Basel, Switzerland, 1 tablet per 50 mL).

2.2 Vectors

1. Shuttle vector pEBP18 (Fig. 1a): this 10.6 kb shuttle vector replicates in *E. coli* (ori_{Ec}) and in *P. putida* (ori_{Pp}) as episomal plasmid. In *B. subtilis*, the shuttle vector is integrated into the amylase locus of the bacterial chromosome ($amyE'_{Bs}$, '$amyE_{Bs}$) via homologous recombination. Heterologous DNA is inserted into the *Bam*HI cloning site. *Swa*I restriction sites upstream and downstream of the cloning site enable reisolation of DNA fragments. Heterologous genes are expressed from the inducible promoters P_{T7} (T7 RNA polymerase dependent) in *E. coli*, *P. putida* and *B. subtilis* or P_{xyl} (inducible by xylose) in *B. subtilis*. The included GFP gene (*gfp*) can be used to monitor gene expression. The *cos* site allows highly efficient transduction of *E. coli* by phage infection (which is necessary if the shuttle vector carries large inserts increasing its size to 37–52 kb) [52].

2. pUC18: 2.6 kb standard cloning vector for *E. coli* with *ori pMB1*, carrying an ampicillin resistance gene (Thermo Fisher Scientific, Waltham, Massachusetts, USA).

3. pBBR1MCS series (Fig. 1b): pBBR1MCS vectors contain a multiple cloning site, a *mob* site for conjugational transfer and a broad-host-range origin of replication which is recognized by Gram-negative bacteria like *E. coli* and *B. glumae*. For the protocols in this chapter, the 4.7 kb plasmid pBBR1MCS [53] is used which harbors a chloramphenicol resistance marker. Other plasmids of the pBBR1MCS series [54] can also be used, namely pBBR1MCS-2 (kanamycin), pBBR1MCS-3 (tetracycline), and pBBR1MCS-5 (gentamycin).

4. pIC20H-RL (Fig. 2c): The 9.5 kb plasmid pIC20H-RL is a pUC19 derived multi copy *E. coli* vector with *ori pMB1* and Ap^R as resistance gene and carries the TREX cassettes [31].

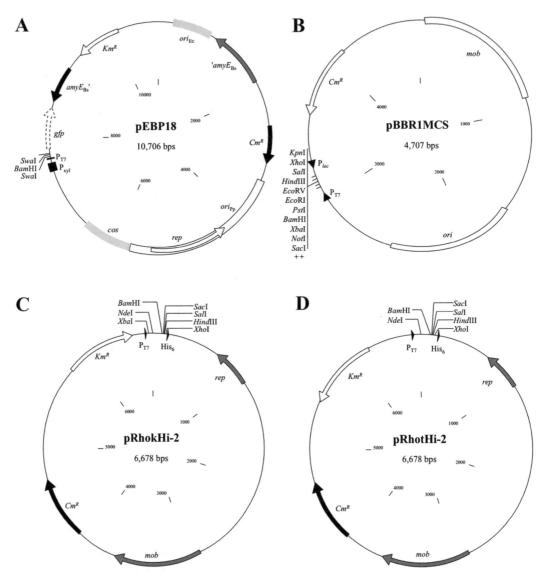

Fig. 1 Vectors for metagenomic library construction and expression in various host organisms. (**a**) Shuttle vector pEBP18 for library construction in *E. coli*, *P. putida*, and *B. subtilis*. (**b**) Expression plasmid pBBR1MCS for *B. glumae* PG1. Additional vectors of the pBBR1MCS series are available which differ in the antibiotic resistance gene and in multiple cloning site composition [43]. (**c**) Plasmid pRhokHi-2 for constitutive expression in *R. capsulatus*. (**d**) Plasmid pRhotHi-2 for T7 RNA polymerase dependent expression in *R. capsulatus*. Km^R kanamycin resistance gene, Cm^R chloramphenicol resistance gene, P_{T7} T7-promoter region, P_{Xyl} Xyl-promoter-region, P*lac* lac-promoter region, ori_{Pp} origin of replication for *P. putida*, ori_{Ec} origin of replication for *E. coli*, *rep* origin of replication, *mob* origin of transfer, $amyE_{Bs}$ integration sites for *B. subtilis*, His_6 6× histidine tag, *cos* transduction site, ++ additional restriction sites available. Drawings are not to scale

These comprise resistance markers (Tc^R and Gm^R, respectively), an *oriT* for conjugational transfer, elements of transposon Tn5, and T7 promoters for T7 RNA polymerase-dependent bidirectional transcription of DNA fragments. The cassettes may be

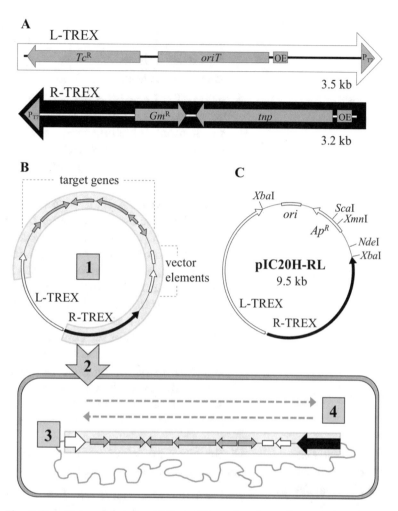

Fig. 2 Structure and function of the pathway *transfer* and *ex*pression system TREX. (**a**) The TREX system consists of two DNA cassettes, the L-TREX (*white*) and R-TREX (*black*) cassette, which comprise all elements for integrating and expressing a DNA fragment with multiple genes in a heterologous bacterial host. (**b**) Schematic depiction of the principle of TREX-mediated transfer and expression, which includes the "labeling" of a DNA fragment with target genes of interest with the TREX cassettes (step 1), the conjugational transfer of the TREX-labeled genes to a Gram-negative bacterial host (step 2), the randomized integration of TREX-labeled genes into the bacterial chromosome by transposition (step 3) (the transposing region of the plasmid construct is indicated by grey shading at step 1), and finally, the bidirectional expression of all genes by T7 RNA polymerase (step 4). (**c**) Plasmid pIC20H-RL carries the TREX cassettes as <L-TREX-R> module encompassing the L-TREX and R-TREX cassettes in an "inside-out" fashion with the T7 promoters pointing outward, flanked by *Xba*I restriction sites. For straight-forward one-step TREX labeling, this module can be inserted into a vector carrying a DNA fragment to be expressed. Alternatively, *Nde*I, *Xmn*I, or *Sca*I sites may be used to introduce target genes in this vector. *Ap*R ampicillin resistance gene, *Gm*R gentamicin resistance gene, *Tc*R tetracycline resistance gene, *oriT* origin of transfer, OE outside end of transposon Tn5, P$_{T7}$ T7 bacteriophage promoter, *tnp* Tn5 transposase gene

isolated as 6.8 kb *Xba*I fragment and inserted into a vector carrying a DNA fragment that is to be expressed, thereby "labeling" it for further steps of transfer and integration as well as expression in different hosts.

5. pML5-T7: The pML5 derived construct is a broad host range vector with *oriV*, which carries a tetracycline resistance gene and is mobilizable due to an *oriT* element [55]. The 17.7 kb vector carries the T7 RNA polymerase gene under control of the *lacUV5* promoter and the gene encoding the respective repressor lacI [56].

6. pRho vectors (Fig. 1c, d, *see* **Note 4**): Vectors pRhokHi-2 and pRhotHi-2 are used for constitutive and T7-dependent expression, respectively. The 6.7 kb vectors contain a broad-host-range origin of replication suitable for *R. capsulatus*, *P. putida* and *E. coli*, a *mob* site for mobilization of the plasmid to *R. capsulatus* and a kanamycin resistance gene (*Km*^{R}). Both plasmids are distinguished by the orientation of the *Km*^{R} gene. Target genes cloned into the multiple cloning site of pRhokHi-2 are under control of the constitutive P*aphII* promoter, while in pRhotHi-2 a T7 promoter upstream and a T7 terminator downstream of the multiple cloning site mediate efficient T7 RNA polymerase dependent expression. For easy purification and immunodetection, a His$_6$-tag encoding DNA sequence is present downstream of the target gene [36].

2.3 Preparation of Competent Cells: Solutions and Cuvettes

All chemicals are obtained from Carl Roth GmbH (Karlsruhe, Germany), if not noted otherwise.

1. Electroporation cuvettes: 1 mm gap and 2 mm gap (Bio-Budget Technologies GmbH, Krefeld, Germany).

2. MilliQ water is a registered trademark for water purification systems (Millipore GmbH, Schwalbach, Germany) providing water with a conductance of 18.2 mΩ at 25 °C. Sterilize by autoclaving (121 °C, 2 bar, 20 min) and store at 4 °C.

3. Glycerol solution: 10% (v/v) Rotipuran glycerol (Carl Roth GmbH, Karlsruhe, Germany) in MilliQ water. Sterilize by autoclaving (121 °C, 2 bar, 20 min) and store at 4 °C.

4. Sucrose solution: 300 mM sucrose (Merck KGaA, Darmstadt, Germany) in MilliQ water. Sterilize by autoclaving (121 °C, 2 bar, 20 min) and store at 4 °C.

5. Sucrose–glycerol solution: 300 mM sucrose (Merck KGaA, Darmstadt, Germany) and 10% (v/v) Rotipuran glycerol (Carl Roth GmbH, Karlsruhe, Germany) in MilliQ water. Sterilize by autoclaving (121 °C, 2 bar, 20 min) and store at 4 °C.

6. Paris-Medium: 60 mM potassium hydrogen phosphate (K$_2$HPO$_4$), 40 mM potassium dihydrogen phosphate

Table 3
Concentrations [µg/mL] of antibiotics

	pEBP18 system	*E. coli*	*P. putida*	*B. glumae*	*R. capsulatus*
Ampicillin	150	100	–	–	–
Chloramphenicol	7.5	50	–	200	–
Gentamycin	–	50	25	10	–
Irgasan	–	–	25	–	–
Kanamycin	20	50	–	50	25
Streptomycin	–	–	–	–	200
Tetracycline	–	10	50	40	–

(KH_2PO_4), 3 mM trisodium citrate dihydrate (Na_3-citrat), 20 mM potassium L-glutamate monohydrate (K-L-glutamate, AppliChem GmbH, Darmstadt, Germany), 3 mM magnesium sulfate ($MgSO_4$), 1 % (w/v) α-D(+)-glucose, 0.1 % (w/v) Bacto casamino acids (Becton Dickinson GmbH, Heidelberg, Germany), 20 mg/L L-tryptophan (Merck KGaA, Darmstadt, Germany), 2.2 mg/L ammonium-iron (III) citrate (Fe(III) NH_4-citrate (Fluka, Sigma-Aldrich Chemie GmbH, Munich, Germany)). Prepare the medium from separately sterilized stock solutions (Table 3). Store at 4 °C for up to 2 weeks.

7. $MgCl_2$ solution: 100 mM $MgCl_2$ in MilliQ water. Sterilize at 121 °C (2 bar, 20 min) and store at 4 °C.

8. $CaCl_2$ solution: 100 mM $CaCl_2$ in MilliQ water. After sterilization (121 °C, 2 bar, 20 min) store at 4 °C.

2.4 Solutions for DNA Extraction and Purification

Chemicals were obtained from Carl Roth GmbH (Karlsruhe, Germany) if not noted otherwise.

1. Isopropanol: Rotisolv 2-propanol.

2. Ethanol: Rotisolv ethanol is diluted to 70 % (v/v) with deionized water.

3. Sodium acetate: solution of 3 M sodium acetate in deionized water. Adjust to pH 5.5 with acetic acid (do not use HCl).

4. Solution #1 (for extraction of genomic DNA from a bacterial sample): 345 mM sucrose (Merck KGaA, Darmstadt, Germany), 10 mM Tris–HCl pH 8.0, 1 mM EDTA pH 8.0, and 2 mg/mL lysozyme (Sigma-Aldrich Chemie GmbH, Munich, Germany).

5. Solution #2 (for extraction of genomic DNA from a bacterial sample): 300 mM NaCl, 2 % (w/v) SDS, 100 mM Tris–HCl pH 8.0, and 20 mM EDTA pH 8.0.

6. 2 mM DTT (1,4-dithiothreitol, Carl Roth GmbH, Karlsruhe, Germany): prepare a stock solution of 1 M DTT solubilized in deionized water.

7. 50 µg/mL RNaseA.

8. Phenol–chloroform solution (ready to use): Roti-phenol–chloroform–isoamyl alcohol (25:24:1), pH 7.5–8.

9. Chloroform–isoamyl alcohol solution: Rotisolv chloroform mixed with Rotipuran isoamyl alcohol (24:1).

10. TE buffer: 10 mM Tris–HCl, and 1 mM EDTA, pH 8.0.

11. Loading buffer (6×): 50% (v/v) Rotipuran glycerol, 0.1% (w/v) SDS, 100 mM EDTA pH 8.0, and 0.05% (w/v) bromophenol blue.

12. Agarose gel electrophoresis is performed according to a standard protocol and gels are stained with ethidium bromide (*see* also ref. [50], Vol. 1, Chap. 5).

2.5 Commercial Kits

1. Plasmid DNA preparation: innuPREP Plasmid Mini Kit (Analytik Jena AG, Jena, Germany) or NucleoBond Xtra Midi Kit (Macherey-Nagel GmbH & Co. KG, Dueren, Germany).

2. DNA isolation from agarose gels: innuPrep DOUBLEpure Kit (Analytik Jena AG, Jena, Germany).

2.6 Enzymes

Enzymes are obtained from Thermo Fisher Scientific (Waltham, Massachusetts, USA) unless noted otherwise and applied with buffers at optimal reaction temperature.

1. Restriction enzymes: *Bam*HI (10 U/µL), *Bsp*143I (*Sau*3AI, 10 U/µL), *Nde*I (10 U/µL), *Swa*I (10 U/µL), *Xho*I (10 U/µL).

2. FastAP thermosensitive alkaline phosphatase, 1 U/µL.

3. T4 DNA ligase, 1 U/µL.

4. T4 polynucleotide kinase, 10 U/µL.

5. Lysozyme from chicken egg white (Fluka, Sigma-Aldrich Chemie GmbH, Munich, Germany): 100 mg/mL dissolved in 10 mM Tris–HCl, sterilized by sterile filtration (pore diameter of filter: 0.22 mm), and stored at –20 °C.

6. Proteinase K from *Tritirachium album* (Merck KGaA, Darmstadt, Germany): 10 mg/mL solubilized in deionized water, sterilized by filtration (pore diameter of filter: 0.22 mm), and stored at –20 °C.

7. DNase-free RNaseA is prepared according to ref. [50], Vol. 3, Appendix A4.39. 100 mg/mL Ribonuclease A from bovine pancreas (Fluka, Sigma-Aldrich Chemie GmbH, Munich, Germany) is dissolved in sodium acetate solution (0.01 M sodium acetate; adjust to pH 5.2 with acetic acid). Heat to

100 °C for 15 min and cool slowly to room temperature. Adjust the pH by adding 0.1 volume of 1 M Tris–HCl (pH 7.4). Prepare aliquots of 1 mL each and store at –20 °C.

2.7 DNA Ladder

1. GeneRuler 1 kb DNA ladder (Thermo Fisher Scientific, Waltham, Massachusetts, USA), fragments (in bp): 10,000, 8000, 6000, 5000, 4000, 3500, 3000, 2500, 2000, 1500, 1000, 750, 500, 250.

2. 1 kb DNA extension ladder (Thermo Fisher Scientific, Waltham, Massachusetts, USA), fragments (in bp): 40,000, 20,000, 15,000, 10,000, 8144, 7126, 6108, 5090/5000, 4072, 3054, 2026, 1636, 1018, 517/506.

2.8 Devices and Materials

The devices described here may be replaced by alternative devices with adequate specifications.

1. DNA concentration is measured with a BioPhotometer (Eppendorf AG, Hamburg, Germany) in combination with the quartz cuvette TrayCell (Hellma GmbH & Co. KG, Müllheim, Germany) and a 1 or 0.2 mm lid.

2. For anaerobic cultivation of *R. capsulatus* on solid media: Microbiology Anaerocult A system (Merck KGaA, Darmstadt, Germany), consisting of air-tight containers as well as gas packs to deplete atmospheric oxygen.

3. French Press cell disruptor, with French pressure cell 40K, 1″ piston diameter (Thermo Fisher Scientific, Waltham, Massachusetts, USA).

4. Electroporation Device: MicroPulser (Bio-Rad, Munich, Germany).

5. Cellulose acetate membrane filters: 0.2 μm pore size, 25 mm diameter (GE Healthcare UK Limited, Buckinghamshire, UK).

3 Methods

3.1 Metagenomic Library Construction with the Shuttle Vector pEBP18

3.1.1 Linearization and Dephosphorylation of the Shuttle Vector pEBP18

1. Prepare 50 μg of vector pEBP18 DNA from an overnight culture of *E. coli* DH5α (pEBP18) with the NucleoBond Xtra Midi Kit. Determine DNA concentration photometrically.

2. Hydrolyze 50 μg of vector with 50 U *Bam*HI in a volume of 200–300 μL at 37 °C for 4 h (*see* **Note 5**).

3. Use agarose gel electrophoresis to analyze an aliquot (1–2 μL) of the hydrolyzed DNA and the same amount of undigested vector as control. If linearization is incomplete, add 2.5 μL enzyme buffer (10×), 20 U *Bam*HI, and 20.5 μL deionized water. Mix carefully and incubate for 2 additional hours at 37 °C. Repeat this step until complete linearization of the

vector is achieved, but ensure that concentration of *Bam*HI stock solution in the reaction mix does not exceed 5 % (v/v).

4. Once the vector is completely linearized, remove *Bam*HI: Extract with phenol–chloroform as described in Subheading 3.1.2, **step 6**. Precipitate the DNA by adding 0.1 volume 3 M sodium acetate and 0.7 volume isopropanol (–20 °C). Mix by repeated inversion of the reaction tube. Incubate on ice for 10 min and centrifuge at 16,000×*g* and room temperature for 30 min. Discard supernatant and wash the pellet with 900 µL 70 % chilled ethanol. Centrifuge, discard supernatant, and air-dry. Dissolve DNA pellet in nuclease-free water.

5. Measure DNA concentration photometrically and calculate the concentration of DNA ends (http://www.promega.com/biomath):

$$\text{pmol DNA ends} = \text{g DNA} \times \frac{\text{pmol}}{660\text{pg}} \times \frac{10^6\,\text{pg}}{\text{g}} \times \frac{1}{N} \times 2 \times \frac{\text{kb}}{1000\text{bp}}$$

("*N*": number of nucleotides (bp). "660 pg/pmol": average molecular weight of a single nucleotide pair. "2": number of ends in a linear DNA molecule. "kb/1000 bp": conversion factor for kilobases to base pairs.)

6. Prepare the dephosphorylation reaction as follows: Use 1 pmol of DNA ends with 1 U of FastAP and 2 µL of FastAP buffer (10×). Adjust total volume to 20 µL with nuclease-free water.

7. Incubate dephosphorylation reaction mix at 37 °C for 10 min.

8. Heat-inactivate FastAP by applying 75 °C for 5 min.

9. Purify the dephosphorylated vector by agarose gel electrophoresis and gel extraction (*see* **Note 6**).

10. In order to verify the quality of vector preparation (i.e., efficiency of linearization and dephosphorylation), perform a religation control prior to application of the vector for ligation reactions: Transform competent *E. coli* DH5α cells with 1–2 µL of dephosphorylated vector (*see* Subheading 3.1.5.2) and plate on selective LB agar plates. Incubate overnight at 37 °C. Vector quality is acceptable if no or only a few *E. coli* colonies are visible after incubation.

3.1.2 Isolation of Metagenomic DNA

This method for isolation of metagenomics DNA applies to samples from bacterial cell pellets derived from biofilms or lake water. It is not recommended to use this protocol for extraction of DNA from soil samples, since humic substances, organic compounds, or saline that often contaminate environmental DNA are difficult to remove and interfere with enzyme reactions like restriction digest or ligation.

1. Gently resuspend ~1 g of cells in 3 mL solution #1. Incubate the sample in a water bath at 37 °C for 1.5 h.

2. Mix the solution gently and periodically by inversion of the tube. Do not vortex the preparation at any step of this protocol, as this might result in shearing of the genomic DNA.

3. Add 6 mL solution #2 containing 2 mM DTT and 50 mg/mL RNaseA to each sample and incubate at 55 °C for 30 min repeating **step 2**.

4. Add 100 mg/mL proteinase K. Incubate at 55 °C for 15 min repeating **step 2**.

5. Homogenize the DNA solution by aspiration and gentle ejection through a cannula (diameter of ~0.9 mm) into a new falcon tube (*see* **Note 7**).

6. In order to remove proteins and purify DNA, extract DNA with phenol-chloroform according to ref. [50], Vol. 3, Appendix A8.9 (slightly modified). Be careful to use protection equipment and use an extractor hood as the procedure involves toxic mixtures.

   (a) Add 0.5–1 volume of phenol-chloroform solution to the homogenate.

   (b) Invert the tube until the solution gets turbid. Centrifuge at $3000 \times g$ and 4 °C for 5 min to separate the organic phase (lower phase, yellow color) and aqueous phase (upper phase) (*see* **Note 8**). DNA is usually included into the aqueous phase, but if the pH of the phenol-chloroform solution deviates from 7.8 to 8.0, migration of nucleic acids into the organic phase may occur.

   (c) Transfer the non-colored aqueous DNA phase into a new falcon tube. Be careful not to remove proteins from the interphase (use a modified pipette tip where the end is cut off to widen the opening).

   (d) Add 0.5–1 volume of chloroform-isoamylalcohol solution to aqueous phase and repeat **step b**.

   (e) Collect aqueous phase in several fresh 2 mL reaction tubes.

7. Concentrate the DNA by isopropanol precipitation as described before (*see* Subheading 3.1.1, **step 4**).

8. Dissolve the DNA pellet in 100 μL 65 °C TE buffer by gently pipetting up and down. Incubate at 65 °C for 10 min and subsequently continue incubation at 4 °C and at least overnight to completely solubilize DNA (incubation over several days may enhance elution efficiency). The resulting solution should appear viscous.

9. Determine the DNA concentration and purity photometrically. Purity of DNA is indicated by an $A_{260/230}$ value of 2.0–2.2

and an $A_{260/280}$ value of 1.8. If significant deviations from these values are observed or if the sample smells due to residual phenol, repeat purification procedure.

10. Store the DNA at 4 °C, or at −20 °C for long-term storage.

3.1.3 Fragmentation of Metagenomic DNA

In this protocol, we use enzymatic digestion with *Bsp*143I (a *Sau*3AI isoschizomer) to generate fragmented metagenomic DNA. *Bsp*143I recognizes a 4-bp recognition site and generates *Bam*HI compatible ends. The size of generated DNA fragments should not exceed 10 kb since larger fragments may interfere with efficient performance of activity-based screenings.

1. Analyze the quality and concentration of environmental DNA by agarose gel electrophoresis with a low percentage agarose gel (0.5–0.6% (w/v)), a separation distance of 25–30 cm, and a 1 kb DNA extension ladder as marker. If the DNA is of high molecular weight (>40 kb) continue with **step 2**, otherwise repeat DNA isolation from the habitat sample. If the sample is high in RNA content (indicated by the presence of a high degree of low molecular weight fragments), perform RNA hydrolysis using RNaseA and repeat extraction of DNA with phenol-chloroform (*see* Subheading 3.1.2, **step 6**).

2. For partial hydrolysis of metagenomic DNA, mix 4 μg of isolated DNA and 4 μL enzyme buffer (10×) with 28 μL MilliQ water. Incubate this premix at 37 °C for 10 min.

3. Prepare seven 1.5 mL reaction tubes labeled 0, 2, 4, 6, 8, 10, 12 [min] and pipet 2 μL loading buffer into each. Keep them on ice.

4. Add 4 μL *Bsp*143I (1 U/mL) to the tempered premix and mix by pipetting up and down.

5. Pipet 4 μL of the reaction mix directly into the reaction tube labeled "0 min" and keep it on ice. Incubate the residual reaction mixture at 37 °C.

6. Repeat **step 5** every 2 min by transferring another 4 μL aliquot into the appropriate reaction tube and keep it on ice.

7. Analyze the restriction digest kinetics by agarose gel electrophoresis with a low percentage agarose gel (0.5–0.6% (w/v)) and a separation distance of 10 cm. A successful partial digest is indicated by formation of a "smear" of DNA instead of clearly distinguishable bands. Use the test digest from **step 6** to estimate the optimal incubation time to achieve the highest concentration of mixed size DNA fragments in the range of 3–6 kb. If no adequate incubation time can be discerned, repeat test digest with adjusted enzyme concentrations.

8. For preparative DNA fragmentation, dilute 4 μg of isolated DNA in 36 μL of MilliQ water. Incubate at 37 °C for 10 min.

Add an adequate concentration of *Bsp*143I (as estimated in **step** 7) and adjust the total volume to 40 μL. Incubate at 37 °C for an amount of time indicated by the test digests (**step** 7). Stop the reaction by adding 8 μL loading buffer.

9. Use agarose gel electrophoresis to separate mixed size DNA fragments and cut an agarose block containing DNA fragments ranging from 3 to 6 kb out from the gel. Purify DNA from the gel slice with the innuPREP DOUBLE pure gel extraction kit.

10. Analyze 200–300 ng of purified DNA by gel electrophoresis to verify correct size and sufficient concentration.

3.1.4   Ligation of Metagenomic DNA with Vector pEBP18

1. Photometrically measure the concentration of DNA of both vector and insert.

2. Calculate the amount of DNA needed for ligation with the following formula. For metagenomic DNA, assume an average insert size of your prepared partially digested DNA.

$$\text{Mass fragment}\,[\text{ng}] = \frac{5 \times \text{mass vector}\,[\text{ng}] \times \text{fragment length}\,[\text{bp}]}{\text{vector length}\,[\text{bp}]}$$

3. Combine 1 μL of vector DNA with the calculated amount of insert DNA. Add MilliQ H_2O to a volume of 17 μL as well as 2 μL 10× T4 DNA ligase buffer and 1 μL of T4 DNA ligase (1 U/μL). Gently mix the solution by pipetting up and down.

4. Incubate overnight at 16 °C.

5. Inactivate ligase by heat treatment at 65 °C for 10 min following incubation.

3.1.5   Transformation of Bacterial Hosts with a pEBP18 Metagenomic Library

Preparation of Electrocompetent E. coli Cells

Preparation and transformation of electrocompetent *E. coli* cells were performed according to ref. [50], Vol. 1, Chap. 1, Protocol 26 with modifications.

1. Streak *E. coli* strain on LB agar plates and incubate overnight at 37 °C.

2. Inoculate a single colony into 5 mL LB medium. Incubate the culture overnight at 37 °C under constant shaking (120 rpm).

3. Inoculate 220 mL LB medium with an aliquot of the preculture to a final $OD_{580} = 0.05$. Incubate the culture at 37 °C under permanent shaking (120 rpm). Determine the cell density of the growing culture (OD_{580}) until an optical density of $OD_{580} = 0.4$–0.5 is reached.

4. Transfer cell suspension into four 50 mL falcon tubes and incubate on ice for 20 min. Prepare 25 1.5 mL reaction tubes on ice. Cool down solutions for cell preparation on ice.

5. Harvest cells by centrifugation (4 °C, 10 min, 3000×*g*).

6. Discard supernatant and gently resuspend each pellet in 50 mL MilliQ water.

7. Repeat **steps 5** and **6**, but this time resuspend each pellet in 25 mL MilliQ water. Pool the suspension from two falcon tubes.

8. Repeat **steps 5** and **6**, but resuspend each pellet in 2 mL glycerol solution. Pool the suspension from two falcon tubes.

9. Repeat **steps 5** and **6**, but resuspend the pellet in 0.5 mL glycerol solution and prepare aliquots of 25 μL. Incubate aliquots at −20 °C for 1 h, then store at −80 °C.

10. Test quality of electrocompetent cells by performing a test transformation (*see* Subheading 3.1.5.2) with 1 μL of pUC18 and incubation at 37 °C for 1 h after electroporation.

Transformation of Electrocompetent *E. coli* Cells

1. Thaw one aliquot of electrocompetent *E. coli* cells on ice and cool an electroporation cuvette (1 mm gap) on ice.

2. Add 1 μL ligation mixture to electrocompetent *E. coli* cells. Mix gently by pipetting up and down.

3. Pipet suspension into an electroporation cuvette. Carefully dry the electrodes on the outside of the cuvette with a paper towel. Place the cuvette in the electroporation device and perform electroporation with Bio-Rad MicroPulser using program EC1 (1.8 kV).

4. Quickly add 600 μL EM1 medium to the cells and transfer solution to a reaction tube. Incubate at 37 °C for 3 h (120 rpm).

5. Plate serial dilutions of transformation mixture on selective EM1 agar plates and incubate overnight at 37 °C. Store remaining transformation mixture at 4 °C.

6. Calculate number of transformants on each plate to estimate the optimal dilution factor. Dilute the remaining transformation mixture accordingly, plate on selective EM1 agar plates and incubate at 37 °C overnight.

7. Total count of single colonies should be >200,000. If this number is not achieved, repeat transformation with ligation mixture.

8. Cultivate 40 clones separately in 5 mL selective liquid LB medium overnight at 37 °C and isolate plasmid DNA. Hydrolyze 5 μg recombinant DNA from each sample with *Swa*I in a total reaction volume of 50 μL (*see* Subheading 3.1.1, **steps 2–4**).

9. Analyze restriction pattern by agarose gel electrophoresis. Successful cloning is indicated by one or more additional bands as compared to hydrolyzed empty pEBP18 vector. Inserts should be about 3–6 kb in size. If more than a single insert band is present (indicating that *Swa*I cuts within the inserts), estimate total insert size by adding the sizes of the respective insert fragments. The ratio of clones without insert should not exceed 10 %.

10. Pick individual clones and replate them to agar plates with an appropriate substrate to screen for the desired enzyme activity.

Preparation of Electrocompetent P. putida KT2440 Cells

1. Streak *P. putida* KT2440 on EM1 agar plates. Incubate overnight at 30 °C.

2. Inoculate a single colony into 100 mL EM medium in a vented Erlenmeyer flask with baffled bottom. Incubate overnight at 30 °C under constant shaking (120 rpm).

3. Transfer overnight culture into four 50 mL falcon tubes, dilute each fraction 1:1 with MilliQ water (*see* **Note 9**) and cool on ice.

4. Harvest cells by centrifugation ($3000 \times g$, 4 °C, 10 min). Wash each pellet three times with 50 mL, 25 mL and 5 mL of sucrose solution, respectively. Pool the suspensions, harvest cells by centrifugation, and resuspend pellets in 600 μL sucrose solution. Prepare aliquots of ~130 μL competent cells from the resuspension.

5. If desired, test preparation quality of competent cells by electroporation (as described under Subheading 3.1.5.4) with 1 μL of pEBP18 plasmid DNA.

Library Construction in P. putida KT2440

1. For electroporation, mix electrocompetent *P. putida* cells with or 1 μL pEBP18 metagenomic library DNA (*see* Subheading 3.1.4) (*see* **Note 10**). Transfer suspension to electroporation cuvettes (2 mm gap). Wipe electrodes on the outside of the cuvette with a paper towel and place in the electroporation device. Perform electroporation with Bio-Rad MicroPulser using program EC2 (2.5 kV).

2. Quickly resuspend cells in 600 μL EM1 by pipetting up and down. Transfer solution into a test tube and incubate cells at 30 °C for 3 h (120 rpm).

3. Plate serial dilutions of transformants on selective EM1 agar plates. If the total number of single clones is <200,000 repeat transformation to obtain more clones.

4. Inoculate 40 *P. putida* clones separately in 5 mL selective EM medium each and cultivate at 37 °C overnight. Isolate plasmid DNA, digest with *Swa*I and perform agarose gel electrophoresis to analyze insert DNA. Inserts should be 3–6 kb in size. The ratio of clones without insert should not exceed 10 % (for more detailed information *see* Subheading 3.1.5.2, **step 9**).

Transformation of B. subtilis TEB1030

B. subtilis TBE1030 should be transformed utilizing its natural competence to ensure optimal integration efficiency into the genome by homologous recombination at the amylase gene locus. *B. subtilis* TBE1030 cannot be transformed with ligation mixtures.

Thus, single plasmids or plasmid pools obtained from the *E. coli* or *P. putida* libraries will be used.

1. Streak *B. subtilis* TEB1030 on EM1 agar plates. Incubate overnight at 37 °C.

2. Inoculate a single colony in 5 mL Paris-Medium in a vented Erlenmeyer flask with baffled bottom. Incubate this preculture overnight at 37 °C and 120 rpm.

3. Inoculate 10 mL Paris-Medium in an Erlenmeyer flask with baffled bottom with 200 μL of the preculture. Determine cell density (OD_{580}) of the growing culture at intervals of 15–30 min. Continue work with the next step when the culture reaches an optical density of $OD_{580} = 1$.

4. Prepare two 500 μL aliquots of the *B. subtilis* culture. Add 1 μg plasmid DNA and 1 μg empty vector (control), respectively. Further incubate the aliquots at 37 °C and 120 rpm for 6 h.

5. Plate aliquots of 200 and 300 μL of the transformed cells on selective EM1 agar plates and incubate at 37 °C overnight. A few transformants should be obtained after 24–36 h with the aliquots containing plasmid DNA, while no colonies should appear in the controls.

6. Transposition can occur via either Campbell-type integration (single cross over) or homologous recombination. To distinguish between both types of integration, check amylase activity. Streak colonies on a master plate and a starch indicator plate and incubate overnight at 37 °C. The next day, color starch plate with 5 mL iodine solution, incubate at room temperature for 2 min, and remove iodine solution. Homologous recombination disrupts the amylase gene, resulting in a black colony. If instead a halo appears around the colony, amylase activity is still present, indicating that transposition has occurred via Campbell-type integration.

7. Correct transformants (Cm^R, $\Delta amyE$) can be transferred from the master plate to agar plates with substrates to perform activity-based assays.

3.2 Expression of Clustered Genes with TREX

The TREX system enables the expression of native gene clusters in diverse bacterial hosts [30, 31]. It consists of two DNA cassettes (L-TREX and R-TREX cassette) and is handled including the following key steps (Fig. 2).

(1) A plasmid is constructed which carries a DNA fragment containing the target gene cluster and the TREX cassettes. (2) Conjugational transfer to a host organism and transposon integration of the construct into the host genome are employed to produce stable expression strains. (3) Expression of clustered genes is

carried out using T7 RNA polymerase which convergently transcribes the DNA fragment from two T7 promoters. The system can thus be used for metagenome mining of gene clusters encoding biosynthetic pathways or complex multi-subunit proteins [57–59].

The TREX system is versatile with respect to the application protocols which can be easily adapted to a large variety of different DNA fragments and expression host strains. In the following, we first provide general guidelines for TREX application (Subheading 3.2.1) and thereafter describe as an example for application the expression of a carotenoid biosynthesis gene cluster in *P. putida* (Subheading 3.2.2).

3.2.1 General Guidelines for the Application of the TREX Expression System

Principle: As a first step, the TREX cassettes and the target DNA fragment are combined on a plasmid, the "TREX expression construct" (*see* Fig. 2b, step 1). The target DNA fragment containing the gene cluster of interest is thus labeled with the TREX cassettes to enable delivery and expression.

Construction of the TREX Expression Construct

Construction procedure: TREX expression constructs can be assembled by various methods including restriction/ligation cloning, Gibson assembly, or homologous recombination in yeast.

1. A "carrier vector" containing the target DNA fragment can be constructed and TREX cassettes that can be obtained as a 6.8 kb *Xba*I fragment from pIC20H-RL (*see* Subheading 2.2, **item 4**, Fig. 2c) inserted into a unique *Xba*I site of the vector (as described in ref. [31]).

2. In case *Xba*I is not applicable because it hydrolyzes the inserted DNA fragment or the chosen vector, any appropriate unique endonuclease restriction site in the carrier vector can be chosen and TREX cassette inserted by blunting DNA ends (using for example the Fast End Repair Kit from Thermo Fisher Scientific™).

3. Alternatively, the *E. coli* vector pIC20H-RL which carries the TREX cassettes can be used as the vector element and the DNA fragment to be expressed inserted into one of the unique endonuclease restriction sites *Xmn*I, *Sca*I, or *Nde*I. Note that use of *Xmn*I and *Sca*I will disrupt the ampicillin resistance gene and hence requires use of tetracycline for selection of cells carrying this vector.

Size of insert DNA fragment: As shown experimentally, DNA fragments up to ca. 20 kb can be inserted into host chromosomes and successfully expressed [30, 31]. Theoretically, there is no size limit known for the TREX application, and thus transfer and expression also of larger DNA fragments may be envisaged.

Choice of replicon: It is important to use a narrow host range *E. coli* replicon for the TREX expression construct, as present in e.g., pUC vectors. After transfer to an expression host other than *E. coli*, this enables selection of clones which do not propagate the plasmid but carry the TREX transposon stably integrated in the chromosome. In case that *E. coli* will be used as expression host, a suitable suicide plasmid system harboring a replicon with specific characteristics like temperature sensitivity should be used to enable plasmid curing and specific selection of clones with the TREX transposon stably integrated in the chromosome, as described in ref. [31].

Transfer to Expression Host and TREX-Transposon Integration

Principle: The TREX expression construct is introduced into an expression host of choice (Fig. 2b, step 2) where it does not replicate but is integrated into the bacterial chromosome to produce stable expression strains (Fig. 2b, step 3).

Transfer of TREX construct: The TREX expression construct can be transferred to any Gram-negative host which is accessible via conjugation (e.g., *P. putida* or *R. capsulatus*) or may alternatively be introduced by any method of choice like electroporation (e.g., *E. coli* or *P. putida*). For screening of metagenome libraries, the use of expression strains with chromosomally integrated T7 polymerase gene is preferable as opposed to plasmid-based expression of the T7 polymerase (see below) to enable enhanced throughput by one-step construction of expression clones that can then directly be subjected to an appropriate screening assay.

Transposon integration: The use of a suicide vector and selection with gentamycin enables straightforward selection of clones with the TREX-transposon stably integrated in the host chromosome (*see* **Note 11**). Notably, elements of transposon Tn5 enabling this step convey non-directed integration. Therefore, a library of different strains with individual transposon insertion sites is generated. It was shown that each individual insertion site of the TREX transposon affects the induced gene expression mediated by T7 RNA polymerase [31]. Furthermore, it was shown, that the insertion site can facilitate constitutive T7 RNA polymerase-independent gene expression mediated by a chromosomal promoter [30]. Therefore, the investigation of multiple clones for functional gene expression is recommended to identify clones providing optimal expression conditions and product yields.

Expression of Gene Clusters

Principle: To enable transcription of all genes in a given DNA fragment, T7 RNA polymerase is employed which is capable of efficiently transcribing large DNA regions and functions largely independent of bacterial regulatory elements like transcription terminators [60, 61]. Additionally, bidirectional expression of the DNA fragment from two sides enables transcription of all enclosed genes, independent of their orientation [31] (Fig. 2b, step 4).

Expression of T7 RNA polymerase: T7 RNA polymerase can be implemented in different host systems by plasmid-based expression of the respective polymerase gene, e.g., from broad-host-range vectors such as pML5-based plasmids [36, 55, 56] which enable induction of expression from promoters P*lac*- or P*fru* in different bacterial hosts. Alternatively, strains carrying the T7 polymerase gene in their chromosome like *E. coli* BL21(DE3) can be used [31]. Note that there are tools available enabling the construction of novel T7 expression strains [62].

3.2.2 Application of TREX for the Functional Expression of Carotenoid Biosynthesis Genes in P. putida

Construction of a TREX Vector Carrying Carotenoid Biosynthesis Genes

1. The 6.9 kb carotenoid biosynthesis gene cluster from *Pantoea ananatis* is amplified by PCR using genomic DNA as a template with primers adding appropriate restriction sites (here *Xba*I and *Eco*RI).

2. Hydrolyze 5 μg of both the PCR product and vector pUC18 according to Subheading 3.1.1, **steps 2–4** with *Xba*I and *Eco*RI in a total reaction volume of 50 μL. Incubation is carried out overnight.

3. Purify the DNA by performing agarose gel electrophoresis followed by preparation of DNA from agarose gel slices with the innuPREP Plasmid Mini Kit.

4. Insert the DNA fragment into the vector pUC18 by ligation (*see* Subheading 3.1.4) to construct the carrier vector (*see* Subheading 3.2.2.1, Fig. 2b, step 1).

5. Excise TREX cassettes from vector pIC20H-RL by hydrolysis (*see* Subheading 3.1.1, **steps 2–4**): Use 5 μg plasmid DNA in a total volume of 50 μL with *Xba*I as restriction endonuclease. Proceed with gel extraction purification of the 6.8 kb TREX fragment using the innuPrep DOUBLEpure kit.

6. Linearize the carrier vector with *Xba*I using the same procedure as in **step 5**.

7. Ligate (Subheading 3.1.4) the TREX fragment into the carrier vector to generate the TREX expression construct.

Preparation of Competent *E. coli* Cells and Heat Shock Transformation

1. Cultivate *E. coli* cells from a fresh LB agar plate in 5 mL LB medium. Incubate overnight at 37 °C.

2. Inoculate 100 mL LB medium with 1 mL of the preculture from **step 1** and grow this culture at 37 °C to an OD_{580} of 0.4–0.6. Keep cells on ice during the following steps and only use solutions precooled to 4 °C.

3. Centrifuge at $4000 \times g$ and 4 °C for 3 min to harvest cells. Resuspend the pellet in 10 mL 100 mM cold $MgCl_2$ solution. Incubate on ice for 30 min.

4. Harvest the cells and resuspend them in 5 mL 100 mM $CaCl_2$ solution containing 20% glycerol. Separate the resuspension into 200 μL aliquots and freeze at −80 °C.

5. For heat shock transformation, thaw one aliquot of competent *E. coli* cells on ice. Add a previously prepared ligation mixture or 2–5 µL of pure DNA and mix by gently pipetting up and down.

6. Incubate on ice for 30–60 min. Transfer the reaction tube to a thermo block preheated to 42 °C. Remove the tube after 2 min and incubate on ice for 5 min. Add 700 µL of LB medium without antibiotics.

7. Incubate at 37 °C for 2 h on a shaking or inverting device.

8. Centrifuge at 16,000×*g* for 3 min at room temperature. Decant supernatant and use the reflow to resuspend the cells.

9. Plate the cells on LB agar plates supplemented with an antibiotic suitable for selection for the transformed plasmid.

Creation of *P. putida* Carotenoid Biosynthesis Gene Expression Strains by Conjugational Transfer of the TREX Construct

1. Use heat shock transformation (*see* Subheading 3.2.2.2, **steps 5–9**) to transfer the TREX expression construct from Subheading 3.2.2.1 into *E. coli* S17-1.

2. Streak out recipient strain *P. putida* KT2440 on an LB agar plate without antibiotic.

3. Inoculate separate liquid cultures of *E. coli* S17-1 transformed with the TREX expression construct and *P. putida* in 5 mL LB (supplemented with tetracycline in case of *E. coli*) and incubate shaking overnight at 30 °C.

4. Mix 500 µL of overnight cultures of both donor and recipient, and pellet cells by centrifugation (2 min, 11,000×*g*).

5. To wash out antibiotic, discard supernatant, resuspend cells in 1 mL fresh LB medium, and pellet cells again. Remove supernatant leaving a small volume of ca. 100–200 µL for gentle resuspension of cells.

6. Pipet the cell solution onto a cellulose acetate filter that is placed on an LB agar plate without antibiotic and incubate at 30 °C overnight for conjugational plasmid transfer (*see* Fig. 2b, step 2).

7. After incubation, add 1 mL LB medium to a 2 mL reaction tube and use sterile forceps to transfer the filter into the tube (*see* **Note 12**). Wash cells from filter by vortexing, and remove the filter.

8. Prepare three consecutive 1:10 dilutions from the cell suspension (*see* **Note 13**). Plate 100 µL of each dilution on selection agar containing 25 µg/mL irgasan to prevent growth of *E. coli* and 25 µg/mL gentamycin to select for clones with the TREX transposon (*see* Fig. 2b, step 3).

9. In addition, centrifuge the remaining volume of the initial cell suspension to pellet cells (2 min, 11,000×*g*), remove

supernatant leaving ca. 100 μL to resuspend cells and plate these as well.

10. Incubate plates at 30 °C for 1 or 2 days.

11. After incubation, isolate 3–10 individual clones by streaking on new selection agar plates and incubating at 30 °C overnight.

Expression of Carotenoid Gene Cluster in *P. putida*

1. Transfer plasmid pML5-T7 [56], in separate set-ups into *P. putida* strains with the TREX transposon generated in Subheading 3.2.2.1 via conjugation. Proceed as described above (under Subheading 3.2.2.3) with the following adaptions: Use 10 μg/mL tetracycline to select for the plasmid in *E. coli* S17-1. As opposed to conjugational transfer and transposition, ca. 5 h incubation on the filter membrane is sufficient for plasmid transfer. Use LB agar selection plates with 25 μg/mL irgasan to prevent growth of *E. coli* and 50 μg/mL tetracycline to select for plasmid pML5-T7. Streak a single colony on a new selection plate for further use.

2. For expression (*see* Fig. 2b, step 4), use a single colony of *P. putida* with the TREX transposon and plasmid pML5-T7 to inoculate a 5 mL culture in LB medium with 50 μg/mL tetracycline in a glass reaction tube and incubate rotating at 30 °C overnight.

3. Use this culture to inoculate a 50 mL expression culture with a starting cell density $OD_{580}=0.1$ in LB medium supplemented with tetracycline and incubate shaking at 30 °C. Induce T7 RNA polymerase expression and thus carotenoid biosynthesis gene expression at $OD_{580}=0.5$ after ca. 2 h by addition of IPTG to a final concentration of 0.5 mM and proceed with the cultivation.

4. Harvest cells to assay for functional gene expression by detection of carotenoids by appropriate methods like UV/Vis spectrometry or HPLC [31].

3.3 Expression in Burkholderia glumae

The genome of *B. glumae* PG1 consists of 7.8 Mbp and is organized in two replicons of 4.1 Mbp on chromosome 1 and 3.7 Mbp on chromosome 2 [32]. Several *B. glumae* strains are phytopathogenic and produce virulence factors which are missing in strain PG1 [33]. This strain is already used for the production and secretion of an industrially relevant lipase [34, 35]; thus, it represents an interesting alternative to existing Gram-negative bacterial expression hosts. We describe here the expression of plasmid-derived genes using *B. glumae* PG1.

3.3.1 Construction of pBBR1MCS-Based Plasmids for Expression in B. glumae PG1

1. Plasmid pBBR1MCS [53] does not provide a ribosome binding site (RBS), thus, DNA fragments to be cloned should be amplified by PCR using primers including a RBS as well as restriction sites for cloning and additional 2–4 bases to enable

efficient restriction. The multiple cloning site of pBBR1MCS provides a set of possible single restriction site combinations (*see* **Note 14**). It needs to be secured that the corresponding restriction sites are absent within the DNA fragment itself and that the buffer conditions fit for all enzymes used. If plasmids with a chloramphenicol resistance cannot be used, other plasmids from the pBBR1MCS series are available (*see* Subheading 2.2, **item 3**).

2. Perform hydrolysis of the PCR fragment and vector with chosen restriction enzymes and up to 5 µg DNA in a total volume of 50 µL (*see* Subheading 3.1.1, **steps 2–4**).

3. Separate and purify vector DNA (~4700 bp for pBBR1MCS) and PCR fragment by agarose gel electrophoresis with a gel extraction kit.

4. Ligate the fragment into the vector (*see* Subheading 3.1.4) and transform *E. coli* DH5α with the ligation mixture (*see* Subheading 3.2.2.2, **steps 5–9**). Use appropriate antibiotics for selection of the chosen vector (*see* Subheading 2.1, **item 12**). Verify cloning success as described in Subheading 3.4.1 (**step 7**). Use appropriate antibiotics for selection of the chosen vector (*see* Subheading 2.1, **item 12**).

3.3.2 Transfer of Plasmid DNA into B. glumae PG1 by Conjugation

1. Inoculate 10 mL LB medium with 20 µL of a *B. glumae* PG1 cryo culture (*see* **Note 15**) and incubate at 30 °C under constant shaking (120 rpm) for 24 h. On the same day, transfer pBBR1MCS containing the gene of interest (or any other mobilizable vector) into *E. coli* S17-1 by heat shock transformation (*see* Subheading 3.2.2.2, **steps 5–9**), plate on LB agar plates containing appropriate antibiotics, and incubate overnight at 37 °C.

2. Inoculate 10 mL LB medium with 500 µL of the *B. glumae* PG1 overnight culture and incubate at 30 °C under constant shaking (120 rpm) overnight, but at least for 16 h. Transfer a single *E. coli* S17-1 colony carrying the mobilizable vector into 10 mL LB medium with appropriate antibiotics and incubate at 37 °C under constant shaking (120 rpm) overnight.

3. On the next day, inoculate 10 mL LB medium (with antibiotics) with an appropriate volume of *E. coli* S17-1 preculture to an $OD_{580} = 0.05$ and incubate at 37 °C under constant shaking (120 rpm) until an $OD_{580} = 0.5–0.8$ is reached (*see* **Note 16**).

4. Centrifuge 2 mL of *E. coli* S17-1 culture ($21,000 \times g$, 1 min) and remove supernatant with a pipette.

5. Add 1 mL of *B. glumae* PG1 overnight culture, centrifuge ($21,000 \times g$, 1 min) immediately, and remove supernatant with a pipette.

6. Add 1 mL fresh LB medium and resuspend cell pellet gently by pipetting (do not vortex) and centrifuge again ($21,000 \times g$, 1 min).

7. Remove supernatant with a pipette and resuspend cell pellet gently in 50 µL fresh LB medium.

8. Place a cellulose acetate filter on an LB agar plate, transfer the resuspended cells to the filter, and incubate at 30 °C for 6 h. Cell suspension should not spill from the filter to the agar plate.

9. Prepare a 2 mL reaction tube containing 1 mL LB medium and transfer the filter with sterile forceps (*see* **Note 12**). Vortex the reaction tube for 20 s. Extend vortex time if filter is crumpled to remove all cells from the filter.

10. Plate 100 µL of cell suspension onto a MME agar plate with appropriate antibiotics for *B. glumae* PG1 and incubate at 30 °C for 48 h (*see* **Note 17**) until colonies become visible (*see* **Note 18**).

3.3.3 Transfer of Plasmid DNA into B. glumae PG1 by Electroporation

1. For preparation of electrocompetent *B. glumae* cells, inoculate 10 mL LB medium with 20 µL of a *B. glumae* PG1 cryo culture (*see* **Note 15**) and incubate at 30 °C under constant shaking (120 rpm) for 24 h.

2. Pre-warm 200 mL LB medium at 30 °C, add 2 mL overnight culture and incubate at 30 °C under constant shaking (120 rpm) until an $OD_{580} = 0.2$ is reached (approximately 4–6 h).

3. Centrifuge the culture at 4 °C and $3000 \times g$ for 20 min and remove the supernatant.

4. Resuspend the cell pellet in 100 mL ice-cold sucrose solution with a pipette.

5. Repeat **steps 3** and **4** twice with 50 mL and 25 mL, respectively, of ice-cold sucrose solution.

6. Repeat **steps 3** and **4** twice with 25 mL ice-cold sucrose–glycerol solution.

7. Resuspend the resulting cell pellet in an adequate volume of sucrose–glycerol solution to an $OD_{580} = 50$.

8. Prepare 50 µL aliquots for either direct use or storage at −80 °C for several weeks. Transformation efficiency will decrease upon longer storage.

9. For electroporation of *B. glumae*, add 5 µL DNA (*see* **Note 19**) to an aliquot of competent *B. glumae* cells and mix by pipetting. Transfer the mixture to a precooled electroporation cuvette (2 mm gap) and perform electroporation with Bio-Rad MicroPulser using program EC2 (2.5 kV).

10. Quickly add 1 mL 2× LB medium to the electroporation cuvette, invert multiple times and transfer medium to a fresh 1.5 mL reaction tube (*see* **Note 20**).

11. Incubate reaction tube at 30 °C on a shaking platform for 3 h.

12. Plate 100 μL on a LB agar plate with appropriate antibiotic concentration. If higher amounts of colonies are desired, proceed as described in **Note 17** for conjugation of *B. glumae* PG1 (Subheading 3.3.2).

13. Incubate LB agar plates at 30 °C for 24–48 h until colonies become visible (*see* **Note 18**).

3.3.4 Cultivation and Cell Harvest of B. glumae PG1

1. Precultures (10 mL LB medium with appropriate antibiotic concentration) are inoculated with a single colony of *B. glumae* PG1 derived from either a transformation procedure (*see* Subheadings 3.3.2 and 3.3.3) or with 20 μL of a cryo culture (*see* **Note 15**).

2. Incubate the preculture at 30 °C under constant shaking (120 rpm) for at least 24 h. When starting from a cryo culture, extend the cultivation time to 48 h if necessary.

3. The main culture is inoculated with an appropriate volume of a preculture to an $OD_{580} = 0.05$ and incubated at 30 °C under constant shaking (120 rpm) for 8–16 h.

4. Cells are harvested by centrifugation with $21,000 \times g$ for 1 min or with $3000 \times g$ for 20 min.

5. After transferring the supernatant to another reaction tube, the cell pellet is washed with a buffer of choice (for example 50 mM Tris–HCl, pH 8.0) by resuspension and subsequent centrifugation (*see* **step 4**).

6. Cell-free supernatant and whole-cell-fraction (resuspended in a buffer of choice) can be analyzed by SDS-PAGE or enzyme activity assays.

3.4 Expression in R. capsulatus

R. capsulatus is a phototrophic α-proteobacterium capable of growing either phototrophically in the light under anaerobic conditions, or chemoheterotrophically in the dark under aerobic conditions. *R. capsulatus* is a valuable alternative to conventional bacterial expression hosts for difficult-to-express proteins because it provides an extensive intracytoplasmic membrane system for accommodation of membrane proteins and, in addition, several metal-containing cofactors which are missing in other bacteria (*see* Table 1) [36, 44, 56].

3.4.1 Construction of pRho-Based Expression Plasmids for Rhodobacter capsulatus

1. Use PCR amplification from plasmid or genomic DNA to obtain a DNA fragment containing the gene to be expressed. Design primers with an added *Nde*I site at the start and an added *Xho*I site at the terminus of the gene (*see* **Note 21**). The

*Nde*I site added to the primer must include the start codon as part of the 6-bp *Nde*I recognition site (CAT<u>ATG</u>). The primer designated to bind at the end of the target gene has to be designed without the stop codon in order to fuse the gene product to a His$_6$ short tag peptide.

2. Hydrolyze vector and PCR product separately (as described in Subheading 3.1.1, **steps 2–4**) with 5 μg of plasmid DNA and *Nde*I and *Xho*I in a total reaction volume of 50 μL. Incubation is carried out at 37 °C overnight.

3. Apply the whole mixture to agarose gel electrophoresis.

4. Excise a gel slice containing the DNA fragment of the desired size (~6.6 kb for vectors pRhokHi-2 and pRhotHi-2) and purify DNA from the gel using the innuPrep DOUBLEpure kit.

5. Perform ligation procedure as described in Subheading 3.1.4.

6. Use heat shock transformation (*see* Subheading 3.2.2.2, **steps 5–9**) with the complete reaction mixture to transfer the plasmid DNA into *E. coli* DH5α cells.

7. Inoculate ten single clones separately in 5 mL LB-medium containing kanamycin at 37 °C overnight. Isolate plasmid DNA from harvested cells with the innuPrep Plasmid Mini Kit. Hydrolyze a 5 μL aliquot of each isolated DNA sample with *Nde*I and *Xho*I (*see* Subheading 3.1.1, **steps 2–4**) and perform agarose gel electrophoresis. Successful cloning is indicated by appearance of two bands at appropriate positions for vector (~6.6 kb) and insert.

3.4.2 Conjugational Transfer of Plasmid DNA into R. capsulatus

Transfer of plasmids into *R. capsulatus* is achieved by conjugation as this organism is not susceptible to transformation.

1. Streak *R. capsulatus* recipient strain on a PY agar plate and incubate at 30 °C for 48 h under phototrophic conditions (*see* Subheading 3.4.3.1). One day before conjugation starts, transfer the mobilizable plasmid (e.g., pRho vectors) into *E. coli* S17-1 donor strains by heat shock transformation (*see* Subheading 3.2.2.2, **steps 5–9**).

2. For conjugational transfer completely scrape *R. capsulatus* single colonies off the plate from **step 1** and resuspend cells in 5 mL RCV medium by pipetting up and down. This yields enough cell suspension for four conjugation approaches.

3. Gently resuspend 20–30 single colonies of *E. coli* donor cells in 1 mL iron-free PY medium by repeatedly inverting the reaction tube. Do not handle the cells too roughly since this can reduce conjugation efficiency due to loss of pili.

4. Mix 0.5 mL of *E. coli* suspension and 1 mL of *Rhodobacter* suspension in a 2 mL reaction tube. Centrifuge the mixture at 16,000 × *g* and room temperature for 10 min.

5. During centrifugation, place one sterile cellulose acetate filter per conjugation approach on a PY agar plate without antibiotic. Up to four filters can be placed on a single agar plate.

6. After centrifugation, remove the supernatant by pipetting (do not decant, as the loose structure of the *Rhodobacter* cell pellet might facilitate loss of cell mass), but leave 100–200 μL of supernatant for resuspension. Resuspend the cells in the remaining liquid and remember to treat the cells gently to prevent *E. coli* pili from shearing. Carefully transfer the whole resuspension volume onto the prepared cellulose acetate filters. Avoid spilling of cell suspension from the filter to the agar plate.

7. Incubate the plate at 30 °C in the dark overnight.

8. Prepare a 2 mL reaction tube containing 1 mL of RCV medium without antibiotic. Carefully transfer the filter with the cell suspension into the tube with sterile forceps (*see* **Note 12**). Vortex the tube until the cells have been rinsed off the filter. Remove the filter and break down any remaining cell clumps by pipetting up and down.

9. Plate 200 μL of cell resuspension onto a PY agar plate. The plate must be selective for the transferred plasmid and should also contain streptomycin for counter selection against remaining *E. coli* donor (*see* **Note 22**). Harvest cells from the remaining cell suspension (10 min, 16,000 × *g*) and remove most of the supernatant with a pipette. Resuspend the pellet in the remaining liquid and plate 200 μL of the resuspension on a second PY agar plate.

10. Cultivate the plates under phototrophic growth conditions for 2–3 days until red *R. capsulatus* colonies emerge.

3.4.3 Cultivation of Rhodobacter capsulatus

R. capsulatus is a facultative phototrophic bacterium which can be cultivated either under chemoheterotrophic conditions (i.e., aerobically in the dark) or phototrophic conditions (i.e., anaerobically in the light) (*see* **Note 23**).

Cultivation on Solid Medium

1. Streak a small amount of *R. capsulatus* cell mass onto a selective PY agar plate.

2. For chemoheterotrophic growth, place the plates in a cell incubator in the dark.

3. For phototrophic growth, place the plates in a gas-tight jar (e.g., Microbiology Anaerocult A system, Merck KgaA, Darmstadt, Germany). Wet the powder of a Gas Pack with 15 mL of deionized water, put it in the gas-tight jar and close the lid (*see* **Note 24**). Place the container between six 60 W light bulbs for proper illumination.

4. Under both chemoheterotrophic and phototrophic conditions incubation is carried out at 30 °C for 48–72 h.

Cultivation of *R. capsulatus* in Liquid Medium

1. Prepare a preculture by inoculating 10 mL of RCV medium (supplemented with antibiotics appropriate for the expression plasmid) in a Hungate anaerobic reaction tube with a single colony from a freshly grown *R. capsulatus* agar plate.

2. Incubate the preculture for 2 days at 30 °C between six 60 W light bulbs.

3. After incubation, measure optical density of the preculture at 660 nm (OD_{660}) (*see* **Note 25**). Calculate the inoculation volume to start the main culture at an OD_{660} of 0.02–0.05 (*see* **Note 26**).

4. Supplement a suitable amount of RCV liquid medium with antibiotics to maintain the expression plasmid. For T_7-dependent expression, 12 mM fructose is added to the medium as an inducer (*see* **Note 27**).

5. For chemoheterotrophic growth of liquid cultures use Erlenmeyer flasks of at least five times the size of the culture volume. For cultivation, use a shaking incubator (100 rpm) in complete darkness at 30 °C (*see* **Note 28**).

6. Phototrophic cultivation may be carried out in various kinds of containers suitable for the culture volume, e.g., Hungate reaction tubes, Erlenmeyer flasks or glass bottles. However, it is important for the vessels to allow gas-tight sealing with rubber septa to maintain an anaerobic milieu while still allowing addition of supplements after sealing. Additionally, containers have to be transparent for phototrophic growth. If the width of the jar exceeds 1 cm, the culture has to be kept in motion by stirring or shaking slowly to minimize self-shading. After sealing of the cultivation vessel, flush the gas phase over the culture 5 min with argon to expel oxygen. Cultivation is carried out between six 60 W light bulbs.

7. Fill the cultivation vessels with the appropriate volume of prepared medium (*see* **step 4**) and add an aliquot of the preculture to achieve an inoculation density of 0.02–0.05.

8. Incubate cultures at 30 °C for 2–3 days (*see* **Note 29**) under the conditions specified in **step 5** (for chemoheterotrophic growth) and **step 6** (for phototrophic growth).

9. Cells are harvested by centrifugation at 6000×*g* and room temperature for 20 min.

3.4.4 Preparation of Cells for Protein Analysis

1. Wash cells harvested from *R. capsulatus* expression cultures two times with SP buffer.

2. Use a small volume of SP buffer supplemented with protease inhibitor to resuspend the cell pellet. Dilute to a cell density (OD_{660}) of the cell suspension of 5–10. Lower cell densities will increase disruption efficiency, while higher densities allow for a higher protein concentration in the final homogenate.

3. *Rhodobacter* cells are disrupted by a French Press device with a pressure of 550 bar in setting "high" and five disruption cycles until the sample appears as a transparent reddish solution.

4. Optional step: Soluble, insoluble and membrane bound proteins may be separated by cell fractionation. To this end, cell lysates are first centrifuged at $2500 \times g$ at 4 °C for 5 min. The resulting pellet contains undisrupted cells and other debris as well as inclusion bodies of insoluble proteins. The supernatant, which contains soluble and membrane proteins, can be further subjected to ultracentrifugation ($135,000 \times g$, 4 °C, 1 h) to yield soluble proteins in the supernatant and a pellet containing cell membranes with bound proteins.

5. The separated fractions may be used for further techniques like analysis by SDS-PAGE or protein purification.

4   Notes

1. Ferrieres and coworkers [63] discovered that a Mu phage transposon located in the genome of *E. coli* S17-1 could occasionally integrate into the recipient genome during the conjugation event. If such an event may cause problems, a Mu phage free *E. coli* S17-1 derivative is available.

2. Supplement addition is carried out after cooling down, since the components would precipitate irreversibly otherwise. Serine can be used as an alternative nitrogen source instead of $(NH_4)_2SO_4$, however, this decreases the growth rate of *R. capsulatus* and activates the enzyme nitrogenase, resulting in hydrogen gas production. This might lead to pressure increase in gastight vessels, which may lead to fracturing or explosion. Therefore, when serine is used as a nitrogen source, leave a dead volume of about one third of the culture vessel.

3. It is important to omit iron in the medium since *E. coli* cannot survive at high iron concentrations.

4. In our lab, the use of pRhokHi-2 and pRhotHi-2 with His$_6$ tagging and kanamycin for selection are standard procedures for expression in *R. capsulatus*. However, a set of different derivatives of the pRho vectors exists, featuring alternative selection markers and tags [36]; the available variants are listed in Table 4.

5. Star activity may occur with the restriction enzyme *Bam*HI at high enzyme concentrations and long incubation times. When *Bam*HI is used at low concentrations (1–2 U/µg DNA), usually no star activity occurs.

6. Columns of commercial gel extraction kits usually only bind up to 10 µg of DNA. Hence, at least five columns must be used for gel extraction of 50 µg DNA.

Table 4
Paris-medium composition (from ref. [64])

Solution	[Stock]ᵃ	Sterilizationᵇ	Storage	Volume
K_2HPO_4	0.5 M	121 °C	RT	6 mL
KH_2PO_4	1 M	121 °C	RT	2 mL
Na_3-citrat	0.5 M	121 °C	RT	300 μL
K-L-glutamate	1 M	121 °C	RT	1 mL
$MgSO_4$	1 M	121 °C	RT	150 μL
Glucose	50% (w/v)	121 °C	RT	1 mL
Casamino acids	10% (w/v)	0.22 μm	−20 °C	1 mL
L-tryptophan	5 mg/mL	0.22 μm	−20 °C	200 μL
Fe(III)NH₄-citrate	2.2 g/L	0.22 μm	4 °C	2.5 mL
MilliQ water		121 °C	RT	Add 50 mL

RT room temperature
ᵃIndicates the concentration of stock solutions]
ᵇBy autoclaving at 121 °C, 2 bar, for 20 min or by filtration with a sterile filter of 0.22 μm pore diameter

7. Homogenization is important to simplify the following phenol–chloroform extraction. Without homogenization, genomic DNA sticks to proteins, impeding the removal of the aqueous phase.

8. Note that high salt (>0.5 M) or sucrose (>10%) concentrations can change the density of the aqueous phase. In this case it may form the lower phase.

9. The dilution step is necessary since stationary grown *P. putida* cells usually stick to each other and are difficult to resuspend.

10. It is preferable to use freshly prepared competent cells for electroporation of *P. putida* KT2440 since storage of aliquots at −80 °C can significantly decrease transformation efficiency.

11. It is advantageous to choose strains with a *recA⁺* genotype for TREX application since mutation of the *recA* gene can significantly lower the transposition efficiency [65].

12. Take the filter on one edge with forceps, carefully bend it over to the opposite edge of the filter and grab also this edge. The picked filter should now have a curved shape perfectly fitting into the reaction tube. Try to avoid crumpling the filter as this could decrease resuspension efficiency.

13. The efficiency of conjugational transfer and transposon integration has to be determined experimentally but is typically in the range of 10^{-5} to 10^{-8} in relation to employed recipient cells,

Table 5
Properties of pRho expression vectors (modified from ref. [36])

Promoter	Vector	Antibiotic resistance[a]	Affinity tag[b]
P*aphII* (constitutive)	pRhokHi-2	Km, Cm	His$_6$
	pRhokS-2	Km, Cm	StrepII
	pRhokHi-6	Km, Sp	His$_6$
P$_{T7}$ (inducible)	pRhotHi-2	Km, Cm	His$_6$
	pRhotS-2	Km, Cm	StrepII
	pRhotHi-6	Km, Sp	His$_6$

[a]*Km* kanamycin, *Cm* chloramphenicol, *Sp* spectinomycin
[b]C-terminal fusion of six histidine residues (His$_6$) or Strep tag II peptide WSHPQFEK [66]

resulting in high numbers of clones at the named dilutions. It is important to generate easily distinguishable single colonies since every clone on the selection agar plates will carry the TREX expression cassette at an individual integration locus in the chromosome, which may have an influence on expression and biosynthetic production. To determine the efficiency of gene delivery in your experiment, count the clones obtained on selection agar after conjugation and divide by the number of clones of recipient cells that were subjected to the same conjugation procedure, but without donor cells and plated at different dilutions on LB agar without antibiotics (Table 5).

14. The pBBR1MCS plasmid series comprises a *lac* promoter for constitutive expression as well as a P$_{T7}$ promoter for application in expression strains providing T7 RNA polymerase, both flanking the MCS. Therefore, the orientation of the cloned gene in the MCS must be adjusted according to the respective promoter.

15. Cryo cultures are prepared by adding 135 µL DMSO to 1.8 mL stationary *B. glumae* PG1 culture and stored at –80 °C. Cultures should be thawed on ice until the desired volume can be aspirated and afterwards immediately frozen again.

16. The desired cell density is reached after 3–4 h. For efficient conjugation, it is important to harvest the donor strain in the exponential growth phase.

17. Depending on the chosen plasmid and the gene of interest, 100 µL cell suspension may not result in sufficient colony numbers. In that case, remove the filter with forceps, centrifuge the suspension (21,000×*g*, 1 min), discard the supernatant, resuspend the cell pellet in the remaining LB medium, and plate it on a MME agar plate. For plasmids with a chloramphenicol or tetracycline resistance cassette, the antibiotic concentration is sufficient for counter selection of *E. coli*.

If gentamycin or kanamycin is used, or if a chosen donor strain can cope with higher antibiotic concentrations, additional counter selection with 25 µg/mL irgasan (final concentration) can be applied.

18. For some *B. glumae* PG1 mutants and cloned genes, we observed a drastic decrease in transformation efficiency both with conjugation and electroporation. Thus, both methods may subsequently be tested if necessary.

19. DNA solution should have a low ionic strength. If using innu-PREP Plasmid Mini Kit for plasmid preparation, elute DNA in desalted H_2O instead of provided elution buffer. A pulse time below 4–5 ms in **step 10** indicates remaining salts that will lead to low transformation efficiency. In such cases, DNA should additionally be purified by dialysis.

20. If cell mixture seems viscous or slimy, cells may be damaged by electroporation. As far as our experience goes, this is caused by an extended cultivation time of the culture used for preparation of competent cells (*see* **step 2**). Cell density should not exceed $OD_{580} = 0.2$ and may even be lowered.

21. It is possible to exchange the *Xho*I site for cloning by other singular restriction sites in the MCS (*Bam*HI, *Sac*I, *Sal*I, or *Hind*III) by designing appropriate primers and adapt the restriction protocol to the new enzyme combination.

22. Streptomycin resistance is an inherent feature of *R. capsulatus* strain B10S and its derivative B10S-T7. Therefore, streptomycin is added to PY agar plates for counter-selection against the *E. coli* donor strains after conjugation. It should be noted, however, that streptomycin should not be used for cultivation in RCV minimal medium, as this may severely inhibit growth of *R. capsulatus*.

23. It is important to minimize illumination of *R. capsulatus* in the presence of oxygen, since this stimulates photooxidative processes which might result in cell death.

24. After activation of the gas pack by addition of water, all steps to introduce the package into the vessel and sealing have to be carried out quickly to prevent exhaustion of the gas pack. Once the jar is closed, it must not be reopened to maintain the anaerobic milieu inside.

25. Standard wavelengths for measuring bacterial cell densities ($\lambda = 580–600$ nm) are not suitable for *R. capsulatus*, since photopigments produced by this organism absorb light at these wavelengths, resulting in incorrect determination of cell density.

26. Avoid disturbing the layer of dead cells at the bottom of the cultivation vessel. Ensure to only draw samples for cell density measurements and inoculations from the upper phase of the culture.

27. In some cases (for example, if premature expression might prove toxic to the cells) it is advisable to cultivate expression cultures until they reach a cell density corresponding to an OD_{660} of 0.4–0.6 before addition of fructose. In the case of anaerobic cultures, use an injection needle to add fructose through the rubber septum without disturbing the anaerobic environment in the vessel.

28. If the shaking device cannot be completely darkened, wrap the cultivation flask in aluminum foil.

29. Optimally expression is carried out until cultures reach stationary phase for maximum yield of biomass. However, if proteolytic degradation of heterologously expressed proteins is an issue, cell harvest within the logarithmic growth phase $(OD_{660} \leq 1)$ may allow increased protein yields.

Acknowledgments

Part of this work was funded by the Bioeconomy Science Center which is financially supported by the Ministry of Innovation, Research and Science of North-Rhine Westphalia, Germany, within the framework of the NRW Strategieprojekt BioSC (No. 313/323 - 400 - 00213), and by the Deutsche Forschungsgemeinschaft within CEPLAS—Cluster of Excellence on Plant Sciences (EXC 1028).

We thank Alexander Bollinger (Institute of Molecular Enzyme Technology, Heinrich-Heine-University Düsseldorf, Germany) for his contribution regarding handling of *B. glumae* PG1.

References

1. Sharpton TJ (2014) An introduction to the analysis of shotgun metagenomic data. Front Plant Sci 5:209

2. Monciardini P, Iorio M, Maffioli S, Sosio M, Donadio S (2014) Discovering new bioactive molecules from microbial sources. Microbial Biotechnol 7:209–220

3. Lee MH, Lee SW (2013) Bioprospecting potential of the soil metagenome: novel enzymes and bioactivities. Genomics Inform 11:114–120

4. Lombard N, Prestat E, van Elsas JD, Simonet P (2011) Soil-specific limitations for access and analysis of soil microbial communities by metagenomics. FEMS Microbiol Ecol 78:31–49

5. Anderson RE, Sogin ML, Baross JA (2014) Evolutionary strategies of viruses, bacteria and archaea in hydrothermal vent ecosystems revealed through metagenomics. PLoS One 9:e109696

6. López-López O, Cerdán ME, González Siso MI (2014) New extremophilic lipases and esterases from metagenomics. Curr Protein Pept Sci 15:445–455

7. Cowan DA, Ramond JB, Makhalanyane TP, De Maayer P (2015) Metagenomics of extreme environments. Curr Opin Microbiol 25:97–102

8. Alcaide M, Stogios PJ, Lafraya A, Tchigvintsev A, Flick R, Bargiela R et al (2015) Pressure adaptation is linked to thermal adaptation in salt-saturated marine habitats. Environ Microbiol 17:332–345

9. Tchigvintsev A, Tran H, Popovic A, Kovacic F, Brown G, Flick R et al (2015) The environment shapes microbial enzymes: five cold-active and salt-resistant carboxylesterases from marine metagenomes. Appl Microbiol Biotechnol 99:2165–2178

10. Mhuantong W, Charoensawan V, Kanokratana P, Tangphatsornruang S, Champreda V (2015)

Comparative analysis of sugarcane bagasse metagenome reveals unique and conserved biomass-degrading enzymes among lignocellulolytic microbial communities. Biotechnol Biofuels 8:1–17

11. McCarthy DM, Pearce DA, Patching JW, Fleming GT (2013) Contrasting responses to nutrient enrichment of prokaryotic communities collected from deep sea sites in the southern ocean. Biology (Basel) 2:1165–1188

12. McNamara PJ, LaPara TM, Novak PJ (2015) The effect of perfluorooctane sulfonate, exposure time, and chemical mixtures on methanogenic community structure and function. Microbiol Insights 8:1–7

13. Tan B, Fowler SJ, Abu Laban N, Dong X, Sensen CW, Foght J, Gieg LM (2015) Comparative analysis of metagenomes from three methanogenic hydrocarbon-degrading enrichment cultures with 41 environmental samples. ISME J 9:2028–2045

14. Mori T, Kamei I, Hirai H, Kondo R (2014) Identification of novel glycosyl hydrolases with cellulolytic activity against crystalline cellulose from metagenomic libraries constructed from bacterial enrichment cultures. Springerplus 3:365

15. Ferrer M, Beloqui A, Timmis KN, Golyshin PN (2009) Metagenomics for mining new genetic resources of microbial communities. J Mol Microbiol Biotechnol 16:109–123

16. Saïdani N, Grando D, Valadié H, Bastien O, Maréchal E (2009) Potential and limits of in silico target discovery - case study of the search for new antimalarial chemotherapeutic targets. Infect Genet Evol 9:359–367

17. Galvão TC, Mohn WW, de Lorenzo V (2005) Exploring the microbial biodegradation and biotransformation gene pool. Trends Biotechnol 23:497–506

18. Trindade M, van Zyl LJ, Navarro-Fernández J, Abd Elrazak A (2015) Targeted metagenomics as a tool to tap into marine natural product diversity for the discovery and production of drug candidates. Front Microbiol 6:890

19. Vakhlu J, Sudan AK, Johri BN (2008) Metagenomics: future of microbial gene mining. Indian J Microbiol 48:202–215

20. Coughlan LM, Cotter PD, Hill C, Alvarez-Ordóñez A (2015) Biotechnological applications of functional metagenomics in the food and pharmaceutical industries. Front Microbiol 6:672

21. Ufarté L, Potocki-Veronese G, Laville E (2015) Discovery of new protein families and functions: new challenges in functional metagenomics for biotechnologies and microbial ecology. Front Microbiol 6:563

22. Leis B, Angelov A, Liebl W (2013) Screening and expression of genes from metagenomes. Adv Appl Microbiol 83:1–68

23. Ekkers DM, Cretoiu MS, Kielak AM, Elsas JD (2012) The great screen anomaly—a new frontier in product discovery through functional metagenomics. Appl Microbiol Biotechnol 93:1005–1020

24. Liebl W, Angelov A, Juergensen J, Chow J, Loeschcke A, Drepper T et al (2014) Alternative hosts for functional (meta)genome analysis. Appl Microbiol Biotechnol 98:8099–8109

25. Leis B, Angelov A, Mientus M, Li H, Pham VT, Lauinger B et al (2015) Identification of novel esterase-active enzymes from hot environments by use of the host bacterium *Thermus thermophilus*. Front Microbiol 6:275

26. Jiang PX, Wang HS, Zhang C, Lou K, Xing XH (2010) Reconstruction of the violacein biosynthetic pathway from *Duganella* sp. B2 in different heterologous hosts. Appl Microbiol Biotechnol 86:1077–1088

27. McMahon MD, Guan C, Handelsman J, Thomas MG (2012) Metagenomic analysis of *Streptomyces lividans* reveals host-dependent functional expression. Appl Environ Microbiol 78:3622–3629

28. Liu L, Yang H, Shin HD, Chen RR, Li J, Du G, Chen J (2013) How to achieve high-level expression in microbial enzymes: strategies and perspectives. Bioengineered 4:212–223

29. Troeschel SC, Thies S, Link O, Real CI, Knops K, Wilhelm S et al (2012) Novel broad host range shuttle vectors for expression in *Escherichia coli*, *Bacillus subtilis* and *Pseudomonas putida*. J Biotechnol 161:71–79

30. Domröse A, Klein AS, Hage-Hülsmann J, Thies S, Svensson V, Classen T et al (2015) Efficient recombinant production of prodigiosin in *Pseudomonas putida*. Front Microbiol 6:972

31. Loeschcke A, Markert A, Wilhelm S, Wirtz A, Rosenau F, Jaeger KE, Drepper T (2013) TREX: a universal tool for the transfer and expression of biosynthetic pathways in bacteria. ACS Synth Biol 2:22–33

32. Voget S, Knapp A, Poehlein A, Vollstedt C, Streit W, Daniel R, Jaeger KE (2015) Complete genome sequence of the lipase producing strain *Burkholderia glumae* PG1. J Biotechnol 204:3–4

33. Seo YS, Lim JY, Park J, Kim S, Lee HH, Cheong H et al (2015) Comparative genome analysis of rice-pathogenic *Burkholderia* provides insight into capacity to adapt to different environments and hosts. MBC Genomics 16:349

34. Knapp A, Voget S, Gao R, Zaburannyi N, Krysciak D, Breuer M et al (2016) Mutations improving production and secretion of extracellular lipase by *Burkholderia glumae* PG1. Appl Microbiol Biotechnol 100:1265–1273

35. Boekema BK, Beselin A, Breuer M, Hauer B, Koster M, Rosenau F et al (2007) Hexadecane and Tween 80 stimulate lipase production in *Burkholderia glumae* by different mechanisms. Appl Environ Microbiol 73:3838–3844

36. Katzke N, Arvani S, Bergmann R, Circolone F, Markert A, Svensson V et al (2010) A novel T7 RNA polymerase dependent expression system for high-level protein production in the phototrophic bacterium *Rhodobacter capsulatus*. Protein Expr Purif 69:137–146

37. Nelson KE, Weinel C, Paulsen IT, Dodson RJ, Hilbert H, Martins dos Santos VA et al (2002) Complete genome sequence and comparative analysis of the metabolically versatile *Pseudomonas putida* KT2440. Environ Microbiol 4:799–808

38. Loeschcke A, Thies S (2015) *Pseudomonas putida*-a versatile host for the production of natural products. Appl Microbiol Biotechnol 99:6197–6214

39. Blank LM, Ebert BE, Buehler K, Bühler B (2010) Redox biocatalysis and metabolism: molecular mechanisms and metabolic network analysis. Antioxid Redox Signal 13:349–394

40. Tiso T, Wierckx N, Blank L (2014) Non-pathogenic *Pseudomonas* as a platform for industrial biocatalysis. In: Grunwald P (ed) Industrial biocatalysis. Pan Stanford, Singapore, pp 323–372

41. Fernández M, Duque E, Pizarro-Tobías P, Van Dillewijn P, Wittich RM, Ramos JL (2009) Microbial responses to xenobiotic compounds. Identification of genes that allow *Pseudomonas putida* KT2440 to cope with 2,4,6-trinitrotoluene. Microbial Biotechnol 2:287–294

42. Simon O, Klaiber I, Huber A, Pfannstiel J (2014) Comprehensive proteome analysis of the response of *Pseudomonas putida* KT2440 to the flavor compound vanillin. J Proteomics 109:212–227

43. Eggert T, Brockmeier U, Dröge MJ, Quax WJ, Jaeger KE (2003) Extracellular lipases from *Bacillus subtilis*: regulation of gene expression and enzyme activity by amino acid supply and external pH. FEMS Microbiol Lett 225:319–324

44. Laible PD, Scott HN, Henry L, Hanson DK (2004) Towards higher-throughput membrane protein production for structural genomics initiatives. J Struct Funct Genomics 5:167–172

45. Masepohl B, Hallenbeck PC (2010) Nitrogen and molybdenum control of nitrogen fixation in the phototrophic bacterium *Rhodobacter capsulatus*. Adv Exp Med Biol 675:49–70

46. Kyndt JA, Fitch JC, Berry RE, Stewart MC, Whitley K, Meyer TE et al (2012) Tyrosine triad at the interface between the Rieske iron-sulfur protein, cytochrome c1 and cytochrome c2 in the bc1 complex of *Rhodobacter capsulatus*. Biochim Biophys Acta 1817:811–818

47. Loppnow H, Libby P, Freudenberg M, Krauss JH, Weckesser J, Mayer H (1990) Cytokine induction by lipopolysaccharide (LPS) corresponds to lethal toxicity and is inhibited by nontoxic *Rhodobacter capsulatus* LPS. Infect Immun 58:3743–3750

48. Simon R, Priefer U, Pühler A (1983) A broad host range mobilization system for *in vivo* genetic-engineering-transposon mutagenesis in Gram-negative bacteria. Nat Biotechnol 1:784–791

49. Katzke N, Bergmann R, Jaeger KE, Drepper T (2012) Heterologous high-level gene expression in the photosynthetic bacterium *Rhodobacter capsulatus*. Methods Mol Biol 824:251–269

50. Sambrook J, Russell DW (2001) Molecular cloning: a laboratory manual. Cold Spring Harbor Press, New York

51. Vogel HJ, Bonner DM (1956) Acetylornithase of *Escherichia coli* – partial purification and some properties. J Biol Chem 218:97–106

52. Cronan JE (2003) Cosmid-based system for transient expression and absolute off-to-on transcriptional control of *Escherichia coli* genes. J Bacteriol 185:6522–6529

53. Kovach ME, Phillips RW, Elzer PH, Roop RM 2nd, Peterson KM (1994) pBBR1MCS: a broad-host-range cloning vector. Biotechniques 16:800–802

54. Kovach ME, Elzer PH, Hill DS, Robertson GT, Farris MA, Roop RM 2nd, Peterson KM (1995) Four new derivatives of the broad-host-range cloning vector pBBR1MCS, carrying different antibiotic-resistance cassettes. Gene 166:175–176

55. Labes M, Pühler A, Simon R (1990) A new family of RSF1010-derived expression and lac-fusion broad-host-range vectors for gram-negative bacteria. Gene 89:37–46

56. Arvani S, Markert A, Loeschcke A, Jaeger KE, Drepper T (2012) A T7 RNA polymerase-based toolkit for the concerted expression of clustered genes. J Biotechnol 159:162–171

57. Fischbach M, Voigt CA (2010) Prokaryotic gene clusters: a rich toolbox for synthetic biology. Biotechnol J 5:1277–1296

58. Rocha-Martin J, Harrington C, Dobson AD, O'Gara F (2014) Emerging strategies and integrated systems microbiology technologies for biodiscovery of marine bioactive compounds. Mar Drugs 12:3516–3559

59. Ferrer M, Martinez-Martinez M, Bargiela R, Streit WR, Golyshina OV, Golyshin PN (2016) Estimating the success of enzyme bioprospecting through metagenomics: current status and future trends. Microbial Biotechnol 9:22–34

60. McAllister WT, Morris C, Rosenberg AH, Studier FW (1981) Utilization of bacteriophage T7 late promoters in recombinant plasmids during infection. J Mol Biol 153:527–544

61. Widenhorn KA, Somers JM, Kay WW (1988) Expression of the divergent tricarboxylate transport operon (tctI) of Salmonella typhimurium. J Bacteriol 170:3223–3227

62. Kang Y, Son MS, Hoang TT (2007) One step engineering of T7-expression strains for protein production: increasing the host-range of the T7-expression system. Protein Expr Purif 55:325–333

63. Ferrieres L, Hemery G, Nham T, Guerout AM, Mazel D, Beloin C, Ghigo JM (2010) Silent mischief: bacteriophage Mu insertions contaminate products of Escherichia coli random mutagenesis performed using suicidal transposon delivery plasmids mobilized by broad-host-range RP4 conjugative machinery. J Bacteriol 192:6418–6427

64. Troeschel SC, Drepper T, Leggewie C, Streit WR, Jaeger KE (2010) Novel tools for the functional expression of metagenomic DNA. Methods Mol Biol 668:117–139

65. Kuan CT, Tessman I (1992) Further evidence that transposition of Tn5 in Escherichia coli is strongly enhanced by constitutively activated RecA proteins. J Bacteriol 174:6872–6877

66. Schmidt TG, Skerra A (2007) The Strep-tag system for one-step purification and high-affinity detection or capturing of proteins. Nat Protoc 2:1528–1535

Chapter 11

A Microtiter Plate-Based Assay to Screen for Active and Stereoselective Hydrolytic Enzymes in Enzyme Libraries

Dominique Böttcher, Patrick Zägel, Marlen Schmidt, and Uwe T. Bornscheuer

Abstract

A procedure for the high-throughput screening (HTS) of esterases is described. This includes a pretest for discrimination of active and inactive clones using an agar plate overlay assay, the enzyme expression in microtiter plates and the measurement of activity and enantioselectivity (E) of the esterase variants using acetates of secondary alcohols as model substrates. Acetic acid released is converted in an enzyme cascade leading to the stoichiometric formation of NADH, which is quantified in a spectrophotometer. The method allows screening of several thousand mutants per day and has already been successfully applied to identify an esterase mutant with an $E > 100$ towards an important building block for organic synthesis. This protocol can also be used for lipases and possibly other hydrolases that are expressed in soluble form in conventional *E. coli* strains.

Key words Hydrolase, Esterase, Lipase, High-throughput assay, Enantioselectivity, Directed evolution, Metagenome

1 Introduction

Lipases and esterases are the most frequently used hydrolases (EC 3) in organic synthesis [1, 2]. They are important biocatalysts and especially suitable for industrial applications as they are very stable and also active in organic solvents. Moreover, they very often exhibit high enantioselectivity and are therefore used in the synthesis of optically active compounds, for which more than 1000 examples can be found in literature. Besides a considerable number of commercially available lipases and to a lesser extent esterases, researchers can create optimized enzyme variants using protein engineering [3–5] or identify new esterases or lipases with desired activity/selectivity using the metagenomic approach [6–8]. These methods can create huge numbers of novel biocatalysts, which are

Wolfgang R. Streit and Rolf Daniel (eds.), *Metagenomics: Methods and Protocols*, Methods in Molecular Biology, vol. 1539, DOI 10.1007/978-1-4939-6691-2_11, © Springer Science+Business Media LLC 2017

time-consuming to screen using conventional methods such as gas chromatography or HPLC.

Consequently, a range of high-throughput assay systems has been developed in the past years to allow for a rapid and reliable identification of suitable enzymes [9–12]. As lipases and esterases are often used to produce optically active compounds, the determination of the enantioselectivity of these enzymes is of major interest and several methods have been described [11, 12] and successfully applied to improve the biocatalysts' selectivity [13–15].

The protocol described here was designed to allow the determination of substrate specificity and enantioselectivity of esterases (or other hydrolases such es peptidases and amidase, where acetamide can serve as substrate) towards secondary alcohols and has the advantage that no surrogate substrates (i.e., chromophores like resorufin) have to be used, as acetates are the preferred esters in the resolution of alcohols. In this assay, hydrolysis of the acetate using an esterase (or lipase) releases acetic acid. This is then converted in an enzyme cascade reaction into citrate with stoichiometrical formation of NADH. This increase in NADH concentration is quantified spectrophotometrically at 340 nm [16] (Fig. 1). This assay is very reliable and fast, as the exact determination of activity and enantioselectivity is possible within minutes for an entire 96-well plate. In addition, the acetic acid kit is commercially available (R-Biopharm GmbH, Darmstadt, Germany).

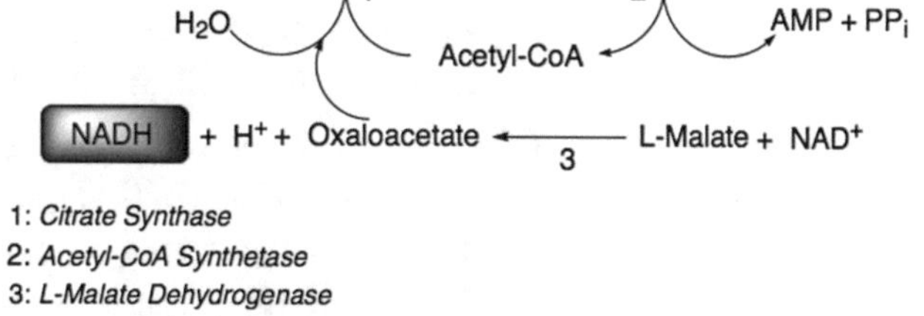
H2O
Hydrolase
Acetic acid
CoA
Citrate
ATP
1
2
H2O
AMP + PPi
Acetyl-CoA
NADH
+ H+ + Oxaloacetate
3
L-Malate + NAD+
1: Citrate Synthase
2: Acetyl-CoA Synthetase
3: L-Malate Dehydrogenase

Fig. 1 Assay based on the conversion of acetic acid released in the hydrolase-catalyzed reaction in a subsequent enzyme cascade yielding an increase in NADH [16]

2 Materials

2.1 Activity Test on Agar Plates (Overlay Agar)

1. Agar plates containing colonies from metagenomic libraries.
2. Replica-plating tool and sterile clothes.
3. Soft agar (0.5 % agar dissolved in water)
4. 1-naphthyl acetate solution: 40 mg/mL in N,N'-dimethyl formamide.
5. Fast Red TR solution: 100 mg/mL in dimethyl sulfoxide.

2.2 Cultivation in Microtiter Plates

1. Lysogeny broth (LB) medium: 10 g tryptone/peptone, 10 g NaCl, 5 g yeast extract, add H_2O to 1000 mL.
2. 60 % glycerol.
3. Antibiotic (e.g., ampicillin, usually 100 µg/mL).
4. Isopropyl-β-D-thiogalactoside (IPTG).
5. 96-well microtiter plates (e.g., Greiner Bio-One, Kremsmunster, Austria).
6. Microtiter plate thermoshaker (e.g., iEMS Microplate Incubator/Shaker HT, Thermo Scientific, Waltham, MA, USA), alternatively use a plastic box with wet tissue placed in a normal incubator.
7. Centrifuge with microtiter plate adapter (e.g., Heraeus Labofuge 400R, Thermo Scientific, Waltham, MA, USA).

2.3 Cell Lysis

1. Lysis buffer: 50 mM NaH_2PO_4, 300 mM NaCl, pH 8.0, 0.1 % (w/v) lysozyme, 1 U/mL DNaseI.

2.4 Enzyme Assay

1. 10 mM sodium phosphate buffer, pH 7.4.
2. Acetate assay reagents (R-Biopharm GmbH, Darmstadt, Germany).

   (a) Bottle 1: 32 mL triethanolamine buffer solution pH 8.4 (see **Note 1**), L-malic acid (134 mg), $MgCl_2 \cdot 6H_2O$, (67 mg) storage at 2–8 °C.

   (b) Bottle 2: lyophilizate containing ATP (175 mg), CoA (18 mg), NAD^+ (86 mg) dissolve in 7 mL distilled water, aliquots are stable at –20 °C for 2 months.

   (c) Bottle 3: suspension of L-malate dehydrogenase (1100 U); citrate synthase (270 U); stable at 2–8 °C.

   (d) Bottle 4: lyophilized acetyl-CoA synthetase (5 U) add 250 µL distilled water, stable at 2–8 °C for 5 days.

3. To prepare the test-kit component mixture use 1000 µL of bottle 1, 200 µL of bottle 2, 10 µL of bottle 3, 20 µL of bottle 4, and 1900 µL distilled water.

4. Racemic (A) or enantiopure (B) acetate substrates 5–50 mM.

5. Multichannel pipette.

6. Microtiter plate spectrophotometer (e.g., Varioskan, Thermo Scientific, Waltham, MA, USA).

Optional

1. Colony picking robot (e.g., Qpix 420 Molecular devices, Sunnyvale, CA, USA).

2. Pipetting robot (Bravo, Agilent Technologies Inc., Santa Clara, CA, USA).

3. 96-pin replicator (Thermo Scientific, Waltham, MA, USA).

3   Methods

The acetic acid assay allows to differentiate active from inactive and enantioselective from nonselective enzyme variants. In the activity test (option A) the resulting graphs will provide only the relative activity of each enzyme variant for the tested substrate (acetate ester). In the selectivity test (option B), one has to calculate the initial reaction rates ($\Delta A/\Delta t$) for each enantiomer separately, and the quotient of the two rates then yields the apparent enantioselectivity E_{app}.

Positive hits from the assay must be verified afterwards using conventional analytical methods, such as chiral GC or HPLC to determine conversion, kinetic parameters, and the true enantioselectivity E_{true}.

3.1 Activity Test on Agar Plates

1. Spread cells containing metagenomic library onto LB agar plates containing an appropriate antibiotic.

2. Incubate the plates overnight at 30 or 37 °C.

3. Transfer colonies by replica plating to LB agar plates containing an appropriate antibiotic and IPTG to induce esterase production.

4. Incubate the plates for 5 h at 37 °C.

5. Prepare overlay soft agar.

6. Prepare solutions of 1-naphthyl acetate and Fast Red TR.

7. Melt the soft agar in a microwave and let it cool down to approximately 40 °C.

8. Mix 100 μL of both solutions with 10 mL soft agar and pour it carefully over the colonies.

9. Active clones will turn brownish in a few seconds.

3.2 Enzyme Production in Microtiter Plates (Fig. 2)

1. Pick single colonies into 96-well microtiter plates containing 200 μL LB medium, supplemented with the required antibiotic, per well. These plates serve as master plates. After cell growth for 4–6 h at 37 °C and 220 rpm, duplicate the master plates by transferring a 1 μL aliquot (*see* **Note 2**) into a new microtiter plate (containing 200 μL LB-antibiotic medium per well) used for the subsequent production of esterase (production plates).

2. Supplement the master plates with glycerol (final concentration 15 % v/v) and store them at –80 °C. These master plates can be also used for future high-throughput assays.

3. Incubate the production plates overnight at 37 °C and 220 rpm and dilute 1:10 the next day with fresh medium (*see* **Note 3**). Cultivate at 37 °C and 220 rpm.

4. After 3 h start enzyme production by addition of inducer solution in an appropriate concentration (e.g., IPTG usually in concentrations from 10 to 1000 μM).

3.3 Cell Lysis in Microtiter Plates

1. After cultivation for approximately 5 h at 30 °C and 220 rpm, centrifuge at $2000 \times g$ for 15 min, discard the supernatant and add 200 μL lysis buffer.

2. Incubate the plates for 30 min at 4 °C, freeze the plates at –80 °C for 1 h and thaw them at 37 °C for approx. 20 min.

3. Centrifuge again at $2000 \times g$ for 15 min and transfer enzyme solution into new microtiter plates (*see* **Note 4**).

3.4 Screening for Activity or Enantioselectivity

1. To a mixture of the test-kit components (150 μL), add 20 μL enzyme solution (*see* **Note 5**) from the production plate. Either an activity test (go on with **step 1** option A) or selectivity test (go on with **step 1** option B) can be performed.

A: Activity Test

1. Start the reaction by adding 20 mL of substrate solution [i.e., racemic acetic acid esters, substrate concentration 5–50 mM dissolved in sodium phosphate buffer (10 mM, pH 7.4)].

2. Monitor the increase of NADH at 340 nm over 10 min (*see* **Note 8**). Use mixtures of the test kit with cell lysates of *Escherichia coli* harboring the empty expression vector without enzyme-encoding gene as negative controls (*see* **Note 7**). A positive control (acetic acid) is included in the test kit.

B: Selectivity Test

1. Transfer 20 μL enzyme solution from one well into two wells of a new microtiter plate (Fig. 2).

2. Add 20 μL of optically pure (*R*)- or (*S*)-acetates alternately into the rows of the plate.

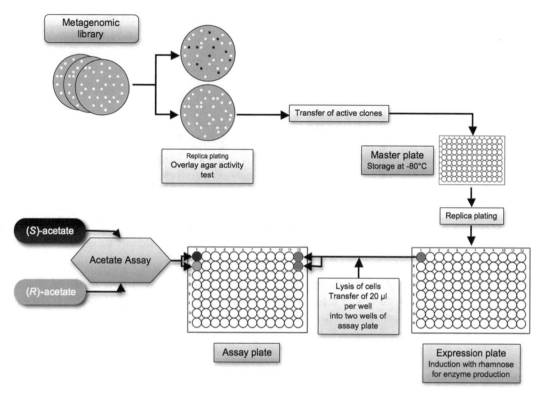

Fig. 2 Enzyme production in microtiter plates and principle of the screening of metagenomic libraries for altered enantioselectivity by adding (*R*)- and (*S*)-substrates to separate wells of a microtiter plate containing the same enzyme variant. If only activity is measured, the enzyme sample must not be split into two wells

3. Measure the increase of absorption at 340 nm for 10 min (*see* **Note 8**) and calculate the initial reaction rates for each enantiomer separately. The quotient of these rates is the apparent enantioselectivity E_{app} (Fig. 3).

4   Notes

1. The acetic acid assay is buffered at pH 8.4. Make sure that your enzyme is active at this pH.

2. This step can be done using a 96-pin replicator or using a liquid handling robot.

3. Dilution with fresh medium is very important to achieve a comparable cell density in each well of the microtiter plate.

4. These plates can be stored at –20 °C, freeze-dried, or directly used for the determination of enantioselectivity/activity. Freeze-dry the enzyme solution if you are expecting only very low activity in the diluted cell extract. Make sure that the enzyme tolerates this procedure.

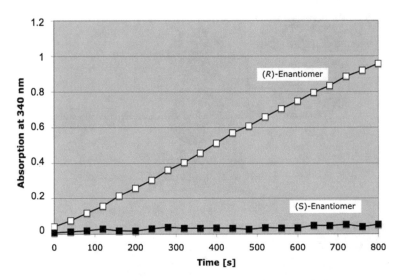

Fig. 3 Initial rates determined by using optically pure (*R*)- or (*S*)-1-phenyl ethyl acetate (5 mg/μL). Reactions were performed by using lyophilized crude cell extract of PFE

5. If you are using freeze-dried enzyme, dissolve it first with 200 μL sodium phosphate buffer per well of the microtiter plate and then transfer 20 μL into each well of the assay plate.

6. Make sure that the absorption increase is in the linear range. In case of nonlinear behavior, the enzyme might be too active and dilution of enzyme solution in a new microtiter plate should solve this problem.

7. Make sure by running appropriate control reactions that no acetic acid is present prior to substrate (acetate) addition. The measurement of crude cell extract containing empty vector with/without substrate are essential, since the *E. coli* cell background may degrade NADH or hydrolyze the substrate.

8. If no activity is measured, an increase of the enzyme amount or prolonged reaction time may exclude false-negative results.

References

1. Bornscheuer UT, Kazlauskas RJ (2006) Hydrolases in organic synthesis: regio- and stereoselective biotransformations, 2nd edn. Wiley-VCH, Weinheim

2. Romano D, Bonomi F, de Mattos MC, Fonseca TD, de Oliveira MDF, Molinari F (2015) Esterases as stereoselective biocatalysts. Biotechnol Adv 33:547–565

3. Schmidt M, Böttcher D, Bornscheuer UT (2010) Directed evolution of industrial biocatalysts. In: Soetaert W, Vandamme E

(eds) Industrial biotechnology. Wiley-VCH, Weinheim, pp 173–205

4. Bornscheuer UT, Huisman G, Kazlauskas RJ, Lutz S, Moore J, Robins K (2012) Engineering the third wave in biocatalysis. Nature 485:185–194

5. Davids T, Schmidt M, Böttcher D, Bornscheuer UT (2013) Strategies for the discovery and engineering of enzymes for biocatalysis. Curr Opin Chem Biol 17: 215–220

6. Handelsman J (2004) Metagenomics: application of genomics to uncultured microorganisms. Microbiol Mol Biol Rev 68:669–685

7. Lopez-Lopez O, Cerdan ME, Siso MIG (2014) New extremophilic lipases and esterases from metagenomics. Curr Protein Pept Sci 15:445–455

8. Kourist R, Krishna SH, Patel JS, Bartnek F, Weiner DW, Hitchman T et al (2007) Identification of a metagenome-derived esterase with high enantioselectivity in the kinetic resolution of arylaliphatic tertiary alcohols. Org Biomol Chem 5:3310–3313

9. Xiao H, Bao ZH, Zhao HM (2015) High-throughput screening and selection methods for directed enzyme evolution. Ind Eng Chem Res 54:4011–4020

10. Reymond J-L (2005) Enzyme assays. Wiley-VCH, Weinheim

11. Bustos-Jaimes I, Hummel W, Eggert T, Bogo E, Puls M, Weckbecker A et al (2009) A high-throughput screening method for chiral alcohols and its application to determine enantioselectivity of lipases and esterases. ChemCatChem 1:445–448

12. Schmidt M, Bornscheuer UT (2005) High-throughput assays for lipases and esterases. Biomol Eng 22:51–56

13. Bornscheuer UT (2013) From commercial enzymes to biocatalysts designed by protein engineering. Synlett 24:150–156

14. Lan D, Popowicz GM, Pavlidis IV, Zhou P, Bornscheuer UT, Wang Y (2015) Conversion of a mono- and diacylglycerol lipase into a triacylglycerol lipase by protein engineering. Chem Biochem 16:1431–1434

15. Schmidt M, Hasenpusch D, Kähler M, Kirchner U, Wiggenhorn K, Langel W et al (2006) Directed evolution of an esterase from *Pseudomonas fluorescens* yields a mutant with excellent enantioselectivity and activity for the kinetic resolution of a chiral building block. Chem Biochem 7:805–809

16. Baumann M, Stürmer R, Bornscheuer UT (2001) A high-throughput-screening method for the identification of active and enantioselective hydrolases. Angew Chem Int Ed Engl 40:4201–4204

Chapter 12

Screening for Cellulase Encoding Clones in Metagenomic Libraries

Nele Ilmberger and Wolfgang R. Streit

Abstract

For modern biotechnology there is a steady need to identify novel enzymes. In biotechnological applications, however, enzymes often must function under extreme and nonnatural conditions (i.e., in the presence of solvents, high temperature and/or at extreme pH values). Cellulases have many industrial applications from the generation of bioethanol, a realistic long-term energy source, to the finishing of textiles. These industrial processes require cellulolytic activity under a wide range of pH, temperature, and ionic conditions, and they are usually carried out by mixtures of cellulases. Investigation of the broad diversity of cellulolytic enzymes involved in the natural degradation of cellulose is necessary for optimizing these processes.

Key words Cellulase, Ionic liquid, Metagenome, Bioethanol, Renewable energy, Biotechnology

1 Introduction

Metagenomics has become a very powerful tool to search for novel enzymes that are useful for biotechnological applications. A number of reviews have summarized the technology [1–3]. Since its first publication and the description of the basic technology [4] a remarkable number of reports have been published providing new enzymes with a high potential for industrial applications [5–8]. Because cellulose is a valuable biopolymer for the production of biofuels (i.e., ethanol) and other biobased products a significant number of publications report on the isolation of metagenome-derived cellulases.

Functional screening of a soil metagenomic library for cellulases revealed a total of eight cellulolytic clones, one of which was purified and characterized [9]. Metagenomic screening of soda-lakes in Africa and Egypt detected more than a dozen cellulases, some of which displayed habitat related halotolerant characteristics [10, 11]. One of the earliest articles presenting metagenome-derived biocatalysts reported the detection of cellulases from a thermophilic, anaerobic digester fueled by lignocellulose [12] and a recent study detected seven cellulases with novel features [13].

While most metagenomic surveys for novel cellulases concentrate on extreme environments, there is sufficient evidence that temperate and therefore highly genetically diverse environments also contain a range of cellulases which are highly stable and suitable for industrial applications [9, 14]. Further examples of successful isolation of metagenome-derived cellulases have been described [15, 16]. It is noteworthy that sequencing based approaches of diverse metagenomes have led to the identification of numerous putative cellulases [17, 18]. Of course functionality of these enzymes has to be affirmed.

Cellulose is next to chitin probably the most abundant renewable energy source, plants usually contain 35–50% (dry weight) cellulose. It can be used as a valuable source for bioethanol and other products. Therefore cellulose, consisting of β-1,4-linked glucose subunits (Fig. 1), must be hydrolyzed into fermentable sugar. Breakdown of cellulose can be performed by chemical treatment or enzymatic hydrolysis. Chemical breakdown has the disadvantage of cost-intensive pollutants. For large scale enzymatic hydrolysis the problem occurs that cellulose is insoluble in water, while cellulases need an aquatic environment to function properly. One solution might be the use of ionic liquids as solvent. These are salts liquid at room temperature, have no detectable vapor pressure and are recyclable. Additionally, some ionic liquids have been described to dissolve cellulose [19–21].

Cellulases are distinguished from other glycoside hydrolases by their ability to hydrolyze β-1,4-glucosidic bonds between glucosyl residues. The enzymatic breakage of the β-1,4-glucosidic bonds in cellulose proceeds through an acid hydrolysis mechanism using a proton donor and nucleophile or base. The hydrolysis can either result in the inversion or retention (double replacement mechanism) of the anomeric configuration of carbon-1 at the reducing end [22–24].

Three major types of enzymatic activity are necessary for complete degradation of cellulose: endoglucanases

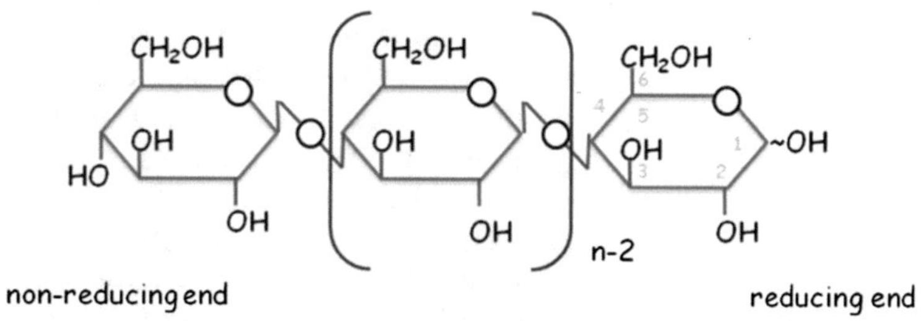

Fig. 1 Celulose structure ᴅ-glucose; linked to large polymers via the β-1,4 glycosidic linkage

(1,4-β-D-glucan-4-glucanohydrolases; EC 3.2.1.4), exoglucanases including cellodextrinases (1,4-β-D-glucan glucanohydrolases; EC 3.2.1.74) and cellobiohydrolases (1,4-β-D-glucan cellobiohydrolases; EC 3.2.1.91), and β-glucosidases (β-glucoside glucohydrolases; EC 3.2.1.21) [25, 26]. The most recent nomenclature describes more than 130 families of glycosyl hydrolases which are organized in 14 clans as listed at the CAZy server (http://afmb. cnrs-mrs.fr/CAZY/).

Cellulases have many industrial applications; next to the generation of bioethanol, a realistic long-term energy source, e.g., the finishing of textiles [27, 28]. These industrial processes require cellulolytic activity under a variety of pH, temperature and ionic conditions, and they are usually carried out by mixtures of cellulases. Investigation of the broad diversity of cellulolytic enzymes involved in the natural degradation of cellulose is necessary for the optimization of these processes.

While there remains much interest in the isolation of cellulases from fungal sources, there has been a recent increase in the isolation of diverse novel cellulases from prokaryotic organisms [24]. The two different structural types of cellulolytic systems found in bacteria are non-complexed and complexed systems. Some anaerobes, e.g., *Clostridium cellulolyticum*, are known to produce an extracellular multi-enzyme complex called cellulosome, which is linked to the cell surface [29]. A cellulosome comprises different hydrolases organized via specific cohesin–dockerin interactions on a non-catalytic scaffolding protein which mediates the attachment to cellulose [29]. The second type of complexed cellulases is produced by Bacteroidetes [30, 31]. The genes encoding the proteins for this complex are organized in a "starch utilization locus" and comprise a transcriptional regulator, a transmembrane protein, a substrate binding protein, hydrolases and proteins with so far unknown function [30, 31]. The cellulases organized in these complexes have only rarely been detected in functional metagenomic screens. In contrast, cellulases from the majority of aerobes, and also of anaerobes, are not organized as complexes but bind directly to cellulose [32]. These non-complexed cellulases can have a modular structure with non-catalytic carbohydrate binding modules (CBMs) and other domains like Ig-like domains connected to the catalytic domain(s) by flexible linkers. CBMs play a role in binding the cellulase to insoluble cellulose [33, 34]. In addition to enzymes with clearly designated carbohydrate-binding domains, a significant number of cellulases have been identified that have no stated CBM and are thus referred to as non-modular cellulases [28]. Cellulases lacking a CBM show reduced activities against insoluble cellulose while retaining the capacity to depolymerize soluble cellulosic substrates [33, 35, 36].

The majority of the so far investigated prokaryotic cellulases have been isolated from cultured microorganisms. Cellulases tend to be active at the pH and temperature conditions corresponding to the environment of the respective organism such as the β-1,4-endoglucanase from the gut bacterium *Cellulomonas pachnodae* which has a pH range between pH 4.8 and pH 6.0 [37] and the endoglucanase from an alkalophilic *Bacillus* species which has a pH range from pH 7.0 to pH 12.0 [38]. Industrial purposes require enzymes that are stable and active under specific conditions of pH, temperature and ionic strength. Many of the cellulases with the industrially relevant characteristics are obtained from extremophile microorganisms [27, 39]. Cultivation of microbes from these or other specific environments is particularly problematic, what results in a large proportion of uncultured bacteria, especially in these habitats. Metagenomics is a cultivation independent analysis of the microbial DNA of a specific habitat and involves direct isolation of DNA from the environment followed by cloning and expression of the metagenome in a heterologous host [40]. This technique has been used to detect a wide range of biocatalysts from uncultured microorganisms [1, 3]. Here we offer some easy to follow protocols for screening microbial cellulases in metagenomes.

2   Materials

2.1   Mineral Salt Medium (MSM)

1. Solution 1 (1 L, 10×): 70 g $Na_2HPO_4 \cdot 2H_2O$, 20 g KH_2PO_4.

2. Solution 2 (1 L, 10×): 10 g $(NH_4)_2SO_4$, 2 g $MgCl_2 \cdot 6H_2O$, 1 g $Ca(NO_3)_2 \cdot 4H_2O$.

3. Trace elements (2000×, 1 L): 5 g EDTA, 3 g $Fe(III)SO_4 \cdot 7H_2O$, 30 mg $MnCl_2 \cdot 4H_2O$, 50 mg $CoCl_2 \cdot 6H_2O$, 20 mg $NiCl_2 \cdot 2H_2O$, 10 mg $CuCl_2 \cdot 2H_2O$, 30 mg $Na_2MoO_4 \cdot 2H_2O$, 50 mg $ZnSO_4 \cdot 7H_2O$, 20 mg H_3BO_4, pH 4.0.

4. Vitamins (1000×, 100 mL): 1 mg biotin, 10 mg nicotinic acid, 10 mg thiamin-HCl (vit. B1), 1 mg *p*-aminobenzoic acid, 10 mg Ca-D(+) pantothenic acid, 10 mg vit. B6 hydrochloride, 10 mg vit. B12, 10 mg riboflavin, 1 mg folic acid.

2.2   Congo Red Plate Assay

1. LB-Agar + CMC (1 L): 15 g agar, 10 g tryptone, 5 g yeast extract, 5 g NaCl, 2 g carboxymethylcellulose (CMC).

2. Congo red solution: 0.2 % Congo red.

2.3   Preparation of Crude Cell Extract

1. LB + CMC (1 L): 10 g tryptone, 5 g yeast extract, 5 g NaCl, 2 g carboxymethylcellulose (CMC).

2. Appropriate antibiotic.

3. 50 mM Tris–HCl pH 8.0.

4. Ultrasonic device (Sonicator UP 200S, Hielscher, Germany).

2.4 DNSA-Assay

1. LB + CMC (1 L): 10 g tryptone, 5 g yeast extract, 5 g NaCl, 2 g carboxymethylcellulose (CMC).

2. DNSA-Reagent (1 L): 10 g 3,5-dinitrosalicylic acid, 2 mL phenol, 0.5 g Na_2SO_3, 200 g K-Na-tartrate, 10 g NaOH. Store at 4 °C (protected from light).

3. McIllvaine-buffer: 0.2 M Na_2HPO_4 (A), 0.1 M citric acid (B). pH 6.5 is adjusted by the addition of (B) to (A) at 65 °C.

2.5 Analysis of Cellulase Reaction Products by Thin-Layer Chromatography

1. Used substrates might be: cellooligosaccharides (1 %, from Sigma, Heidelberg, Germany), lichenan (1 %, from *Cetraria islandica*, Sigma, Heidelberg, Germany) and CMC (1 %, from Sigma, Heidelberg, Germany).

2. Cellulase extract in 50 mM K_2HPO_4.

3. Silica 60 TLC plate (Merck KGaA, Darmstadt, Germany).

4. 5:3:2 (vol/vol/vol) 1-propanol, nitromethane, H_2O.

5. 9:1 (vol/vol) ethanol–concentrated sulfuric acid, prepare fresh.

6. 2:1:1 (vol/vol/vol) ethylacetate, acetic acid, H_2O.

7. Phosphoric acid.

8. Stock solution: 1 g diphenylamine, 1 mL aniline, 100 mL acetone.

9. 6:1:3 (vol/vol/vol) 1-propanol, ethylacetate, H_2O.

2.6 Analysis of Cellulose Breakdown Products by HPLC

1. SepPack cartridge 18 (Waters, Milford, Mass.).

2. HPX-42A carbohydrate column (300 × 7.8 mm; Bio-Rad, Munich, Germany).

3. Differential refractometer.

---

3 Methods

3.1 Enrichment of Highly Cellulolytic Microbial Communities (See Note 1)

From our experience the number of clones that encode cellulases in environmental libraries is rather low. Therefore it is sometimes useful to slightly enrich on a suitable substrate to increase the frequency of cellulolytic organisms and hence enzymes. Therefore usually mineral salt media (*see* Subheading 2.1) are used. The cultures can be run under the desired parameters regarding pH, temperature, oxygen supply, etc. For the enrichment of cellulolytic organisms cellulosic substrates like carboxymethylcellulose (CMC), crystalline cellulose like avicel, cellulosic filter paper or plant material like wood or silage can be used as carbon source.

Once microbial communities are established they can be used for library construction. It is recommended to analyze the microbial community by 16S profiling in order to survey the diversity.

Please note that due to the enrichment steps the diversity is probably significantly reduced, especially when enriching over a long time period.

3.2 Identification of Cellulase-Positive Clones by Screening on Congo Red Plates (See Note 2)

Cellulase-positive clones are usually screened for by using a colorimetric assay on plates containing a cellulosic substrate. The interaction of the direct dye Congo red with intact β-D-glucans provides the basis for a rapid and sensitive screening test for cellulolytic bacteria possessing β-D-glucan-hydrolase activities [41].

1. The *E. coli* clones are stamped or streaked on LB-agar + CMC and incubated overnight at 37 °C, followed by an incubation of 2–7 days at the desired temperature.

2. Colonies are washed off with ddH$_2$O to permit the homogeneous penetration of the staining dye into the medium.

3. Agar plates are stained with Congo red solution for 30 min.

4. The solution is poured off and the agar plates are destained up to three times for 30 min with 1 M NaCl.

5. Cellulase expressing clones exhibit a yellow halo against a red background (*see* Fig. 2).

3.3 Retransformation of Putative Positive Clones

To ensure that the observed catalytic activity of clones is not due to contaminations, the isolation and retransformation of the vector and a subsequent activity assay is recommended.

3.4 Preparation of Crude Cell Extracts of Clones with Cellulolytic Activity

1. For the preparation of crude cell extracts of cellulase positive clones cultures are grown in LB + CMC containing an appropriate antibiotic at 30 °C to an OD of 1.0–1.5.

2. Cells are harvested via mild centrifugation and resuspended in an appropriate volume of 50 mM Tris–HCl pH 8.0 prior to

Fig. 2 Activity staining of metagenome-derived cosmid clones using Congo red staining

cell disruption through sonication at 50% amplitude and cycle 0.5 for 5 min.

3. After centrifuging at $16,000 \times g$ and 4 °C for 30 min the crude cell extract can be stored at 4 °C for several days.

3.5 Enzyme Assays for Cellulase Activities

3.5.1 DNSA-Assay (See Note 3)

Cellulase activity is routinely assayed by measuring the amount of reducing sugar released from CMC using 3,5-dinitrosalicylic acid reagent (*see* Subheading 2.4). The standard assay mixture contains 2 μg of the enzyme or crude cell extract and 1% CMC in a final volume of 0.5 mL with 150 μL McIllvaine buffer (*see* Subheading 2.4). This mixture is incubated at an appropriate temperature for 15 min. During the hydrolysis of cellulose glucose oligomers and monomers are produced and the number of reducing ends increases. These reducing groups react with 3,5-dinitrosalicylic acid forming brown 3-amino-5-nitrosalicylic acid at 100 °C.

The amount of 3-amino-5-nitrosalicylic acid formed is equimolar to the number of reducing ends. Therefore the amount of reducing sugars can be quantified at 546 nm (Fig. 3).

Units of enzyme activity (U) are expressed as micromoles of reducing sugar released per minute per milligram protein. Enzyme activities are formulated by regressing absorbance on concentration following the Beer's law. That describes the relationship between known concentrations and absorbance is linear except at very low or high concentration of the product, in this case reducing sugar. One unit is equal to 1 μmol of reduced sugar per minute.

The enzymatic activity volume is calculated according to the following formula:

$$U / mL = (\Delta E / min \times V) / (\varepsilon \times d \times v)$$

$\Delta E/min$ = Extinction
V = Volume of the test reaction mix.
d = Thickness of the cuvette [cm].
ε = Ascendant of straight calibration line

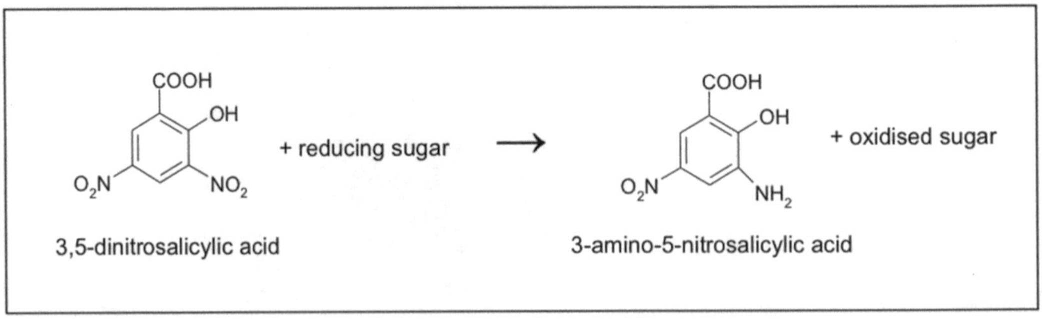

Fig. 3 DNSA assay reaction for the measurement of cellulolytic activity based on the release of reducing sugar ends

v = Sample volume

The specific enzymatic activity [U/mg protein] is defined as the amount of enzyme that liberates 1 μmol of substrate per minute and is calculated as follows:

Specific activity [U/mg protein] = Enzymatic activity volume [U/mL]/protein concentration [mg/mL]

1. The reactions are prepared combining first buffer and enzyme and then adding the substrate.

   Reaction mix:

Sample	100 μL
CMC in ddH$_2$O (2%)	250 μL
McIlvaine-buffer, pH 6.5	150 μL

2. The mixture is incubated for 15 min at 37 °C.

3. After this incubation DNSA reagent is added and the samples are boiled at 100 °C for 15 min.

Sample	100 μL
CMC in ddH$_2$O (2%)	250 μL
McIllvaine-buffer, pH 6.5	150 μL
+ DNSA reagent	750 μL

4. After cooling down on ice the samples are centrifuged at 16,000 × g for 2 min to precipitate falling proteins.

5. The samples are transferred to cuvettes and absorbance is measured at 546 nm.

The pH range of the enzyme is usually determined by measuring standard assay activity between pH 4 and pH 10.5 using 50 mM of appropriate buffers. Acetate buffer is used for pH 4 to pH 6.0, citrate/phosphate buffer (McIllvaine buffer) is used for pH 6 to pH 7.5, Tris–HCl is used for pH 7.5 to pH 9.0, and N-cyclohexyl-3-aminopropanesulfonic acid (CAPS) is used for pH 9.7 to pH 10.5.

For the analysis of the temperature range of the enzyme, activity of the standard assay mixture is assayed at temperatures between 20 and 95 °C.

To analyze substrate specificity, CMC can replaced in the standard assay mixture by lichenan, barley β-glucan, laminarin, oat spelt xylan, or avicel.

Inhibition or enhancement of cellulase activity can be determined for a range of different metal chloride salts, solvents, detergents, and EDTA using in general 1 mM concentrations. The influence of ionic liquids (IL) can be evaluated in the standard assay mixture system when McIllvaine (*see* Subheading 2.4) buffer is replaced by an IL. The assay mixture therefore comprises an IL content of 30% (some ILs that can be used for cellulase activity

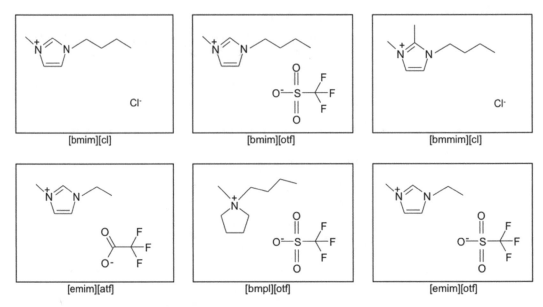

Fig. 4 Ionic liquids that are suitable for cellulase activity assays

assays are shown exemplarily in Fig. 4). This value can be regulated up and down. For ILs as well as other additives long term stability assays might be of interest. Therefore the enzyme is incubated in buffer with the desired additives at the favored conditions for different time periods. At the respective time point the substrate is added and the assay can proceed as described above.

3.5.2 Analysis of Cellulase Reaction Products by Thin-Layer Chromatography (TLC) (See Note 4)

To determine whether a cellulase has an endo or exo mode of action, TLC analyses are an adequate tool (Fig. 5). These analyses can also give a good overview on the substrate range hydrolyzed by the enzyme.

1. Different carbohydrates can be used as substrates, e.g., cello-oligosaccharides, lichenan and CMC. These substrates are co-incubated with cellulase extract in 50 mM K_2HPO_4 at adequate pH and temperature conditions.

2. To determine which reaction products occur first, aliquots from different incubation times can be spotted on a silica 60 TLC plate.

3. The cellooligosaccharide reaction products are developed and separated in 1-propanol–nitromethane–H_2O (5:3:2, vol/vol/vol) for 2 h. After separation, sugars are visualized by spraying the plates with a freshly prepared mixture of ethanol–concentrated sulfuric acid (9:1, vol/vol).

4. The lichenan reaction products are developed in ethylacetate–acetic acid–H_2O (2:1:1, vol/vol/vol) for 3 h. After separation, sugars are visualized by spraying the plates with a freshly

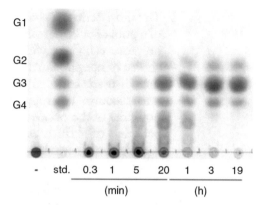

Fig. 5 TLC detection of end products from cellulose degradation: Lane (-) is the sample without the addition of enzyme, (std.) is the standard with glucose (G1), cellobiose (G2), cellotriose (G3), and cellotetraose (G4). The other lanes are different time points of the hydrolysis of lichenan with Cel5A [9]

prepared mixture of 1 mL phosphoric acid and 10 mL stock solution (1 g diphenylamine, 1 mL aniline, 100 mL acetone).

5. The CMC reaction products are separated and developed in 1-propanol–ethylacetate–H_2O (6:1:3, vol/vol/vol) for 2× 3 h, and the sugars are visualized using the same mixture as for visualization of lichenan products.

3.5.3 Analysis of Cellulose Breakdown Products by HPLC

For the investigation of the carbohydrate hydrolysis products, HPLC analysis is an appropriate method.

1. First, enzyme preparation and substrate are co-incubated for 2 h at optimal temperature and pH. As well as for TLC analysis and DNSA assay, different substrates and reaction conditions can be investigated.

2. For stopping the reactions, tubes are incubated at 100 °C for 10 min.

3. The assay mixtures are centrifuged and proteins of the supernatant are removed with a SepPack cartridge 18.

4. There are a lot of different HPLC columns and elution buffers that can be used for the analysis of carbohydrate hydrolysis products. One possibility is the analysis of the samples with a HPX-42A column. Elution is carried out with H_2O at 85 °C; the flow rate is 0.6 mL/min. Detection is performed with a differential refractometer.

4 Notes

Altogether, screening for and assaying cellulases is not that complicated; here we just provide some simple notes.

1. The most "critical" step in this procedure and for the discovery of a pool of enzymes which is adequate for the detection of one or more cellulases with interesting properties might be the choice of sample. Furthermore, the quality of enrichment culture, if used, and of the metagenomic library must be taken into account. We suggest investigating habitats with a high potential of the occurrence of cellulolytic bacteria, like intestinal tracts of herbivores or rotting trees. If an enrichment step is desired or inevitable, it is reasonable to enrich over a rather short time period to keep diversity as broad as possible.

2. Screening for cellulase-active clones on Congo red indicator plates is easy, only the time period for growth of bacteria and expression of cellulolytic activity might be variable. Washing off bacterial cells is critical, when cellulolytic activity is rather low.

3. The same occurs for the DNSA-assay, where gloves should be worn and when samples are boiled, the lid should be stabilized to protect from spraying phenol (in DNSA solution, *see* Subheading 2.3). When ionic liquids are added to the assay mixtures, it is necessary to completely agitate IL and aquatic phase, otherwise results are falsified.

References

1. Streit WR, Schmitz RA (2004) Metagenomics - the key to the uncultured microbes. Curr Opin Microbiol 7:492–498

2. Daniel R (2004) The soil metagenome - a rich resource for the discovery of novel natural products. Curr Opin Biotechnol 15:199–204

3. Schmeisser C, Steele H, Streit WR (2007) Metagenomics, biotechnology with non-culturable microbes. Appl Microbiol Biotechnol 75:955–962

4. Schmidt TM, DeLong EF, Pace NR (1991) Analysis of a marine picoplankton community by 16S rRNA gene cloning and sequencing. J Bacteriol 173:4371–4378

5. Ferrer M, Golyshina OV, Chernikova TN, Khachane AN, Reyes-Duarte D, Santos VA et al (2005) Novel hydrolase diversity retrieved from a metagenome library of bovine rumen microflora. Environ Microbiol 7:1996–2010

6. Ferrer M, Golyshina OV, Plou FJ, Timmis KN, Golyshin PN (2005) A novel alpha-glucosidase from the acidophilic archaeon *Ferroplasma acidiphilum* strain Y with high transglycosylation activity and an unusual catalytic nucleophile. Biochem J 391:269–276

7. Beloqui A, Pita M, Polaina J, Martinez-Arias A, Golyshina OV, Zumarraga M et al (2006) Novel polyphenol oxidase mined from a metagenome expression library of bovine rumen: biochemical properties, structural analysis, and phylogenetic relationships. J Biol Chem 281:22933–22942

8. Voget S, Leggewie C, Uesbeck A, Raasch C, Jaeger KE, Streit WR (2003) Prospecting for novel biocatalysts in a soil metagenome. Appl Environ Microbiol 69:6235–6242

9. Voget S, Steele HL, Streit WR (2006) Characterization of a metagenome-derived halotolerant cellulase. J Biotechnol 126:26–36

10. Grant S, Sorokin DY, Grant WD, Jones BE, Heaphy S (2004) A phylogenetic analysis of Wadi el Natrun soda lake cellulase enrichment cultures and identification of cellulase genes from these cultures. Extremophiles 8:421–429

11. Rees HC, Grant S, Jones B, Grant WD, Heaphy S (2003) Detecting cellulase and esterase enzyme activities encoded by novel genes present in environmental DNA libraries. Extremophiles 7:415–421

12. Healy FG, Ray RM, Aldrich HC, Wilkie AC, Ingram LO, Shanmugam KT (1995) Direct isolation of functional genes encoding cellulases from the microbial consortia in a thermophilic, anaerobic digester maintained on

lignocellulose. Appl Microbiol Biotechnol 43:667–674

13. Feng Y, Duan CJ, Pang H, Mo XC, Wu CF, Yu Y et al (2007) Cloning and identification of novel cellulase genes from uncultured microorganisms in rabbit cecum and characterization of the expressed cellulases. Appl Microbiol Biotechnol 75:319–328

14. Pottkamper J, Barthen P, Ilmberger N, Schwaneberg U, Schenk A, Schulte M et al (2009) Applying metagenomics for the identification of bacterial cellulases that are stable in ionic liquids. Green Chem 11:957–965

15. Guo H, Feng Y, Mo X, Duan C, Tang J, Feng J (2008) Cloning and expression of a beta-glucosidase gene umcel3G from metagenome of buffalo rumen and characterization of the translated product. Sheng Wu Gong Cheng Xue Bao 24:232–238

16. Pang H, Zhang P, Duan CJ, Mo XC, Tang JL, Feng JX (2009) Identification of cellulase genes from the metagenomes of compost soils and functional characterization of one novel endoglucanase. Curr Microbiol 58:404–408

17. Warnecke F, Luginbuhl P, Ivanova N, Ghassemian M, Richardson TH, Stege JT et al (2007) Metagenomic and functional analysis of hindgut microbiota of a wood-feeding higher termite. Nature 450:560–565

18. Ilmberger N, Güllert S, Dannenberg J, Rabausch U, Torres J, Wemheuer B et al (2014) A comparative metagenome survey of the fecal microbiota of a breast- and a plant-fed Asian elephant reveals an unexpectedly high diversity of glycoside hydrolase family enzymes. PLoS One 9:e106707

19. Heinze T, Schwikal K, Barthel S (2005) Ionic liquids as reaction medium in cellulose functionalization. Macromol Biosci 5:520–525

20. Swatloski RP, Spear SK, Holbrey JD, Rogers RD (2002) Dissolution of cellulose [correction of cellose] with ionic liquids. J Am Chem Soc 124:4974–4975

21. Wu J, Zhang J, Zhang H, He J, Ren Q, Guo M (2004) Homogeneous acetylation of cellulose in a new ionic liquid. Biomacromolecules 5:266–268

22. Beguin P, Aubert JP (1994) The biological degradation of cellulose. FEMS Microbiol Rev 13:25–58

23. Birsan C, Johnson P, Joshi M, MacLeod A, McIntosh L, Monem V et al (1998) Mechanisms of cellulases and xylanases. Biochem Soc Trans 26:156–160

24. Hilden L, Johansson G (2004) Recent developments on cellulases and carbohydrate-binding modules with cellulose affinity. Biotechnol Lett 26:1683–1693

25. Bayer EA, Chanzy H, Lamed R, Shoham Y (1998) Cellulose, cellulases and cellulosomes. Curr Opin Struct Biol 8:548–557

26. Kumar R, Singh S, Singh OV (2008) Bioconversion of lignocellulosic biomass: biochemical and molecular perspectives. J Ind Microbiol Biotechnol 35:377–391

27. Ando S, Ishida H, Kosugi Y, Ishikawa K (2002) Hyperthermostable endoglucanase from *Pyrococcus horikoshii*. Appl Environ Microbiol 68:430–433

28. Lynd LR, Zhang Y (2002) Quantitative determination of cellulase concentration as distinct from cell concentration in studies of microbial cellulose utilization: analytical framework and methodological approach. Biotechnol Bioeng 77:467–475

29. Schwarz WH (2001) The cellulosome and cellulose degradation by anaerobic bacteria. Appl Microbiol Biotechnol 56:634–649

30. Pope PB, Mackenzie AK, Gregor I, Smith W, Sundset MA, McHardy AC et al (2012) Metagenomics of the Svalbard reindeer rumen microbiome reveals abundance of polysaccharide utilization loci. PLoS One 7:e38571

31. Flint HJ, Scott KP, Duncan SH, Louis P, Forano E (2012) Microbial degradation of complex carbohydrates in the gut. Gut Microbes 3:289–306

32. Zhang YH, Lynd LR (2004) Toward an aggregated understanding of enzymatic hydrolysis of cellulose: noncomplexed cellulase systems. Biotechnol Bioeng 88:797–824

33. Bolam DN, Ciruela A, McQueen-Mason S, Simpson P, Williamson MP, Rixon JE et al (1998) *Pseudomonas* cellulose-binding domains mediate their effects by increasing enzyme substrate proximity. Biochem J 331(Pt 3):775–781

34. Carvalho AL, Goyal A, Prates JA, Bolam DN, Gilbert HJ, Pires VM et al (2004) The family 11 carbohydrate-binding module of *Clostridium thermocellum* Lic26A-Cel5E accommodates beta-1,4- and beta-1,3-1,4-mixed linked glucans at a single binding site. J Biol Chem 279:34785–34793

35. Coutinho JB, Gilkes NR, Kilburn DG, Warren RAJ, Miller RC Jr (1993) The nature of the cellulose-binding domain effects the activities of a bacterial endoglucanase on different forms of cellulose. FEMS Microbiol Lett 113:211–217

36. Fontes CM, Clarke JH, Hazlewood GP, Fernandes TH, Gilbert HJ, Ferreira LM (1997) Possible roles for a non-modular, thermostable and proteinase-resistant cellulase from the mesophilic aerobic soil bacterium *Cellvibrio mixtus*. Appl Microbiol Biotechnol 48:473–479

37. Cazemier AE, Verdoes JC, Op den Camp HJ, Hackstein JH, van Ooyen AJ (1999) A beta-1,4-endoglucanase-encoding gene from *Cellulomonas pachnodae*. Appl Microbiol Biotechnol 52:232–239

38. Sanchez-Torres J, Perez P, Santamaria RI (1996) A cellulase gene from a new alkalophilic *Bacillus* sp. (strain N186-1). Its cloning, nucleotide sequence and expression in *Escherichia coli*. Appl Microbiol Biotechnol 46:149–155

39. Solingen P, Meijer D, Kleij W, Barnett C, Bolle R, Power S, Jones B (2001) Cloning and expression of an endocellulase gene from a novel streptomycete isolated from an East African soda lake. Extremophiles 5:333

40. Handelsman J, Rondon MR, Brady SF, Clardy J, Goodman RM (1998) Molecular biological access to the chemistry of unknown soil microbes: a new frontier for natural products. Chem Biol 5:R245–R249

41. Teather RM, Wood PJ (1982) Use of Congo red-polysaccharide interactions in enumeration and characterization of cellulolytic bacteria from the bovine rumen. Appl Environ Microbiol 43:777–780

Chapter 13

Liquid Phase Multiplex High-Throughput Screening of Metagenomic Libraries Using p-Nitrophenyl-Linked Substrates for Accessory Lignocellulosic Enzymes

Mariette Smart, Robert J. Huddy, Don A. Cowan, and Marla Trindade

Abstract

To access the genetic potential contained in large metagenomic libraries, suitable high-throughput functional screening methods are required. Here we describe a high-throughput screening approach which enables the rapid identification of metagenomic library clones expressing functional accessory lignocellulosic enzymes. The high-throughput nature of this method hinges on the multiplexing of both the *E. coli* metagenomic library clones and the colorimetric p-nitrophenyl linked substrates which allows for the simultaneous screening for β-glucosidases, β-xylosidases, and α-L-arabinofuranosidases. This method is readily automated and compatible with high-throughput robotic screening systems.

Key words Metagenomics, High-throughput screening, Liquid-phase screening, Multiplex screening, Colorimetric substrates, Lignocellulosic enzymes, β-Glucosidases, β-Xylosidases, α-L-Arabinofuranosidases, p-Nitrophenyl substrates, Function-driven screening

1 Introduction

Metagenomic gene discovery involves the direct cloning of DNA isolated from environmental samples followed by the generation of large clone libraries for subsequent screening using functional- or sequence-based approaches [1–5]. The high degree of microbial diversity associated with environmental samples means that a large number of clones (typically between 10^5 and 10^7 clones depending on the vector used) from a metagenomic library need to be screened in order to access a large proportion of the genetic potential contained within the sample. High-throughput screening (HTS) methods are essential to effectively identify library clones harboring low frequency or rare genes [6]. Performing function-driven HTS, as an alternative to sequence driven screening, allows the identification of genes with low sequence homology to previously identified genes [4, 7] and makes it possible to screen for specific functional and performance properties.

Wolfgang R. Streit and Rolf Daniel (eds.), *Metagenomics: Methods and Protocols*, Methods in Molecular Biology, vol. 1539, DOI 10.1007/978-1-4939-6691-2_13, © Springer Science+Business Media LLC 2017

HTS of metagenomic libraries can be performed using either solid- and liquid-phase screens. The suitability of using either of these for a specific enzyme class is dependent on the availability of substrates for the identification of desired enzyme activities. Solid-phase screens generally rely on the use of chemical dyes and insoluble or chromophore-linked derivatives of substrates, supplemented into the growth media. High-throughput screening methods have been validated for a relatively small group of enzymes including: cellulases, chitinases, DNA polymerases, proteases, and lipolytic enzymes (references within [7]). HTS for these enzyme classes, excluding the DNA polymerases, is mostly performed using solid media based assays; see examples of screening methods described in Chapter 1 [8], and relies on performing the screening under conditions which are optimal for the growth of, and protein expression from, the host strain (generally *Escherichia coli*) used for metagenomic library construction. This imposes numerous limitations on the ability to screen for biocatalysts with desired biochemical properties, such as thermal stability and pH optima which differ from that which is optimal for the host's cultivation.

The use of alternative host expression systems, more suited to expression of genes within the environmental DNA from which libraries are constructed, may increase the access to the genetic potential contained within the metagenomic DNA. In general, more than 60% of the genes from environmental DNA are not compatible with the *E. coli* translation and transcription system [9, 10]. Alternative host systems for which vector and transformation systems have been developed include the gram positive Actinomycete, *Streptomyces lividans* (described in refs. 6, 11), improving access to the genetic potential within sources rich in Actinomycetes and other organisms containing high GC content DNA [12]. For archaea-rich environmental DNA the archaeal host *Sulfolobus solfataricus* (described in refs. 7, 13) may be preferential, while the extreme thermophile *Thermus thermophilus* is a favored host for thermophilic source material [14]. When expressing soil-derived metagenomic DNA, the use of expression hosts such as *Agrobacterium tumefaciens*, *Burkholderia graminis*, *Caulobacter vibrioides*, *Pseudomonas putida*, and *Cupriavidus metallidurans* has demonstrated differing production levels of specific metabolites compared to that achieved from an *E. coli* host [15]. The use of these and other host systems may improve access to the genetic diversity contained within the metagenome, but is still dependent on an ability to perform the functional screen under conditions optimal for the host expression. This makes the use of cell free protein extracts an attractive alternative to screen libraries under conditions closely related to those of the industrial applications for which biocatalysts are required [16]. Thus the development of robust, reliable and validated HTS methods for screening metagenomic libraries contained within *E. coli* host systems is key to accessing the genetic potential contained within these cloned metagenomes.

Here we present a liquid-phase, cell-free, and HTS approach suitable for use with *p*-nitrophenyl (*p*NP) linked substrates for the functional screening of metagenomic libraries. We have successfully used this technique to screen metagenomic libraries for accessory lignocellulosic enzymes (β-glucosidases, β-xylosidases, and α-L-arabinofuranosidases) for which no pre-existing HTS was available [17]. Multiplexing of both the *E. coli* library clones and substrates targeting the three enzyme classes resulted in an efficient and higher throughput process for the functional screening of the metagenomic libraries. Three libraries were used for the validation of the method: (1) compost metagenomic DNA cloned into the fosmid vector pCCFOS™ and expressed in *E. coli* EPI300™-T1ᴿ cells as described in [18], (2) a second library derived from different compost-sourced metagenomic DNA using the fosmid vector pCCFOS™, prepared as for the above, and (3) a library constructed using the SuperBAC1 Bacterial Artificial Chromosome [19] suitable for expression in both *E. coli* and *Bacillus* spp. hosts. The protocol presented here, which employs a QPix2 robotic system (Molecular Devices), is suitable for simultaneous screening of up to 50,000 clones for three different enzyme classes, with the identification and confirmation of the enzyme activities of positive clones within a 7 day working period. By multiplexing eight library clones into the single well of a 96-well screening plate, we condensed the screening of two 384-well microtiter plates containing library clones into a single 96-well microtiter plate for screening, thus reducing the cost and increasing the throughput of liquid-phase screening. We further reduced the cost and increased the throughput of this method by multiplexing substrates to simultaneously screen for three enzyme classes.

2   Materials

All solutions should be prepared using deionized or distilled water using analytical grade reagents. Autoclaving, where indicated, should be performed at 121 °C for 20 min.

2.1   Library Clone Culturing and Expression

1. Lysogeny broth (also known as Luria–Bertani, abbreviated as LB, medium): For a liter of medium add 5 g yeast extract, 10 g tryptone, and 5 g NaCl to 800 mL water. Mix using a magnetic stirrer bar and plate until dissolved and adjust pH to 7.5 with NaOH if required. Adjust volume to 1 L and autoclave.

2. LB agar: Prepare LB as described above and supplement with 15 g of agar per liter medium before autoclaving.

3. Chloramphenicol: Prepare a 15 mg/mL stock solution by adding 150 mg to 9 mL water in a graduated 15 mL falcon tube or 10 mL volumetric flask. Dissolve and adjust volume to 10 mL. Filter-sterilize using a 0.22 μm nitrocellulose syringe filter. Store as 1 mL aliquots at –20 °C.

4. L-Arabinose: 10% (w/v) solution in water: Make up 10 mL by adding 1 g L-arabinose to 9 mL water in a graduated 15 mL falcon tube or 10 mL volumetric flask. Dissolve and adjust volume to 10 mL. Filter-sterilize and store as for chloramphenicol.

5. Growth and induction medium: LB supplemented with 15 μg/mL chloramphenicol and 0.01% (w/v) L-arabinose. Prepare a master mix of the LB containing the antibiotic and L-arabinose by adding 100 μL 15 mg/mL chloramphenicol and 100 μL 10% (w/v) L-arabinose to each 100 mL of LB.

6. 96-well mitrotiter plates.

7. QPix2 robotic system (Molecular Devices) or 96 pin hedgehog for colony picking from a 96-well plate format.

8. Multichannel pipette (100 μL volume) or automated liquid handling platform.

9. Breathable sealing films for microtiter plates (Sigma).

10. Shaking incubator set to 37 °C.

2.2 p-Nitrophenyl Liquid Assays

1. BugBuster® 10× Protein Extraction Reagent (Novagen).

2. Multichannel pipette (10 μL volume).

3. Sodium phosphate buffer: For a 0.1 M sodium phosphate buffer at pH 7 prepare a solution containing 0.061 M Na_2HPO_4 and 0.039 M NaH_2PO_4. For 1 L of buffer, add 8.7 g Na_2HPO_4 anhydrous salt and 4.7 g NaH_2PO_4 anhydrous salt to 900 mL water and adjust pH to 7 with HCl or NaOH if required. Make volume up to 1 L and autoclave.

4. pNP-α-L-arabinofuranoside (Sigma or Carbosynth): To prepare a 0.11 M stock solution add 0.3 g of substrate to 10 mL methanol. Heat to 37 °C to dissolve. This substrate is light sensitive and stock solution tubes should be covered in foil and stored at –20 °C until required. Before use, heat to 37 °C to allow any substrate that has precipitated to dissolve.

5. pNP-β-D-xylopyranoside (Sigma or Carbosynth): Prepare as described for pNP-α-L-arabinofuranoside.

6. pNP-β-D-glucopyranoside (Sigma or Carbosynth): Prepare a 0.11 M stock solution in water by adding 0.33 g substrate into 10 mL water and heating to 37 °C to dissolve. Cover in foil, store and use as described for pNP-α-L-arabinofuranoside.

7. Substrate and buffer mixture: 0.1 M sodium phosphate buffer (pH 7), 4 mM pNP-α-L-arabinofuranoside, 4 mM pNP-β-D-xylopyranoside, 4 mM pNP-β-D-glucopyranoside. To prepare

100 mL of the substrate and buffer mixture, add 3.6 mL of each of the 0.11 M *p*NP substrate stocks, prepared as described above, to 100 mL 0.1 M sodium phosphate buffer. For a substrate buffer mixture containing a single substrate add only 3.6 mL of the desired substrate to 100 mL 0.1 M sodium phosphate buffer.

8. Transparent microplate sealing film (Sigma).

3 Methods

This section is divided into three subsections. In Subheading 3.1 a method for the multiplexing of the metagenomic library clones is described, Subheading 3.2 describes the methodology for performing the *p*NP-linked substrate assay on these multiplexed clones, while Subheading 3.3 covers the identification of the specific clone carrying the gene of interest and the enzyme activity thereof. A schematic diagram outlining the methodology is provided in Fig. 1. The method described below is suitable for the high-throughput screening of metagenomic fosmid pCC1FOS™ clones harbored in *E. coli* EPI300™-T1^R cells (*see* **Note 1**).

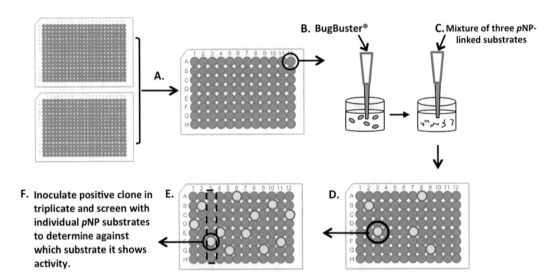

Fig. 1 Schematic representation of the liquid-phase high-throughput screening method. (**a**) Multiplex eight *E. coli* EPI300™-T1^R fosmid (pCCFOS) library clones into one well of a 96-well microtiter plate containing 100 μL LB supplemented with 15 μg/mL chloramphenicol and 0.1 % L-arabinose. Culture at 37 °C for 48 h with shaking (200 rpm) and lyse by the addition of 10 μL BugBuster® protein extraction reagent (Novagen) (**b**). (**c**) Perform enzyme assays in 50 mM sodium phosphate buffer (pH 7) supplemented with 2 mM of *p*NP-α-L-arabinofuranoside, *p*NP-β-D-xylopyranoside and *p*NP-β-D-glucopyranoside. Incubate enzyme reactions at 37 °C for 4 h before identifying wells containing positive clones (**d**). (**e**) Inoculate each of the eight clones contained within a positive well singularly to identify the clone harboring the enzyme activity by repeating the enzyme assay with the mixed substrates. Upon identification of the positive clone, inoculate it in triplicate and screen it with individual substrates to determine specific enzyme activity (**f**)

**3.1 Multiplexing
of Library Clones**

1. Prepare a sufficient number of 96-well microtiter plates so that each well contains 100 µL growth and induction medium using a multichannel pipette or automated liquid handling platform.

2. Using a QPix2 robotic system (Molecular Devices) or hedgehog with 96 pin format corresponding to a standard 96-well microtiter plate, multiplex eight metagenomic library clones (*see* **Note 2**) into each well of the prepared 96-well microtiter plates. Clones may be inoculated from either stored liquid cultures, should the library be stored as glycerol stocks, or from colonies grown on solid medium should plating of the library be preferred before screening (*see* **Note 3**).

3. Cover inoculated plates with a breathable film to limit evaporation and incubate at 37 °C for 48 h with shaking (200 rpm).

**3.2 Liquid
pNP Assays**

1. Add 10 µL BugBuster® Protein Extraction Reagent (Novagen) to each well of the microtiter plates to be screened and incubate for a further 30 min at 37 °C.

2. To the resulting protein extracts, add 100 µL of substrate and buffer mixture (*see* **Note 4**), cover with transparent microplate sealing film and incubate at 37 °C for 4 h (*see* **Note 5**).

3. Identify positive clones visually upon development of a yellow color (Fig. 2).

**3.3 Identifying
Clones Harboring
Enzymes of Interest**

1. Determine which of the multiplexed clones harbor the enzyme activity of interest by locating the clones of interest from the master plates (*see* **Notes 2** and **3**), and inoculating each of the eight clones originally multiplexed into the well which showed positive activity individually into separate wells of a 96-well secondary screening plate. Use 96-well microtiter plates with 100 µL growth and induction medium as described in **step 1** of Subheading 3.1.

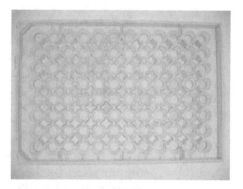

Fig. 2 High-throughput screening plate showing the *yellow* color produced after the addition of the *p*NP-linked substrates to the multiplexed fosmid metagenomic library clones

2. Cover the inoculated plates with breathable sealing film and incubate at 37 °C for 48 h with shaking (200 rpm).

3. Add 10 μL BugBuster® (Novagen) to each well of the microtiter plate to be screened and incubate for a further 30 min at 37 °C.

4. To the resulting protein extracts add 100 μL of substrate mixture, cover the plates with transparent sealing film and incubate at 37 °C for 4 h.

5. Identify which of the library clones harbor the enzyme activities of interest by the visual confirmation of the development of a yellow color.

6. Inoculate the positive library clones (as described in **step 1** of Subheading 3.1) in triplicate.

7. Incubate inoculated plates at 37 °C for 48 h with shaking (200 rpm).

8. Add 10 μL BugBuster® Protein Extraction Reagent (Novagen) to each well of the microtiter plate to be screened and incubate for a further 30 min at 37 °C.

9. For each of the positive clones, add 100 μL of substrate buffer mix containing either pNP-α-L-arabinofuranoside, pNP-β-D-xylopyranoside, or pNP-β-D-glucopyranoside to each of the triplicate protein extracts and incubate at 37 °C for 4 h (*see* **Note 4**).

10. The development of a yellow color following the addition of the substrate will indicate the specific enzyme activity expressed from the metagenomic fosmid clone (*see* **Note 5** and **6**).

4   Notes

1. This method has been validated using pCC1FOS™ fosmid vector metagenomic library clones expressed in *E. coli* Epi300™ cells. It has also been used for the high throughput screening of a bacterial artificial chromosome library constructed in the SuperBac1 vector and mutant fosmid clones generated using the HyperMu™ <Kan-1> insertion kit (Epicentre). All of these clones were also expressed in *E. coli* Epi300™ cells. The success of this method for the screening of metagenomic libraries constructed using bacterial host systems other than *E. coli* has not been validated; however, we expect these to be successful should there be a methodology to successfully lyse the cells without affecting the proteins contained in the resulting cellular extract. Alternative hosts such as *S. lividans* may also be engineered to have the added advantage of secreting proteins into the growth medium [20], thus not requiring lysis of the

bacteria to release the cellular extract prior to the assay step. Another *Streptomyces* sp., *S. albus*, is also readily lysed in 0.1% Triton X-100 (v/v) and 2 mg/mL lysozyme in the presence of a physiological buffer (e.g., phosphate buffer) and a protease inhibitor such as dithiothreitol (DTT) at 37 °C for 30 min [21]. Such a lysis step could readily be included in the assay protocol described above. Reagents such as B-PER Bacterial Protein Extraction Reagent (Thermo Scientific) have been successfully used for the lysis of both gram positive and gram negative bacterial cells and may therefore be good alternatives to the BugBuster® Protein Extraction Reagent used in this method. Alternatively, a specialized 96-well sonicator head can be used if available, although prevention of overheating the cell lysates, which may result in protein denaturation and subsequent loss of enzyme activity, is critical.

2. The metagenomic library clones subjected to HTS using the method described in this chapter were contained within 384 well microtiter plates and were multiplexed into 96-well microtiter plates using a QPix2 robotic system (Molecular Devices). This was achieved by using the 96 pin-head assembly and setting the A1 position of this head sequentially to positions A1, A2, B1, and B2 in the 384-well microtiter plate to allow the screening of all fosmid clones contained within the plate. Therefore, two metagenomic library 384 well microtiter plates, containing the metagenomic library clones, were multiplexed into a single 96-well microtiter plate to obtain eight fosmid clones per well. The number of metagenomic library clones multiplexed into a single well can be optimized for the system to be tested. Here we successfully multiplexed eight clones and achieved a sufficiently high hit rate (1:270) in the primary screening phase as eight clones were simultaneously screened for activity on three different pNP-linked substrates. A similar multi-substrate approach was followed by Maruthamuthu et al. [22] when screening metagenomic libraries for lignocellulosic enzymes, although six chromogenic substrates were mixed using a solid phase screening and a significantly lower hit rate was achieved; 1:1157 for a library created from microorganisms enriched on untreated wheat straw. Should the enzyme activity of interest be expected at a lower frequency, a larger number of clones could be multiplexed to obtain a sufficiently high hit rate; such a modification would also increase the throughput of the method. Up to 96 library clones were pooled in primary screens by Rabausch et al. [23] when screening environmental libraries for flavonoid-modifying enzymes. However, the chance of "missing" low expression clones when multiplexing a large number of clones may be increased and detection of these clones may be dependent on the sensitivity of the assay used.

3. Care should be taken to prevent cross contamination of wells and the orientation of the plates need to be clearly marked to allow the identification of clones containing proteins of interest following screening.

4. This approach to HTS has been successfully used to screen for accessory lignocellulosic enzymes using colorimetric *p*NP-linked substrates; however, it could be employed to identify any number of enzyme classes provided suitable substrates are available. Suitable substrates would need to be stable under the specific assay conditions and either produce a product which could be visualized, such as the colorimetric assay described here, or spectrophotometrically measured, such as fluorescent or chemiluminescent products. The use of the latter requires that a microtiter plate reader with suitable excitation and emission filters is available. Spectrophotometric detection of positive clones may require the removal of cell debris following the lysis of the host expression cells, and can be achieved by centrifuging the 96-well screening plates in an Eppendorf benchtop centrifuge, or similar device, fitted with a swing-bucket rotor and adapters for 96-well plates.

5. The temperature and duration of incubation of cell lysates/protein extracts preceding the enzyme assay may be altered to allow the selection of functional proteins with different degrees of intrinsic thermal stability. In our study we identified three α-arabinofuranosidases with differing thermal stabilities by preincubating the protein extracts at temperatures ranging from 25 to 90 °C before performing the enzyme assay. Subsequent cloning, purification and characterization of the proteins of interest showed similar thermal stabilities to those achieved using the "crude" cellular extract in this high-throughput method [17]. Similarly, the enzymatic reaction may be performed at elevated temperatures to select for proteins with higher enzyme thermophilicity. This allows the screening for functional enzymes to be performed under application-relevant conditions.

6. A subset of the positive clones (288) obtained from the primary screening of 46,000 clones from library 1 was subjected to secondary screening. As eight clones were multiplexed for the primary screening, we expected to obtain 36 fosmid clones positive for either of the enzyme activities tested during HTS. However, only 31 positive clones were recovered with 13 α-L-arabinofuranosidase, 9 β-glucosidase, and 9 β-xylosidase activities identified.

Following identification of positive fosmid or BAC clones, we either performed next generation sequencing on an equimolar mixture of fosmid DNA from 12 to 16 fosmid clones, or identified the gene of interest by transposon mutagenesis using a HyperMu™ <Kan-1> insertion kit (Epicentre).

References

1. Schloss PD, Handelsman J (2003) Biotechnological prospects from metagenomics. Curr Opin Biotechnol 14:303–310

2. Streit WR, Schmitz RA (2004) Metagenomics–the key to the uncultured microbes. Curr Opin Microbiol 7:492–498

3. Cowan D, Meyer Q, Stafford W, Muyanga S, Cameron R, Wittwer P (2005) Metagenomic gene discovery: past, present and future. Trends Biotechnol 23:321–329

4. Simon C, Daniel R (2011) Metagenomic analyses: past and future trends. Appl Environ Microbiol 77:1153–1161

5. Ferrer M, Martínez-Martínez M, Bargiela R, Streit WR, Golyshina OV, Golyshin PN (2015) Estimating the success of enzyme bioprospecting through metagenomics: current status and future trends. Microb Biotechnol 9:22–34

6. Handelsman J, Rodon MR, Brady SF, Clardy J, Goodman RM (1998) Molecular biological access to the chemistry of unknown soil microbes: a new frontier for natural products. Chem Biol 5:R242–R249

7. Simon C, Daniel R (2009) Achievements and new knowledge unraveled by metagenomic approaches. Appl Microbiol Biotechnol 85:265–276

8. Vieites JM, Gauzzaroni M-E, Beloqui A, Golyshin PN, Ferrer M (2010) Molecular methods to study complex microbial communities. Methods Mol Biol 668:1–37

9. Schmeisser C, Steele H, Streit WR (2007) Metagenomics, biotechnology with non-culturable microbes. Appl Microbiol Biotechnol 75:955–962

10. Liebl W, Angelov A, Juergensen J, Chow J, Loeschcke A, Drepper T et al (2014) Alternative hosts for functional (meta)genome analysis. Appl Microbiol Biotechnol 98:8099–8109

11. Vrancken K, Van Mellaert L, Anné J (2010) Cloning and expression vectors for a Gram-positive host, *Streptomyces lividans*. Methods Mol Biol 668:97–107

12. McMahon MD, Guan C, Handelsman J, Thomas MG (2012) Metagenomic analysis of *Streptomyces lividans* reveals host-dependent functional expression. Appl Environ Microbiol 78:3622–3629

13. Angelov A, Liebl W (2010) Heterologous gene expression in the hyperthermophilic Archaeon *Sulfolobus solfataricus*. Methods Mol Biol 668:109–116

14. Hildalgo A, Berenguer J (2013) Biotechnological applications of *Thermus thermophilus* as host. Curr Biotechnol 2:304–312

15. Craig JW, Chang F-Y, Kim JH, Obiajulu SC, Brady SF (2010) Expanding small-molecule functional metagenomics through parallel screening of broad-host-range cosmid environmental DNA libraries in diverse Proteobacteria. Appl Environ Microbiol 76:1633–1641

16. Burton S, Cowan DA, Woodley JM (2002) The search for the ideal biocatalyst. Nat Biotechnol 30:35–46

17. Fortune BM (2014) Cloning and characterization of three compost metagenome-derived α-L-arabinofuranosidases with differing thermal stabilities. Dissertation, University of the Western Cape

18. Ohlhoff CW, Kirby BM, Van Zyl L, Mutepfab DLR, Casanuevaa A, Huddya RJ et al (2015) An unusual feruloyl esterase belonging to family VIII esterases and displaying a broad substrate range. J Mol Catal B Enzym 118:79–88

19. Handelsman J, Liles M, Mann D, Riesenfeld C, Goodman RM (2002) Cloning the metagenome: culture-independent access to the diversity and functions of the uncultivated microbial world. Methods Microbiol 33:241–255

20. Anné J, Vrancken K, Van Mellaert L, Van Impe J, Bernaerts K (2014) Protein secretion biotechnology in Gram-positive bacteria with special emphasis on *Streptomyces lividans*. Biochim Biophys Acta 1843:1750–1761

21. Horbal L, Fedorenko V, Luzhetskyy A (2014) Novel and tightly regulated resorcinol and cumate-inducible expression systems for *Streptomyces* and other actinobacteria. Appl Microbiol Biotechnol 98:8641–8655

22. Maruthamuthu M, Jiménez DJ, Stevens P, van Elsas JD (2016) A multi-substrate approach for functional metagenomics-based screening for (hemi)cellulases in two wheat straw-degrading microbial consortia unveils novel thermoalkaliphilic enzymes. BMC Genomics 17:86

23. Rabausch U, Juergensen J, Ilmberger N, Böhnke S, Fischer S, Schubach B et al (2013) Functional screening of metagenome and genome libraries for detection of novel flavonoid-modifying enzymes. Appl Environ Microbiol 76:4551–4563

Chapter 14

Screening Glycosyltransferases for Polyphenol Modifications

Nele Ilmberger and Ulrich Rabausch

Abstract

Glycosyltransferases offer the opportunity to glycosylate a variety of substrates including health beneficial molecules like flavonoids in a regiospecific manner. Flavonoids are plant secondary metabolites that have antimicrobial, antioxidative, and health beneficial effects. Glycosylation often has impact on these properties and furthermore enhances the water solubility, the stability, and the bioavailability of the molecules. To detect flavonoid glycosylating enzymes we established a metagenome screen for the discovery of modifying clones. This function based screening technique can furthermore detect other modifications like methylations. The method relies on analysis of the culture supernatant extracts from biotransformation reactions in a thin layer chromatography (TLC) approach.

Key words Glycosyltransferase, Flavonoid, META, Biotransformation, TLC

1 Introduction

Metagenomics is a powerful tool to search for novel enzymes that are useful for biotechnological applications. Since the conception of the technology a remarkable number of articles were published describing novel enzymes with high potential for industrial applications [1]. Interestingly, the majority of identified and characterized enzymes belong to the group of hydrolases, probably due to the high industrial demand and the simple high throughput screening tools. Thereby other groups like ligases, isomerases, and transferases are underrepresented [2].

Transferases (EC 2) catalyze the transfer of functional groups from a donor to an acceptor molecule and are subclassified by the chemical group they transfer [3]. These enzymes have attracted much attention as they present a tool to specifically introduce desired groups into bioactive molecules.

Glycosyltransferases (GTs) (EC 2.4) specifically transfer sugar moieties from activated sugar molecules to a saccharide or non-saccharide acceptor, forming a glycosidic bond [3]. The sugar

Wolfgang R. Streit and Rolf Daniel (eds.), *Metagenomics: Methods and Protocols*, Methods in Molecular Biology, vol. 1539, DOI 10.1007/978-1-4939-6691-2_14, © Springer Science+Business Media LLC 2017

transfer can either result in the inversion or retention of the configuration at the anomeric carbon atom [4]. The most recent nomenclature describes almost 100 families of glycosyltransferases as listed at the CAZy server (http://www.cazy.org/ GlycosylTransferases.html), mainly distinguished by amino acid sequence similarities. Glycosyltransferases are of particular interest for natural product and drug design [5]. For example polyphenols like flavonoids can be substrates of glycosyltransferases and are auspicious candidates as they have a variety of beneficial effects on human health. Flavonoids are plant-derived secondary metabolites that can have, among others, anti-carcinogenic, antimicrobial, antiviral, anti-inflammatory, antioxidative, and hormonal properties [6]. The addition and substitution of functional groups causes dramatic changes in the physicochemical properties of a molecule [7], e.g., flavonoid glycosylation enhances the water solubility and therefore the bioavailability of the molecule [8]. In nature a broad diversity of flavonoids exists, exhibiting a variety of backbones. The glycosylation of flavonoids at free hydroxyl groups therefore allows an enormous diversification of the substrate. Thereby O-glycosylation is the most often occurring type of glycosylation (Fig. 1).

Glycosyltransferases active on polyphenols in general belong to family GT 1 [9]. All enzymes of this family catalyze an inverting reaction mechanism and possess a GT-B fold, meaning a typical structure containing two similar Rossmann-like domains [10]. Altogether the N-terminal domain binds the acceptor substrate and the C-terminal domain of the enzyme binds the donor substrate [9]. Interestingly, next to glycosyltransferases, some glycoside hydrolases have been shown to glycosylate polyphenols via a transglycosylation mechanism [11, 12].

One explanation for the limited information on transferases from metagenomic libraries is due to the lack of described function driven screening methods. Nevertheless, suitable assays may be taken from other applications. For example, there are several assays for measuring the activity of glycosyltransferases [13–16]. These assays can also be applied to screen metagenomic libraries; however, they are likely cost-intensive. Recently, we developed a sensitive, medium throughput screen for glycosyltransferases

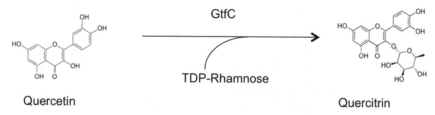

Fig. 1 Exemplary reaction of the glycosyltransferase GtfC [17]. The enzyme glycosylates quercetin at the OH group at C3 by transferring rhamnose from the nucleotide sugar dTDP-rhamnose. The reaction product is quercitrin

active on polyphenols using TLC (thin layer chromatography) designated META (*Me*tagenome *E*xtract *TLC A*nalysis) [17].

Glycosylation and other modifications alter the characteristics of the polyphenol like solubility and therefore its behavior in the TLC eluent. The polyphenols can easily be detected on the TLC plate with UV light as these molecules absorb UV light and often emit fluorescence. Furthermore, the UV absorbance spectrum is altered by modifications of the molecule. With this screen positive clones can be discovered in pools of 96 metagenomic clones and quantities of only 4 ng modified flavonoid can be detected. Several enzymes have been discovered with this screen so far [17, 18].

2   Materials

2.1   Biotrans formation Reactions

1. MSM (Mineral Salt Medium):

    (a) Solution 1 (10×): 70 g $Na_2HPO_4 \cdot 2H_2O$, 20 g KH_2PO_4, H_2O *ad* 1000 mL

    (b) Solution 2 (10×): 10 g $(NH_4)_2SO_4$, 2 g $MgCl_2 \cdot 6H_2O$, 1 g $Ca(NO_3)_2 \cdot 4H_2O$, H_2O *ad* 1000 mL

    (c) Trace element stock solution (2000×): 5 g EDTA, 3 g $Fe(III)SO_4 \cdot 7H_2O$, 30 mg $MnCl_2 \cdot 4H_2O$, 50 mg $CoCl_2 \cdot 6H_2O$, 20 mg $NiCl_2 \cdot 2H_2O$, 10 mg $CuCl_2 \cdot 2H_2O$, 30 mg $Na_2MoO_4 \cdot 2H_2O$, 50 mg $ZnSO_4 \cdot 7H_2O$, 20 mg H_3BO_4, H_2O *ad* 1000 mL. pH 4.0. Filter sterilized.

    (d) Vitamin stock solution (1000×): 1 mg biotin, 10 mg nicotinic acid, 10 mg thiamin-HCl (vit. B1), 1 mg *p*-aminobenzoic acid, 10 mg Ca-d(+) pantothenic acid, 10 mg vit. B6 hydrochloride, 10 mg vit. B12, 10 mg riboflavin, 1 mg folic acid, H_2O *ad* 1000 mL. Filter sterilized.

    (e) Solution 1 and 2 are autoclaved. After the solutions have cooled down, 100 mL of each stock solution is combined and 1 mL vitamin and 1 mL trace element stock solution are added. Furthermore a suitable carbon source must be added. Then sterile water is added to a final volume of 1 L.

2. RM (Rich Medium): 10 g Bacto peptone (Difco), 5 g yeast extract, 5 g casamino acids (Difco), 2 g meat extract (Difco), 5 g malt extract (Difco), 2 g glycerol, 1 g $MgSO_4 \cdot 7H_2O$, 0.05 g Tween 80, H_2O ad 1000 mL, pH 7.2

3. LB (Lysogeny Broth): 10 g peptone, 5 g yeast extract, 5 g NaCl, H_2O *ad* 1000 mL

4. TB (Terrific Broth): 12 g casein, 24 g Yeast extract, 12.5 g K_2HPO_4, 2.3 g KH_2PO_4, H_2O *ad* 1000 mL, pH 7.2

5. PBS (phosphate buffer saline): 50 mM sodium phosphate, 150 mM NaCl, pH 7.0

2.2 Analysis of Biotransformation Products by Thin-Layer Chromatography

1. TLC eluent: "Universal Pflanzenlaufmittel" [19]: ethyl acetate (EtOAc)/–acetic acid–formic acid–H_2O (100:11:11:27)

2. "Naturstoff reagent A" [20]: diphenyl boric acid β-aminoethyl ester

3. TLC plate: Merck silica gel 60 F_{254} TLC plate

3 Methods

3.1 Biotrans formation Reactions of Metagenome Library Clones

For the identification of glycosyltransferase encoding metagenomic clones whole cell catalysis is chosen, as glycosyltransferases need NDP-activated sugar as a co-substrate, e.g., UDP-glucose. These molecules are very cost-intensive and in a biotransformation approach activated sugars are produced by the host.

1. To screen metagenomic libraries, multiple clones are tested in parallel, e.g., the 96 clones from one microtiter plate. Initially the clones are grown individually either

   (a) in liquid culture (e.g., LB, TB, RM, and MSM are suitable media) in 96-well plates or

   (b) on agar plates (e.g., LB agar).

2. After overnight growth at 37 °C the single clones are pooled.

   (a) Liquid cultures are united and jointly harvested by centrifugation at $4500 \times g$ for 10 min.

   (b) From agar plates the colonies are washed off with 50 mM sodium phosphate buffer saline (PBS) using a Drigalski spatula. Then the cells are harvested as outlined above.

   The cell pellet is resuspended in 50 mL liquid medium containing the appropriate antibiotic(s), 100 μM of the flavonoid substrate. Depending on the vector/host system gene/copy number induction can be performed simultaneously.

3. The biotransformation reactions are performed in 300 mL Erlenmeyer flasks at 28 °C while shaking at 175 rpm.

4. Samples of 2 mL are taken from the reaction after 16, 24, and 48 h for TLC analysis (Subheadings 3.2 and 3.3).

5. Positive pools are verified in a second biotransformation.

6. Subsequently smaller pools are tested until the single active clone is identified.

7. Single clones are tested analogously but pre-cultured in 5 mL LB medium overnight at 37 °C. This culture is then used to inoculate 20 mL of biotransformation medium 1:100–1:1000 in 100 mL Erlenmeyer flasks. After an OD_{600} of 0.8–1.0 is reached the substrate is added and, if possible, induction is initiated.

3.2 Metagenome Extract Sample Preparation for TLC Analysis (See Note 1)

1. For flavonoid extraction from biotransformation reactions 2 mL samples are centrifuged for 2 min at maximum speed.

2. The supernatant is mixed with the equal volume ethyl acetate and shaken thoroughly.

3. Then the samples are centrifuged for 5 min at 4 °C and $3000 \times g$.

4. The upper phase is used for TLC analysis (Subheading 3.3).

3.3 Analysis of Biotransformation Products by TLC (See Notes 2 and 3)

1. The ethyl acetate extracts (Subheading 3.2) from biotransformation reactions (Subheading 3.1) or enzyme assays (Subheading 3.4) are transferred into HPLC flat bottom vials and used for TLC analysis. Samples of 20 µL are applied on 20×10 cm^2 (HP)TLC silica 60 F_{254} plates (Merck KGaA, Germany) versus 200 pmol of reference flavonoids with the ATS 4 (CAMAG, Switzerland). If this device is not available, samples can be applied with a micropipette tip by hand.

2. The sampled TLC plates are developed in TLC eluent and dried in hot air for 1 min, e.g., with a hair-dryer.

3. The chromatograms are read depending on the absorbance maximum of the respective educt flavonoid at 285–370 nm by the TLC Scanner 3 (CAMAG, Switzerland) (Fig. 2). Next to the comparison of R_f (retardation factor, *aka* retention factor) values, the TLC scanner allows the scanning of UV absorbance spectra in single bands. This enables a more distinct identification

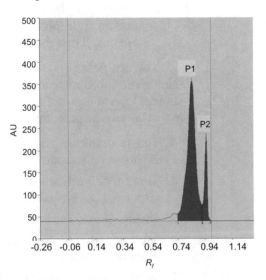

Fig. 2 TLC chromatogram. Culture extract in EtOAc from a biotransformation reaction of GtfC [17] after 40 h with 100 µM quercetin was applied on a Merck silica gel 60 F_{254} TLC plate. The chromatogram is displayed in relative absorbance units (AU) versus the R_f value measured at 330 nm on a TLC Scanner 3 (CAMAG, Switzerland). Peak 2 (P2) is the remaining quercetin substrate, peak 1 (P1) is the reaction product quercitrin

of substances if reference substances are available. In alternative, plates can also be analyzed with a UV-lamp that emits at 285–370 nm.

4. Subsequently, the substances on developed TLC plates can be derivatized by either spraying with or dipping the plates in a 1 % (wt/vol) methanolic solution of "Naturstoff reagent A".

5. After immediate drying in hot air, the TLC plates are dipped in or sprayed with a 5 % (wt/vol) solution of polyethylene glycol 4000 in ethanol (70 %, vol/vol). For dipping, a chromatogram immersion device (CAMAG, Switzerland) is used.

6. After complete drying the fluorescence of the bands is determined by the TLC Scanner 3. Also, the bands are visualized with a UV-lamp as stated above and photographed (Fig. 3).

3.4 Enzyme Assay

For the determination of kinetic parameters or characteristics like pH and temperature optima the enzyme's activity must be measured directly.

1. Biocatalytic reaction mixtures of 1 mL contained 5 µg purified enzyme.

2. Reactions are performed in 50 mM sodium phosphate buffer, at appropriate pH and temperature.

3. The respective activated sugar (UDP-glucose) is added to defined concentrations from 50 mM stock solutions in 50 mM

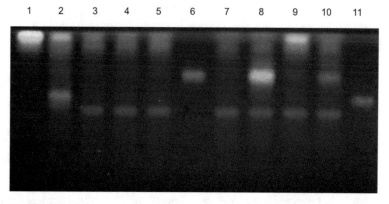

Fig. 3 Photography of a UV irradiated, developed TLC plate. Samples of 20 µL extract from biotransformation reactions with 100 µM quercetin of single metagenome clones from a six clone pool after 24 h were applied on a Merck silica gel 60 F_{254} TLC plate. The TLC plate was derivatized with "Naturstoff Reagent A" and documented at 365 nm. Quercetin, quercitrin and isoquercitrin were used as reference substrates (2 µL of 100 µM solution, lanes 1, 6, and 11, respectively). Lanes 2 and 10 were positive controls (*Bacillus cereus* ATCC 10987 and the clone pool preliminarily verified positive, respectively). One band in lane 8 showed the same R_f value as in lane 10, both with equal R_f to quercitrin (lane 6)

sodium phosphate buffer, pH 7.0. Final concentrations of 500 μM are used to determine K_m/kcat for the acceptor substrate, pH and temperature optima.

4. Acceptor substrates are used in specific concentrations from stock solutions of 100 mM in DMSO. Final concentrations of 100 μM are used to obtain the K_m/kcat of the donor substrate, pH and temperature optima.

5. After an appropriate time period the reactions are stopped by dissolving 100 μL reaction mixture 1/10 in ethyl acetate–acetic acid (3:1).

6. These samples are centrifuged for 2 min at maximum speed in a microcentrifuge.

7. Supernatants are used directly for quantitative TLC analysis (Subheading 3.3).

4 Notes

1. At this point it is very important to use only the upper phase, as protein contaminations can plug the syringe used for applying the samples on the TLC plate.

2. To avoid carryover of substances, i.e., prevent false positives, samples are spotted with double syringe rinsing in between.

3. The incubation time after "Naturstoff Reagent A" and polyethylene glycol 4000 is important for the fluorescence intensity. A time period of 2–15 min is optimal.

References

1. Perner M, Ilmberger N, Köhler HU, Chow J, Streit WR (2011) Metagenomics in different habitats. In: Bruijn FJD (ed) Handbook of molecular microbial ecology II. John Wiley and Sons, Inc., Hoboken, NJ, pp 481–498

2. Taupp M, Mewis K, Hallam SJ (2011) The art and design of functional metagenomic screens. Curr Opin Biotechnol 22:465–472

3. Boyce S, Tipton KF (2001) Enzyme classification and nomenclature. In: Encyclopedia of life sciences. John Wiley and Sons, Ltd., Hoboken, NJ

4. Lairson LL, Henrissat B, Davies GJ, Withers SG (2008) Glycosyltransferases: structures, functions, and mechanisms. Annu Rev Biochem 77:521–555

5. Luzhetskyy A, Bechthold A (2008) Features and applications of bacterial glycosyltransferases: current state and prospects. Appl Microbiol Biotechnol 80:945–952

6. Xiao ZP1, Peng ZY, Peng MJ, Yan WB, Ouyang YZ, Zhu HL (2011) Flavonoids health benefits and their molecular mechanism. Mini Rev Med Chem11(2):169–177

7. Kren V, Martinkova L (2001) Glycosides in medicine: "The role of glycosidic residue in biological activity". Curr Med Chem 8:1303–1328

8. Graefe EU, Wittig J, Mueller S, Riethling AK, Uehleke B, Drewelow B et al (2001) Pharmacokinetics and bioavailability of quercetin glycosides in humans. J Clin Pharmacol 41:492–499

9. Osmani SA, Bak S, Møller BL (2009) Substrate specificity of plant UDP-dependent glycosyltransferases predicted from crystal structures and homology modeling. Phytochemistry 70:325–347

10. Breton C, Snajdrova L, Jeanneau C, Koca J, Imberty A (2006) Structures and mechanisms of glycosyltransferases. Glycobiology 16:29–37

11. Noguchi A, Inohara-Ochiai M, Ishibashi N, Fukami H, Nakayama T, Nakao M (2008) A novel glucosylation enzyme: molecular cloning, expression, and characterization of *Trichoderma viride* JCM22452 alpha-amylase and enzymatic synthesis of some flavonoid monoglucosides and oligoglucosides. J Agric Food Chem 56:12016–12024

12. Shimoda K, Hamada H (2010) Production of hesperetin glycosides by *Xanthomonas campestris* and cyclodextrin glucanotransferase and their anti-allergic activities. Nutrients 2:171–180

13. Aharoni A, Thieme K, Chiu CP, Buchini S, Lairson LL, Chen H et al (2006) High-throughput screening methodology for the directed evolution of glycosyltransferases. Nat Methods 3:609–614

14. Collier AC, Tingle MD, Keelan JA, Paxton JW, Mitchell MD (2000) A highly sensitive fluorescent microplate method for the determination of UDP-glucuronosyl transferase activity in tissues and placental cell lines. Drug Metab Dispos 28:1184–1186

15. Northen TR, Lee JC, Hoang L, Raymond J, Hwang DR, Yannone SM et al (2008) A nanostructure-initiator mass spectrometry-based enzyme activity assay. Proc Natl Acad Sci U S A 105:3678–3683

16. Yang M, Brazier M, Edwards R, Davis BG (2005) High-throughput mass-spectrometry monitoring for multisubstrate enzymes: determining the kinetic parameters and catalytic activities of glycosyltransferases. Chembiochem 6:346–357

17. Rabausch U, Juergensen J, Ilmberger N, Bohnke S, Fischer S, Schubach B et al (2013) Functional screening of metagenome and genome libraries for detection of novel flavonoid-modifying enzymes. Appl Environ Microbiol 79:4551–4563

18. Rabausch U, Ilmberger N, Streit WR (2014) The metagenome-derived enzyme RhaB opens a new subclass of bacterial B type alpha-L-rhamnosidases. J Biotechnol 191:38–45

19. Wagner H, Bladt S, Zgainski EM (1983) Drogenanalyse, Dünnschichtchromatographische Analyse von Arzneidrogen. Springer, Berlin, p 321

20. Neu R (1957) Chelate von Diarylborsäuren mit aliphatischen Oxyalkylaminen als Reagenzien für den Nachweis von Oxyphenyl-benzo-γ-pyronen. Naturwissenschaften 44:181–182

Chapter 15

Methods for the Isolation of Genes Encoding Novel PHA Metabolism Enzymes from Complex Microbial Communities

Jiujun Cheng, Ricardo Nordeste, Maria A. Trainer, and Trevor C. Charles

Abstract

Development of different PHAs as alternatives to petrochemically derived plastics can be facilitated by mining metagenomic libraries for diverse PHA cycle genes that might be useful for synthesis of bioplastics. The specific phenotypes associated with mutations of the PHA synthesis pathway genes in *Sinorhizobium meliloti* and *Pseudomonas putida*, allows the use of powerful selection and screening tools to identify complementing novel PHA synthesis genes. Identification of novel genes through their function rather than sequence facilitates the functional proteins that may otherwise have been excluded through sequence-only screening methodology. We present here methods that we have developed for the isolation of clones expressing novel PHA metabolism genes from metagenomic libraries.

Key words PHA/PHB pathway, *Sinorhizobium meliloti*, *Pseudomonas putida*, Microbial community gene libraries, Phenotypic complementation

1 Introduction

It is now well recognized that the majority of microbial community members is not represented in the culturable fraction. Metagenomic analyses of complex microbial communities necessitates a multifaceted approach that involves both sequence-based analyses and phenotypic selection. The use of phenotypic selection techniques represents a powerful tool for the isolation of truly novel genes that would not otherwise be identified on the basis of sequence alone [1].

Polyhydroxyalkanoates (PHA) represent a class of microbial polyesters composed of hydroxyacyl monomers, of which polyhydroxybutyrate (PHB) is the best-studied member [2]. In the bacterial cell, PHAs are synthesized as cytoplasmically localized, electron-transparent granules under conditions of abundant carbon when growth is limited by the availability of another key nutrient [3]. The elastomeric and biodegradative properties of PHAs have

Wolfgang R. Streit and Rolf Daniel (eds.), *Metagenomics: Methods and Protocols*, Methods in Molecular Biology, vol. 1539, DOI 10.1007/978-1-4939-6691-2_15, © Springer Science+Business Media LLC 2017

generated considerable interest as potentially economically competitive, environmentally benign replacements to petrochemically derived plastics [4]. Additionally, the potential use of PHAs in the medical field as materials for bio-compatible surgical implants is promising [5, 6]. Indeed, the potential commercial value of PHAs has generated the interest that has driven much of the research in this field.

The mechanical and physical properties of PHAs vary depending on the nature of the hydroxyacyl monomers [7]. A range of properties, including melting point, elasticity, and tensile strength, may be altered by changing the composition of the monomer subunits (reviewed in [2]). The type of PHA synthesized by a given bacterial species depends on a multitude of factors, including the precursors provided to the polymerase enzyme responsible for construction of the polymer as well as the nature of the polymerase enzyme itself. The regulation of PHA accumulation and degradation has also been shown to involve a class of proteins called phasins [8]. Phasins are involved in PHA granule formation, specifically in determining the size and number of PHA granules [8].

The cellular role of PHB, although not fully understood, is known to extend further than simply acting as an intracellular carbon store that can be mobilized to provide a bacterium with a competitive advantage over other soil microbes. PHAs have been shown to protect the cell from a wide range of stresses including heat shock, UV irradiation, exposure to oxidizing agents, and osmotic shock [9]. PHB metabolism is also tightly linked to the redox state of the cell; previous studies have shown that in some bacteria, large quantities of PHB are accumulated under conditions of oxygen limitation [10–12]. Furthermore, it has been suggested that PHB synthesis may act as an alternative electron acceptor under conditions of oxygen limitation; NAD(P)H is channeled into PHB formation to relieve inhibition of isocitrate dehydrogenase and citrate synthase in order to allow continued operation of the TCA cycle [10, 13, 14].

The isolation of novel PHA metabolism genes by phenotypic complementation of S. meliloti [15] and P. putida [16] is potentially useful for production of PHA with a range of useful properties.

The PHA pathways elucidated in Sinorhizobium meliloti (Fig. 1 and Fig. 2), the nitrogen-fixing symbiont of alfalfa, is compared with the PHA pathway of Pseudomonas putida (Fig. 2), which produces medium chain length PHA. Mutants of several of these PHA pathway enzymes have demonstrated interesting and informative phenotypes [16–19] that may be exploited as easy selection methods for the recovery of complementing clones from metagenomic libraries. Such clones could contain genes with

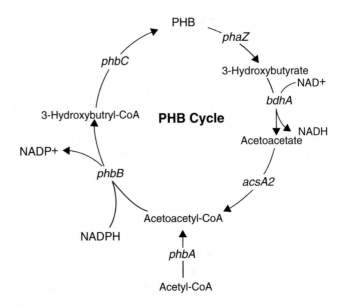

Fig. 1 PHB cycle of *S. meliloti*

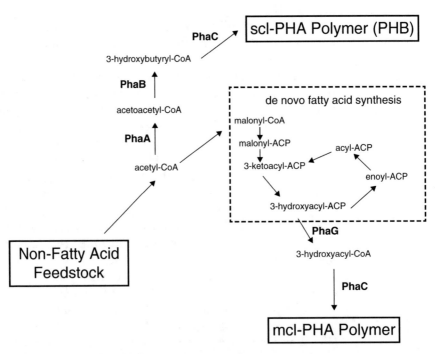

Fig. 2 PHB/PHA synthesis pathways of *S. meliloti* and *P. putida*. Note that *phaA*, *phaB*, and *phaC* gene designations are often used interchangeably with *phbA*, *phbB* and *phbC* in the *scl*-PHA pathway

interesting or valuable properties. Phenotypic screens that have been previously described include exopolysaccharide synthesis [20], staining with lipophilic dyes [21], fatty acid detoxification [22], and nutritional auxotrophy [19, 23].

2 Materials

2.1 Bacterial Growth Media

1. Luria–Bertani medium (LB) [24]: 5 g yeast extract, 10 g tryptone, 5 g NaCl, 1 L dH$_2$O, (15 g agar).

2. Tryptone yeast extract medium (TY) [25]: 5 g tryptone, 3 g yeast extract, 0.5 g CaCl$_2$, 1 L dH$_2$O, (15 g agar).

3. Modified M9 medium for *Rhizobium* (*see* **Note 1**) [26]: 7 g Na$_2$HPO$_4$, 3 g KH$_2$PO$_4$, 1 g NH$_4$Cl, 1 g NaCl, (15 g Agar). This is autoclaved, cooled to 55 °C, and the following are added sterilely: 1 mL 0.5 M MgSO$_4$, 0.1 mL 1 M CaCl$_2$.

4. *Rhizobium* minimal medium (RMM) [27]: Solutions A, B, C, and D are prepared and sterilized separately. RMM is made by adding 1 % (v/v) each of RMM A and RMM B and 0.1 % (v/v) each of RMM C and RMM D.

(a) RMM A: 145 g KH$_2$PO$_4$, 205 g K$_2$HPO$_4$, 15 g NaCl, 50 g NH$_4$NO$_3$, 1 L dH$_2$O.

(b) RMM B: 50 g MgSO$_4$·7H$_2$O, 1 L dH$_2$O.

(c) RMM C: 10 g CaCl$_2$·2H$_2$O, 1 L dH$_2$O.

(d) RMM D: 123.3 g MgSO$_4$·7H$_2$O, 87 g K$_2$SO$_4$, 0.247 g H$_3$BO$_3$, 0.1 g CuSO$_4$·5H$_2$O, 0.338 g MnSO$_4$·H$_2$O, 0.288 g ZnSO$_4$·7H$_2$O, 0.056 g CoSO$_4$·7H$_2$O, 0.048 g Na$_2$MoO$_4$·2H$_2$O, 1 L dH$_2$O.

5. Yeast Mannitol Medium (YM): 0.4 g yeast extract, 10 g mannitol, 0.5 g K$_2$HPO$_4$, 0.2 g MgSO$_4$·7H$_2$O, 0.1 g NaCl, 1 L dH$_2$O, pH to 7.0, 18 g agar.

6. Yeast mannitol medium with Nile Red (YM-NR): 0.4 g yeast extract, 10 g mannitol, 0.5 g K$_2$HPO$_4$, 0.2 g MgSO$_4$·7H$_2$O, 0.1 g NaCl, 1 L dH$_2$O, pH to 7.0, 18 g agar, 0.5 µg/mL Nile Red.

2.2 Molecular Biology Reagents

1. Gigapack III XL Lambda packaging extract (Stratagene).

2. EpiCentre™ EZ-Tn5 Insertion Kit (Epicentre).

3. Small-scale plasmid preparation solution I: 50 mM glucose, 25 mM Tris–HCl pH 8.0, 10 mM EDTA pH 8.0.

4. Small-scale plasmid preparation solution II: 0.2 N NaOH, 1 % SDS.

5. Small-scale plasmid preparation solution III: 60 mL 5 M potassium acetate, 11.5 mL glacial acetic acid, 28.5 mL dH$_2$O, store at 4 °C.

6. T$_{10}$E$_{25}$: 10 mM Tris–HCl pH 8.0, 25 mM EDTA pH 8.0.

7. T$_{10}$E$_1$: 10 mM Tris–HCl pH 8.0, 1 mM EDTA pH 8.0.

8. TAE buffer: 40 mM Tris-Acetate, 1 mM EDTA.

9. 40× TAE buffer: 242 g Tris base, 57.1 mL glacial acetic acid, 100 mL 0.5 M EDTA, pH 8.0.

10. Phage dilution buffer: 10 mM Tris–HCl pH 8.3, 100 mM NaCl, 10 mM MgCl$_2$.

3 Methods

3.1 Bacterial Growth and Storage Conditions

1. *Escherichia coli* strains are routinely grown at 37 °C using Luria–Bertani (LB) medium [24]. *S. meliloti* strains are routinely cultured at 30 °C in either LB [24] or TY [25] medium. *P. putida* strains are routinely cultured at 30 °C in LB [24]. When *S. meliloti* is grown in modified M9 [26] or Rhizobium minimal medium (RMM) [27] the medium is supplemented with 15 mM glucose, D-3-hydroxybutyrate (D3HB), L-3-hydroxybutyrate (L3HB), DL-3-hydroxybutyrate (DLHB), acetoacetate (AA), or acetate as the carbon source. For growth under high carbon conditions, *S. meliloti* is cultured in Yeast Mannitol (YM) medium.

2. Antibiotics are used in the growth medium where appropriate. Concentrations for *E. coli* are as follows: ampicillin 100 μg/mL, chloramphenicol 25 μg/mL, gentamycin 10 μg/mL, kanamycin 25 μg/mL, nalidixic acid 5 μg/mL, tetracycline 10 μg/mL. Concentrations for *S. meliloti* are as follows: gentamicin 75 μg/mL, neomycin 200 μg/mL, spectinomycin 100 μg/mL, streptomycin 200 μg/mL, tetracycline 10 μg/mL, trimethoprim 400 μg/mL.

3. All bacterial cultures are stored at –70 °C in glass cryovials containing 7 % dimethyl sulfoxide (DMSO).

3.2 Construction of Metagenomic Libraries from Soil

1. High molecular weight total DNA from soil samples is isolated as described by Cheng et al. [28].

2. Cosmid libraries are constructed by cloning fragments from BamHI partial digests (*see* **Note 2**) into the BamHI site of the IncP Tc^R plasmid pRK7813 [29] or pJC8 [28] followed by packaging with Gigapack III XL Lambda packaging extract and transduction of *E. coli* HB101 [30].

3. Tc^R colonies are selected and representative library clones are analyzed by restriction digest.

4. Colonies are pooled and subcultured. The resultant libraries are maintained at –70 °C as aliquots in LB containing 7 % DMSO.

3.3 Transfer of a Metagenomic Library into S. meliloti and P. putida by Triparental Conjugation

Conjugation is typically performed by triparental mating between *E. coli* donors carrying the metagenomic library, an *E. coli* strain carrying a helper plasmid, and an *S. meliloti* or *P. putida* recipient.

1. Wash all strains in 0.85 % NaCl to remove antibiotics.
2. Combine 1 mL saturated broth culture of the *S. meliloti* or *P. putida* recipient with 500 µL each of the *E. coli* donor and helper strains.
3. Recover cells by centrifugation, resuspend in 20 µL 0.85 % NaCl, spot onto a non-selective LB or TY plate.
4. Incubate overnight at 30 °C.
5. Resuspend mating spot in 1 mL 0.85 % NaCl.
6. Prepare serial dilutions of the resuspended mating spot in 0.85 % NaCl; plate 100 µL of the appropriate dilutions onto selective medium and incubate overnight at 30 °C.

3.4 Transfer of Putative Complementing Clones from S. meliloti or P. putida into E. coli

1. Wash all strains in 0.85 % NaCl to remove antibiotics.
2. Combine 1 mL saturated broth culture of the *S. meliloti* or *P. putida* recipient with 500 µL each of the *E. coli* donor and helper strains.
3. Recover cells by centrifugation, resuspend in 20 µL 0.85 % NaCl, spot onto a non-selective LB or TY plate.
4. Incubate overnight at 30 °C.
5. Resuspend mating spot in 1 mL 0.85 % NaCl.
6. Prepare serial dilutions of the resuspended mating spot in 0.85 % NaCl; plate 100 µL of the appropriate dilutions onto selective medium and incubate overnight at 37 °C.
7. Restreak transconjugants onto selective medium and isolate the cosmid DNA by standard plasmid isolation techniques [24].

3.5 Genetics and Molecular Biology

In vitro Tn5 mutagenesis of plasmid DNA is used to generate transposon mutations that facilitate the subsequent determination of plasmid DNA sequence. These mutageneses are performed using the Epicentre™ EZ-Tn5 Insertion Kit as per manufacturer's instructions.

3.6 PHA Accumulation

PHB content is conveniently determined using a modified version of the colorimetric assay developed by Law and Slepecky [31]. This assay is based in the hydrolysis of PHB and subsequent conversion of the monomer to crotonic acid by concentrated H_2SO_4. Crotonic acid has an absorption maximum at 235 nm. The amount of crotonic acid can be used to determine PHB content of the initial sample. PHB content is expressed as a percentage of total cellular dry mass. Do not use any plasticware in this protocol (*see* **Note 3**).

1. Pellet cells in screw-capped Pyrex centrifuge tubes at 7000 rcf in an IEC 21000R centrifuge with a 7685c rotor (or equivalent) for 10 min.

2. Wash cell pellet in dH$_2$O and pellet again.

3. Resuspend pellet in 2.0 mL of 5.25 % NaOCl and incubate at 37 °C for 1 h to allow for complete cell lysis to occur.

4. Pellet samples at 7000 rcf for 15 min and wash in 5 mL dH$_2$O followed by 5 mL EtOH and finally 5 mL acetone.

5. The pellet, which should be white in color, should be allowed to dry before the PHB is extracted.

6. PHB is extracted by the addition of 10 mL of cold chloroform. The tubes should be capped, vortexed, and transferred to a boiling water bath. The tubes are removed from the water bath and vortexed every 1–2 min for 10 min before cooling to room temperature. The PHB should now be dissolved in the chloroform.

7. Once cool, the tubes are vortexed again and 1 mL is removed and transferred to a glass test tube.

8. The chloroform should be allowed to evaporate completely at room temperature (*see* **Note 4**) (should take 24–48 h) before addition of 10 mL concentrated H$_2$SO$_4$.

9. The tubes are then capped with marbles (to prevent entry of water and pressure build up) and transferred to a boiling water bath for 10 min, after which time they are removed and allowed to cool to room temperature.

10. After mixing well by vortex, OD from 220 to 280 nm is measured and PHB is quantified by comparison to data generated by a standard curve (*see* **Note 5**).

PHA deposits may also be visualized by transmission electron microscopy:

1. Samples are prepared from 100 mL stationary phase YM cultures.

2. Cells are harvested by centrifugation, suspended in phosphate buffer (pH 6), and collected by centrifugation.

3. The cells are then suspended in 1 mL of 2.5 % glutaraldehyde in phosphate buffer, and kept at 4 °C for 1 h, followed by three series of centrifugation and resuspension in 1 mL of phosphate buffer.

4. The washed cells are suspended in 1 mL of 0.5 % OsO$_4$ in phosphate buffer and kept at room temperature for 16 h, then diluted to 8 mL in phosphate buffer.

5. The cells are collected by centifugation and resuspended in 2 % agar, a drop of which is then allowed to harden on a microscope slide.

6. The agar-suspended cells are then dehydrated in a series from 50 % acetone to 100 % acetone washes, embedded in eponaraldite, sectioned at a thickness of 60–90 nm on a Reichert Ultracut E ultramicrotome (or equivalent), stained with uranyl acetate and lead citrate, and examined on a Philips CM10 transmission electron microscope (or equivalent) using an accelerating voltage of 60 kV.

3.7 Screening of Metagenomic Libraries for PHA Synthesis Clones

The distinct, non-mucoid colony morphology exhibited by PHB synthesis mutants of *S. meliloti* on YMA, and less opaque colony morphology of PHA synthesis mutant of *P. putida* on LB supplemented with 0.5 % octanoate provides a powerful screen for complementation by PHA synthesis genes [20, 30]. This screen may be further enhanced by the inclusion of 0.5 μg/mL Nile Red into the YM agar (YM-NR) or LB agar (LB-NR); PHB-synthesizing colonies will stain pink, while non-synthesizing colonies remain unpigmented (*see* **Note 6**).

3.7.1 Complementation

1. The metagenomic libraries are introduced *en masse* into *S. meliloti* Rm11476 or *P. putida* PpUW2 containing a deletion of the *phaC1-phaZ-phaC2* region by triparental conjugation.

2. Transconjugants are selected on YM-NR or LB-NR agar supplemented with an appropriate antibiotic—Tc for libraries constructed in pRK7813; Nm for selection in Rm11476; Km for selection in PpUW2—and the resultant colonies are screened for pink coloration and mucoidy or opacity.

3. Clones from pink, mucoid/opaque colonies are transferred to *E. coli* DH5α by triparental conjugation.

4. The complementing cosmids are then reintroduced into *S. meliloti phbC* mutants to confirm the associated colony and growth.

5. Cosmid DNA from complementing clones is analyzed to identify clones exhibiting unique restriction patterns.

6. PHB accumulation is confirmed in the transconjugants by PHB assay and by transmission electron microscopy.

3.7.2 Sequence Analysis of Complementing Clones

1. Complementing clones exhibiting unique restriction patterns are subcloned into pBBR1MCS-5 [32]; complementing clones are identified by complementation analysis on YM-NR.

2. The complementing region is localized by EZ-Tn-Kan-2 in vitro mutagenesis and subsequent subcloning steps; the

DNA sequence of the complementing clones is facilitated by the transposon insertions.

3. The resultant DNA sequence is compared to other sequences by BLASTX analysis [33].

3.8 Utilization of Nutritional Auxotrophy to Facilitate the Isolation of PHB Cycle Genes from Metagenomic Libraries

S. meliloti mutants of different PHB cycle genes exhibit nutritional auxotrophies that represent powerful selection tools for the isolation of complementing clones from metagenomic libraries. These are summarized in Table 1.

3.8.1 Complementation

1. The metagenomic libraries are introduced *en masse* into the appropriate *S. meliloti* mutant.

2. Transconjugants are selected on RMM or M9 agar supplemented with appropriate antibiotic to counterselect the *E. coli* donor and an appropriate carbon source.

3. Isolated clones are screened for the presence of a cosmid by patching onto LB or TY medium containing the appropriate antibiotic (Tc for libraries constructed in pRK7813 or pJC8).

4. Cosmids from the resulting colonies are transferred to *E. coli* DH5α by triparental conjugation.

Table 1
Nutritional auxotrophies and colony phenotypes of *S. meliloti* PHB cycle mutants

ORF	Auxotrophy	Nile Red	Mucoidy	Reference
WT	None	+	+	[34]
phbA	No growth on acetoacetate	–	–	(unpublished)
phbB	Poor growth on D-3-hydroxybutyrate and acetoacetate	–	–	[20]
phbC	Poor growth on D-3-hydroxybutyrate and acetoacetate	–	–	[19, 35]
phaZ	None	+	++	(unpublished)
bdhA	No growth on D-3-hydroxybutyrate	+	+	[36]
acsA2	Poor growth on acetoacetate	+	+	[35]
phaP1	Slow growth on succinate	+	+	[37]
phaP2	Slow growth on succinate	+	+	[37]
phaP1/P2	Slow growth on succinate	–	++	[37]

5. Complementing cosmids are then reintroduced into the appropriate *S. meliloti* PHB cycle mutant to confirm complementation on the appropriate carbon source.

6. Cosmid DNA from complementing clones is analyzed to identify clones exhibiting unique restriction patterns.

3.8.2 Sequence Analysis of Complementing Clones

1. Complementing clones exhibiting unique restriction patterns are subcloned into pBBR1MCS-5 [32]; complementing clones are identified by selection for growth on the appropriate carbon source.

2. The complementing region is localized by EZ-Tn-Kan-2 in vitro mutagenesis and subsequent subcloning steps; the DNA sequence of the complementing clones is facilitated by the transposon insertions.

3. The resultant DNA sequence is compared to other sequences by BLASTX analysis [33].

4   Notes

1. To facilitate the growth of rhizobial species, M9 medium is modified to include 0.25 mM $CaCl_2$, 1 mM $MgSO_4$, and 0.3 mg/L biotin.

2. Partial digestion of genomic DNA is optimized by gradient digest. In a tube, 15 μL genomic DNA (15 ng/μL) is mixed with 100 μL 10× digest buffer in a final volume of 500 μL. This mixture is incubated on ice for 30 min. The reaction mix is then aliquoted into 15 tubes (60 μL is added to the first tube; 30 μL is added to the remaining 14) and 5 units of the Sau3AI is added to the first tube. A concentration gradient is established by transferring 30 μL from the first tube into the second, mixing, then transferring 30 μL from tube 2 into tube 3 and so on. 30 μL is removed from the final tube and discarded. The reactions are incubated at 37 °C for 30 min and the reactions are stopped by the addition of 1 μL 0.5 M EDTA mixed with 6× loading dye. The digests are run on an agarose gel and the enzyme concentration that gives fragments of approx. 25–50 kb is selected for subsequent use.

3. Following the initial cell harvest, no plasticware should be used in the PHB extraction protocol; all glassware used must be washed thoroughly in boiling chloroform and rinsed in EtOH prior to use, to remove any traces of plasticizers.   4 .
Evaporation of the chloroform can be expedited by gentle heating at 40 °C.

5. A standard curve is obtained by assaying known quantities of PHB. Standard solutions are prepared from a 1 mg/mL PHB

stock, made by adding 10 mg PHB to 10 mL cold chloroform and heating in a boiling water bath to dissolve, as above. From this, a 100 µg/mL stock is prepared. Aliquots of 0–100 µg PHB are transferred to test tubes and the chloroform is allowed to evaporate before addition of 10 mL H_2SO_4 and processing, as described above.

6. The *exoY*::Tn5 mutant Rm7055 [38, 39], in which the extracellular polysaccharide succinoglycan is not produced, forms non-mucoid colonies that fluoresce brightly under UV illumination. Strain Rm11476, containing both *exoY*::Tn5 and *phbC*::Tn5-233 mutations, forms non-mucoid colonies that do not stain or fluoresce. This is the best genetic background for the detection of clones that complement for PHB accumulation, especially on densely populated plates.

References

1. Henne A, Daniel R, Schmitz RA, Gottschalk G (1999) Construction of environmental DNA libraries in *Escherichia coli* and screening for the presence of genes conferring utilization of 4-hydroxybutyrate. Appl Environ Microbiol 65:3901–3907

2. Anderson AJ, Dawes EA (1990) Occurrence, metabolism, metabolic role, and industrial uses of bacterial polyhydroxyalkanoates. Microbiol Rev 54:450–472

3. Zevenhuizen LPTM (1981) Cellular glycogen, β-1,2-glucan, poly-3-hydroxybutyric acid and extracellular polysaccharides in fast-growing species of Rhizobium. Antonie Van Leeuwenhoek 47:481–497

4. Madison LL, Huisman GW (1999) Metabolic engineering of poly(3-hydroxyalkanoates): from DNA to plastic. Microbiol Mol Biol Rev 63:21–53

5. Shishatskaya EI, Voinova ON, Goreva AV, Mogilnaya OA, Volova TG (2008) Biocompatibility of polyhydroxybutyrate microspheres: *in vitro* and *in vivo* evaluation. J Mater Sci Mater Med 19:2493–2502

6. Shishatskaya EI, Volova TG, Puzyr AP, Mogilnaya OA, Efremov SN (2004) Tissue response to the implantation of biodegradable polyhydroxyalkanoate sutures. J Mater Sci Mater Med 15:719–728

7. Holmes PA (1985) Applications of PHB -- a microbially produced biodegradable thermosplastic. Phys Technol 16:32–36

8. Pötter M, Steinbüchel A (2005) Poly(3-hydroxybutyrate) granule-associated proteins: impacts on poly(3-hydroxybutyrate) synthesis and degradation. Biomacromolecules 6:552–560

9. Kadouri D, Jurkevitch E, Okon Y (2003) Involvement of the reserve material poly-β-hydroxybutyrate in *Azospirillum brasilense* stress endurance and root colonization. Appl Environ Microbiol 69:3244–3250

10. Senior PJ, Beech GA, Ritchie GAF, Dawes EA (1972) The role of oxygen limitation in the formation of poly-3-hydroxybutyrate during batch and continuous culture of *Azotobacter beijerinckii*. Biochem J 128:1193–1201

11. Stam H, van Verseveld HW, de Vries W, Stouhamer AH (1986) Utilization of poly-β-hydroxybutyrate in free-living cultures of *Rhizobium* ORS571. FEMS Microbiol Lett 35:215–220

12. Stockdale H, Ribbons DW, Dawes EA (1968) Occurence of poly-3-hydroxybutyrate in the Azotobacteriaceae. J Bacteriol 95:1798–1803

13. Senior PJ, Dawes EA (1971) Poly-3-hydroxybutyrate biosynthesis and the regulation of glucose metabolism in *Azotobacter beijinkereii*. Biochem J 125:55–66

14. Page WJ, Knosp O (1989) Hyperproduction of poly-3-Hydroxybutyrate during exponential growth of *Azotobacter vinelandii* UWD. Appl Environ Microbiol 55:1334–1339

15. Schallmey M, Ly A, Wang C, Meglei G, Voget S, Streit WR et al (2011) Harvesting of novel polyhydroxyalkanaote (PHA) synthase encoding genes from a soil metagenome library using phenotypic screening. FEMS Microbiol Lett 321:150–156

16. Aneja P, Charles TC (1999) Poly-3-hydroxybutyrate degradation in *Rhizobium* (*Sinorhizobium*) *meliloti*: isolation and characterization of a gene encoding 3-hydroxybutyrate dehydrogenase. J Bacteriol 181:849–857

17. Aneja P, Dziak R, Cai GQ, Charles TC (2002) Identification of an acetoacetyl coenzyme-A synthetase-dependent pathway for utilization of L-(+)-3-hydroxybutyrate in *Sinorhizobium meliloti*. J Bacteriol 184:1571–1577

18. Charles TC, Cai GQ, Aneja P (1997) Megaplasmid and chromosomal loci for the PHB degradation pathway in *Rhizobium* (*Sinorhizobium*) *meliloti*. Genetics 146: 1211–1220

19. Willis LB, Walker GC (1998) The phbC (poly-β-hydroxybutyrate synthase) gene of *Rhizobium* (*Sinorhizobium*) meliloti and characterization of phbC mutants. Can J Microbiol 44:554–564

20. Aneja P, Dai M, Lacorre DA, Pillon B, Charles TC (2004) Heterologous complementation of the exopolysaccharide synthesis and carbon utilization phenotypes of *Sinorhizobium meliloti* Rm1021 polyhydroxyalkanoate synthesis mutants. FEMS Microbiol Lett 239:277–283

21. Ostle AG, Holt JG (1982) Nile blue as a fluorescent stain for poly-β-hydroxybutyrate. Appl Environ Microbiol 44:238–241

22. Kranz RG, Gabbert KK, Madigan MT (1997) Positive selection systems for discovery of novel polyester biosynthesis genes based on fatty acid detoxification. Appl Environ Microbiol 63:3010–3013

23. Povolo S, Tombolini R, Morea A, Anderson AJ, Casella S, Nuti MP (1994) Isolation and characterization of mutants of *Rhizobium meliloti* unable to synthesize poly-3-hydroxybutyrate (PHB). Can J Microbiol 40:823–829

24. Sambrook J, Russell DW (2001) Molecular cloning: a laboratory manual. Cold Spring Harbor Press, Cold Spring Harbor, NY

25. Beringer JE (1974) R factor transfer in *Rhizobium leguminosarum*. J Gen Microbiol 84:188–198

26. Miller JH (1972) Experiments in molecular genetics. Cold Spring Harbor Laboratory, Cold Spring Harbor, NY

27. Dowling DN, Samrey U, Stanley J, Broughton WJ (1987) Cloning of *Rhizobium leguminosarum* genes for competitive nodulation blocking on peas. J Bacteriol 169:1345–1348

28. Cheng J, Pinnell L, Engel K, Neufeld JD, Charles TC (2014) Versatile broad-host-range cosmids for construction of high quality metagenomic libraries. J Microbiol Methods 99:27–34

29. Jones JD, Gutterson N (1987) An efficient mobilizable cosmid vector, pRK7813, and its use in a rapid method for marker exchange in *Pseudomonas fluorescens* strain HV37a. Gene 61:299–306

30. Wang C, Meek DJ, Panchal P, Boruvka N, Archibald FS, Driscoll BT, Charles TC (2006) Isolation of poly-3-hydroxbutyrate metabolism genes from complex microbial communities by phenotypic complementation of bacterial mutants. Appl Environ Microbiol 72:384–391

31. Law J, Slepecky R (1961) Assay of poly-3-hydroxybutyric acid. J Bacteriol 82:33–36

32. Kovach ME, Elzer PH, Hill DS, Robertson GT, Farris MA, Roop RM, Peterson KM (1995) Four new derivatives of the broad-host-range cloning vector pBBR1MCS, carrying different antibiotic-resistance cassettes. Gene 166:175–176

33. Altschul SF, Madden TL, Schäffer AA, Zhang Z, Miller W, Lipman DJ (1997) Gapped BLAST and PSI-BLAST: a new generation of protein database search programs. Nucleic Acids Res 25:3389–3402

34. Meade HM, Long SR, Ruvkun GB, Brown SE, Ausubel FM (1982) Physical and genetic characterization of symbiotic and auxotrophic mutants of *Rhizobium meliloti* induced by transposon Tn5 mutagenesis. J Bacteriol 149: 114–122

35. Cai G, Driscoll BT, Charles TC (2000) Requirement for the enzymes acetoacetyl coenzyme-A synthetase and poly-3-hydroxybutyrate (PHB) synthase for growth of *Sinorhizobium meliloti* on PHB cycle intermediates. J Bacteriol 182:2113–2118

36. Aneja P, Zachertowska A, Charles TC (2005) Comparison of the symbiotic and competition phenotypes of *Sinorhizobium meliloti* PHB synthesis and degradation pathway mutants. Can J Microbiol 51:599–604

37. Wang CX, Sheng XY, Equi RC, Trainer MA, Charles TC, Sobral BWS (2007) Influence of the poly-3-hydroxybutyrate (PHB) granule-associated proteins (PhaP1 and PhaP2) on PHB accumulation and symbiotic nitrogen fixation in *Sinorhizobium meliloti* Rm1021. J Bacteriol 189:9050–9056

38. Leigh JA, Signer ER, Walker GC (1985) Exopolysaccharide-deficient mutants of *Rhizobium meliloti* that form ineffective nodules. Proc Natl Acad Sci U S A 82:6231–6235

39. Miller-Williams M, Loewen PC, Oresnik IJ (2006) Isolation of salt-sensitive mutants of *Sinorhizobium meliloti* strain Rm1021. Microbiology 152:2049–2059

Chapter 16

Function-Based Metagenomic Library Screening and Heterologous Expression Strategy for Genes Encoding Phosphatase Activity

Genis A. Castillo Villamizar, Heiko Nacke, and Rolf Daniel

Abstract

The release of phosphate from inorganic and organic phosphorus compounds can be mediated enzymatically. Phosphate-releasing enzymes, comprising acid and alkaline phosphatases, are recognized as useful biocatalysts in applications such as plant and animal nutrition, bioremediation and diagnostic analysis. Metagenomic approaches provide access to novel phosphatase-encoding genes. Here, we describe a function-based screening approach for rapid identification of genes conferring phosphatase activity from small-insert and large-insert metagenomic libraries derived from various environments. This approach bears the potential for discovery of entirely novel phosphatase families or subfamilies and members of known enzyme classes hydrolyzing phosphomonoester bonds such as phytases. In addition, we provide a strategy for efficient heterologous phosphatase gene expression.

Key words Phosphatases, Phytases, Metagenomic libraries, Phosphorus, Function-based screening

1 Introduction

Phosphorus is essential for growth, metabolism, and reproduction [1]. Due to enhanced demand and fertilization of agricultural land for food and biofuel production the consumption of phosphorus increased significantly during the last century. However, phosphate rock reservoirs renew in time scales of thousands to millions of years. Thus, mineral phosphorus resources are limited or will be even exhausted within the next 50–100 years [2]. Phosphorus is abundant in soil but present in its insoluble form or bound to organic compounds [3]. Consequently, this has led to the exploration of alternatives for obtaining phosphorus. The release of phosphorus in the form of phosphate can be mediated by a diverse group of enzymes. These enzymes, designated phosphatases, are considered as important biocatalysts for efficient phosphorus solubilization and release [4, 5]. Phosphatases showing phytase activity (phytases) are used to release phosphate from

Wolfgang R. Streit and Rolf Daniel (eds.), *Metagenomics: Methods and Protocols*, Methods in Molecular Biology, vol. 1539, DOI 10.1007/978-1-4939-6691-2_16, © Springer Science+Business Media LLC 2017

phytate, the most abundant organic phosphorus compound in soil [6]. The released phosphate can then be utilized by for example agricultural crops as natural phosphorus fertilizer. Phosphatases catalyzing the hydrolysis of phytic acid also play an important role as supplement in animal nutrition, as they release phosphate from phytate present in cereal grains and oilseeds. Furthermore, phosphatases have broad applications in pharmaceutical industry and clinical diagnostics [7].

The almost exclusive use of cultivable microorganisms was a limiting factor with respect to the discovery of new enzymes exhibiting phosphatase activity. Within many recent culture-based approaches, degenerated primers were used to identify phosphatase genes carried by single microorganisms [8–10]. Taking into account that currently less than 1% of microbial taxa can be cultured under laboratory conditions, only a tiny fraction of the existing phosphatase gene pool has been mined by culture-based methods [8, 11–14]. In principle, culture-independent metagenomic approaches provide access to the entire phosphatase gene pool. In this way, novel phosphatases with valuable characteristics such as high stability and catalytic activity under harsh conditions can be identified. The different phosphatase types exhibit a high level of sequence divergence, and different substrate preferences and spectra [15]. These differences point to the employment of function-based screening strategies for the discovery of novel phosphatase-encoding genes from complex metagenomic libraries [11, 13, 16]. In contrast to sequence-based identification of target genes based on conserved DNA regions, the function-based strategy allows identification of enzymes that represent entirely novel phosphatase families.

Here, we describe a rapid function-based metagenomic library screening approach for phosphatase genes, which is based on chromogenic substrate-containing medium. Sarikhani and colleagues [11] used a similar medium for the discovery of phosphatase-encoding genes derived from *Pseudomonas putida*. We successfully tested phytic acid as well as other phosphorus sources such as β-glycerol phosphate in function-based screens of small- and large-insert metagenomic libraries. The number of retrieved phosphatase genes can vary depending on the source of environmental DNA used for the construction of metagenomic libraries. In addition, we present a strategy for efficient heterologous expression of genes conferring phosphatase activity. This strategy allows a moderate instead of a high level heterologous gene expression and the periplasmic localization of the heterologous phosphatase gene products. In this way the risk of detrimental interactions of the produced proteins with host proteins or cell metabolites in the cytoplasm is reduced.

2 Materials

2.1 Identification of Phosphatase Genes by Function-Based Screening of Metagenomic Libraries

2.1.1 Metagenomic Libraries

The function-based screening approach presented here has been tested using small-insert and large-insert metagenomic libraries derived from soil, compost, volcano sediments, glacial samples, and microbial mats. Metagenomic library construction was performed according to protocols described by Simon and Daniel [17]. Small-insert metagenomic libraries were constructed using the plasmid pCR-XL-TOPO (Thermo Fisher Scientific, Waltham, MA, USA) as vector. Large-insert metagenomic libraries were generated using the fosmid vector pCC1FOS™ (Epicentre Biotechnology, Madison, WI, USA).

2.1.2 Medium for Small-Insert Metagenomic Library Screening

1. Modified Sperber medium (SpM): 16 g/L agar, 10 g/L glucose or 2% glycerol, 500 mg/L yeast extract, 100 mg/L CaCl$_2$, and 250 mg/L MgSO$_4$, supplemented with a phosphorus source such as 2.5 g/L phytic acid, β-glycerol phosphate disodium salt pentahydrate, or D-fructose 6-phosphate disodium salt hydrate, 5-bromo-4-chloro-3-indolyl phosphate (BCIP) stock solution: 25 mg/mL in dimethylformamide.

2. Kanamycin stock solution: 50 mg/mL in H$_2$O.

3. NaOH solutions for pH adjustment.

2.1.3 Medium for Large-Insert Metagenomic Library Screening

The materials listed for small-insert metagenomic library screening medium can be used by considering the following modifications and extensions:

1. Chloramphenicol instead of kanamycin stock solution: 12.5 mg/mL in ethanol.

2. L-arabinose stock solution: 1% (w/v) in H$_2$O.

2.1.4 Function-Based Metagenomic Library Screening

1. *E. coli* DH5 alpha electrocompetent cells [18].

2. Super Optimal Broth with Catabolic repressor (SOC).

3. Bio-Rad GenePulser II (Bio-Rad, Munich, Germany) and 1 mm electroporation cuvettes.

4. Heat block with mixing function.

2.1.5 Analysis of Metagenomic DNA Fragments Carried by Positive Clones

1. Lysogeny broth (LB) (autoclaved).

2. Stock solution of antibiotic (kanamycin: 50 mg/mL, when pCR-XL-TOPO is used as vector or chloramphenicol: 12.5 mg/mL, when pCC1FOS is used as vector).

3. L-arabinose stock: 1% (w/v) or CopyControl™ Induction Solution (1000×, Epicentre Biotechnology) (required when pCC1FOS is used as vector).

4. Plasmid mini prep kit (Macherey-Nagel GmbH & Co. KG, Düren, Germany).

5. *Hin*dIII restriction enzyme.

6. Sequencing primers: pCR-XL-TOPO vector: Forward 5′-GTAAAACGACGGCCAG-3′, Reverse 5′-CAGGAAA CAGCTATGAC-3′, pCC1FOS: Forward 5′-GGATGTGCTG CAAGGCGATTAAGTTGG-3′, Reverse 5′-CTCGTATGT TGTGTGGAATTGTGAGC-3′ (other appropriate primers can also be used).

2.2 Heterologous Expression of Phosphatase Genes

2.2.1 Cloning of Putative Phosphatase-Encoding Genes into Expression Vector

1. Phusion High-Fidelity DNA Polymerase PCR kit (Thermo Fisher Scientific GmbH, Schwerte, Germany) (other polymerases with proofreading activity can also be used).

2. pET-20b(+) Novagen vector (Merck KGaA, Darmstadt, Germany).

3. Gel extraction kit (Qiagen, Hilden, Germany).

4. Antarctic phosphatase (New England Biolabs GmbH, Frankfurt am Main, Germany).

5. DNA ligation kit (Thermo Fisher Scientific GmbH, Schwerte, Germany).

6. *E. coli* DH5 alpha electrocompetent cells.

7. Bio-Rad GenePulser II (Bio-Rad) and 1 mm electroporation cuvettes.

8. LB agar plates supplemented with 100 mg/L ampicillin.

9. LB broth (autoclaved).

10. Ampicillin stock solution: 100 mg/mL H_2O.

2.2.2 Heterologous Expression of Genes Encoding Phosphatase Activity

1. *E. coli* BL21 one shot cells (Thermo Fisher Scientific GmbH, Schwerte, Germany).

2. LB agar plates supplemented with 100 mg/L ampicillin.

3. Minimal medium is prepared from stock solution of 5× salts solution (50 g $Na_2HPO_4 \cdot 7H_2O$, 30 g KH_2PO_4, 5 g NaCl, 5 g NH_4Cl) in 1 L water. For 1 L media, add 200 mL of the 10× salt solution to 500 mL of water supplemented with 0.20 % glycerol, adjust the volume and sterilize by autoclaving. Supplement the media by adding 1 mL of $MgSO_4$ (1 M), 1 mL $CaCl_2$ (1 M), and 1 mL $FeSO_4 \cdot 7H_2O$ (0.01 mM). The solutions should be sterilized separately by filtration.

4. 50 mM Hepes buffer pH 8.

5. Shaker with temperature control.

6. French press or any other effective cell disruption device.

2.2.3 Verification of Heterologous Target Gene Expression Based on Phosphatase Activity Test	1. 50 mM sodium acetate buffer (pH 6.0).
	2. Acetone.
	3. 5 N H_2SO_4.
	4. 10 mM ammonium molybdate.
	5. 1 M citric acid.

3 Methods

3.1 Identification of Phosphatase Genes by Function-Based Screening of Metagenomic Libraries

The screening approach presented here is based on a chromogenic substrate (BCIP)-containing medium. This screening medium allows rapid identification of phosphatase activity encoded by small-insert and large-insert metagenomic libraries. We employed metagenomic libraries, which were constructed using plasmids or fosmids as vectors. In general, the described screening can also be performed using cosmid-based or bacterial artificial chromosome-based metagenomic libraries with modifications (e.g., use of appropriate antibiotics). Positive clones carrying potential phosphatase genes and exhibiting phosphatase activity show intense blue color after incubation on solidified screening medium. Sequencing and analysis of the metagenomic inserts derived from the isolated recombinant vectors of the positive clones allow prediction and identification of candidate genes responsible for the detected phosphatase activity.

3.1.1 Preparation of Screening Medium

1. To prepare screening medium, 500 mg/L yeast extract, 100 mg/L $CaCl_2$, 250 mg/L $MgSO_4$, and 2.5 g/L selected phosphorus source (*see* **Note 1**) are solubilized in water. Subsequently, pH is adjusted to 7.2 using NaOH solutions. To solidify the medium 16 g/L agar is added.

2. Autoclave the prepared mixture. After removing from the autoclave, allow cooling to approximately 55 °C and add filter-sterilized (0.22 μm filter) glucose (final concentration: 10 g/L) or autoclaved glycerol solution (final concentration: 2%). With respect to large-insert metagenomic library screening medium, filter-sterilized L-arabinose (0.22 μm filter) in a final concentration of 0.001% or copy control induction solution is also added (*see* **Note 2**).

3. Add 1 mL/L of 25 mg/mL BCIP solution and appropriate antibiotic (kanamycin, final concentration: 50 mg/L or chloramphenicol, final concentration: 12.5 mg/L) to select for clones bearing small-insert or large-insert metagenomic libraries.

4. Pour the media into petri dishes. After solidification store at 4 °C and dark until use. Plates can be stored for up to 1 month under these conditions.

3.1.2 Function-Based Metagenomic Library Screening

1. Prechill the electroporation cuvette on ice.

2. Thaw *E. coli* DH5 alpha electrocompetent cells on ice and transfer 40 μL to the 1 mm electroporation cuvette.

3. Add 1 μL prepared metagenomic library DNA (DNA concentration approximately 350 ng/μL) and mix gently. Do not mix by pipetting the cells up and down.

4. Wipe electrodes on the outside of cuvette with a paper towel to remove condensate and carefully eliminate air bubbles.

5. Electroporate the cells. We use a Bio-Rad Gene Pulser II with the following settings: 25 μF, 200 Ω and 1.25 kV.

6. Immediately add 500 μL of room temperature SOC medium.

7. Transfer the mix into a sterile 2 mL microcentrifuge tube and shake for 60 min at 37 °C and 150 rpm.

8. Spread 100 μL undiluted as well as diluted (tenfold, 100-fold, and 1000-fold) transformed cell suspension on separate screening medium plates containing the appropriate antibiotic. Store the remaining suspension of transformed cells at 4 °C.

9. Incubate the plates at 37 °C overnight. Analyze number of colonies formed on screening medium plates (*see* **Note 3**).

10. Spread the appropriate remaining undiluted or diluted suspension of transformed cells onto screening medium plates containing an appropriate antibiotic to obtain a sufficient number of colonies for detection of target clones.

11. Positive clones will appear after 24–72 h of incubation and show intense blue colony color resulting from reaction of phosphatase with the indicator BCIP (*see* **Note 4**).

3.1.3 Analysis of Metagenomic DNA Fragments Carried by Positive Clones

1. Pick single positive colonies and grow them individually in 5 mL LB broth (*see* **Note 2**) supplemented with the appropriate antibiotic (kanamycin, final concentration: 50 mg/L or chloramphenicol, final concentration: 12.5 mg/L).

2. Shake overnight at 37 °C and 150 rpm.

3. Extract, digest with restriction endonucleases, e.g., *Hin*dIII or any other enzyme present in the used vector and analyze insert DNA by using standard techniques.

4. Determine the insert sequences of vector DNA extracted from positive clones.

5. After the insert DNA sequences have been determined, identify open reading frames (ORFs). An initial prediction of ORFs can be performed using the ORF finder tool provided by the National Center for Biotechnology Information [19, 20].

6. To identify ORFs potentially conferring phosphatase activity, examine coding sequences for similarities to protein families

and domains, e.g., by performing searches against the CDD databases [21]. Consider that the described function-based screening approach allows identification of members of previously unknown phosphatase families. In some cases, the similarity of identified ORFs to known phosphatase sequences might be very low.

3.2 Efficient Heterologous Expression of Phosphatase Genes

Enzymes hydrolyzing phosphomonoester bonds play an important role in regulation of cell metabolism. The heterologous expression strategy described here has been developed to minimize interactions of recombinant phosphatases with host cell molecular activities and putative toxic effects. Metagenomic library-derived target genes are cloned into an expression vector encoding a signal sequence for periplasmic localization to reduce reactions of recombinant phosphatases with biomolecules in the cytoplasm of the host cell. To further reduce potential detrimental effects of phosphatase activity, we recommend conditions that lead to a moderate instead of a high level heterologous gene expression. These conditions include e.g., the use of an appropriate minimal medium rather than complex medium during heterologous phosphatase gene expression and protein production. To verify heterologous production of the enzyme, a phosphatase activity assay should be performed.

3.2.1 Cloning of Putative Phosphatase-Encoding Genes into Expression Vector

1. Design primers for amplification of a putative phosphatase gene. In order to clone the gene into expression vector pET-20b(+), add restriction sites occurring in the multiple cloning site (MCS) of this vector to the primers (one restriction site per primer). To allow directional cloning, each primer should contain a different restriction site. Within the MCS, the different selected restriction sites should be separated by at least 10 bp. Ensure that the selected restriction sites are not present in the gene region encoding the putative phosphatase.

2. Check if the designed primers allow cloning of the PCR product in frame with the His_6 tag and the signal sequence for periplasmic localization encoded by plasmid pET-20b(+).

3. Perform a PCR to amplify the putative phosphatase gene using the primers containing the added restriction sites. We use Phusion High Fidelity Hot Start DNA polymerase to obtain PCR products. The PCR reaction mixture (50 µL) contains 10 µL of fivefold Phusion GC buffer, 200 µM of each dNTP, 1.5 mM $MgCl_2$, 2 µM of each of the primers, 2.5 % DMSO, 0.5 U Phusion High Fidelity Hot Start DNA polymerase (*see* **Note 5**), and approximately 25 ng recombinant plasmid or fosmid DNA extracted from a positive clone.

4. The thermal cycling scheme should be adjusted by considering the size of potential phosphatase genes and annealing temperature of selected primers. A gradient PCR is recommended to

quickly identify an appropriate annealing temperature. The following thermal cycling scheme can be used to test different annealing temperatures: initial denaturation at 98 °C for 2 min, 29 cycles of denaturation at 98 °C for 45 s, annealing gradient ranging from 58 to 68 °C for 45 s, and extension at 72 °C for 30 s per kb, followed by a final extension at 72 °C for 5 min. Check the PCR products by agarose gel electrophoresis. Further PCR reactions using the selected annealing temperature can be performed to obtain a higher amount of the PCR product.

5. Subject the PCR product to agarose gel electrophoresis (0.8 %) and purify it using a gel extraction kit, e.g., QIAquick (Qiagen, Hilden, Germany).

6. Digest the PCR product and pET-20b(+) vector separately using the restriction enzymes selected for directional cloning. Due to the loss of DNA during the following gel purification step, it is important to digest at least 1 µg PCR product and 3 µg pET-20b(+) vector.

7. Dephosphorylation of pET-20b(+) vector. In order to prevent re-circularization of the vector pET-20b(+), the digested plasmid should be treated with a phosphatase prior to the following gel purification step. Add a maximum of 2 U Antarctic phosphatase (1 U/µL) to the pET-20b(+) vector restriction digest. The Antarctic phosphatase is stable and active in most restriction digestion buffers. Incubate for 15 min at 37 °C.

8. Load the digested PCR product and plasmid DNA separately on a 0.8 % agarose gel and purify both using a gel extraction kit.

9. Ligation: the ligation mix (20 µL) contains 2 µL 100 mM DTT, 1 µL 10 mM ATP, 2 µL 10× T4 Ligase buffer, approximately 200 ng pET-20b(+) (digested, dephosphorylated and purified), PCR product (digested and purified), and 1 µL T4 ligase (1 U/µL). A molar ratio 1:3 of vector to PCR product is recommended. Incubate at 16 °C overnight. In order to improve the ligation efficiency the T4 ligase is subsequently inactivated by incubation at 65 °C for 10 min.

10. Transform E. coli DH5 alpha electrocompetent cells with 5 µL ligation reaction via electroporation. Spread diluted (tenfold and 100-fold) suspension of the transformed cells on LB plates containing ampicillin and incubate overnight at 37 °C. Pick six single colonies and grow them in 5 mL LB broth with ampicillin (final concentration: 100 mg/L) overnight at 37 °C and 150 rpm. Extract the plasmid DNA using standard techniques.

11. Digest extracted plasmids, using the restriction enzymes selected for directional cloning, and check for the presence of the insert by agarose gel electrophoresis.

12. Sequence plasmid DNA carrying the desired insert to verify that the putative phosphatase gene has been cloned in the correct orientation and the sequence is error-free.

3.2.2 Heterologous Expression of Genes Encoding Phosphatase Activity

1. Transform *E. coli* BL21 one shot cells. Thaw one tube of *E. coli* BL21 one shot cells on ice and subsequently add 1 µL of the constructed expression plasmid harboring the target gene (maximum of 30 ng). Incubate on ice for 30 min. Perform transformation of the recombinant plasmids into the cells by heat shock treatment at 42 °C for 30 s in a temperature-controlled water bath. Immediately transfer the tube to ice and subsequently add 250 µL SOC medium. Incubate the tube at 37 °C for 45 min. Spread 100 as well as 150 µL suspension of transformed cells on LB plates containing ampicillin (*see* **Note 6**). Incubate plates overnight at 37 °C.

2. Pick 3–4 colonies and grow each in 30 mL minimal medium containing ampicillin (final concentration: 100 mg/L) overnight at 30 °C and 150 rpm.

3. Use the overnight culture to inoculate 250 mL of minimal medium (resulting OD_{600} should be approximately 0.1). Incubate the culture with shaking (150 rpm) at 30 °C until it reaches log phase (OD_{600} 0.4–0.8). Induce the production of the recombinant protein by adding IPTG to a final concentration of 0.25 mM and incubate with shaking (150 rpm) at 30 °C until OD_{600} of approximately 3.2 (*see* **Note 7**).

4. Harvest the cells by centrifugation at $10,000 \times g$ and 4 °C for 20 min. Suspend the resulting cell pellet in chilled lysis buffer 50 mM HEPES pH 7.5. Use a ratio of 1:2 w/v of pellet to buffer (*see* **Note 8**). Disrupt the cells using a prechilled French Press cell (1.38×10^8 Pa).

5. Clarify the cell lysate by centrifugation for 20 min at $9000 \times g$ and 4 °C. The supernatant (crude extract) should be cleared by filtration using a 0.2 µm syringe filter. *Note*: Subsequent purification methods of the crude extract can be applied to purify the target protein but a check for phosphatase activity should be performed using the crude extract.

3.2.3 Verification of Heterologous Target Gene Expression Based on Phosphatase Activity Test

1. To identify activity of target proteins, released inorganic phosphate can be measured according to the ammonium molybdate method [22] with modifications. Add 10 µL of diluted crude extract or purified enzyme to 350 µL of 50 mM sodium acetate buffer (pH 5.0) and incubate for 3 min at 40 °C. Add 10 µL of 100 mM phosphorus source used for function-based screening (some commercial substrates contain traces of free phosphorus causing background coloring). For blanks, use 10 µL lysis buffer (for purified potential phosphatase) or crude extract derived from *E. coli* BL21 carrying empty pET-20b(+) vector (for non-purified samples).

2. After 30 min of incubation at 40 °C, add 1.5 mL of a freshly prepared solution of acetone/5 N H_2SO_4/10 mM ammonium molybdate (2:1:1 v/v) and 100 μL of 1 M citric acid. All assays should be performed in triplicate. When phosphorus has been released in presence of molybdate, a bright yellow phosphomolybdate complex is formed and extracted by acetone. It is possible that the yellow color is directly visible. However, a spectrophotometer measurement at 355 nm is recommended [22].

4   Notes

1. We successfully tested all three phosphorus sources phytic acid, β-glycerol phosphate disodium salt pentahydrate, and D-fructose 6-phosphate disodium salt hydrate with respect to function-based identification of phosphatase genes from small-insert and large-insert metagenomic libraries. However, phosphorus source selection will depend on the research approach and target group of phosphatases. For example, to increase probability of identifying phytases during function-driven screens the phosphorus source phytic acid should be selected as screening substrate. In the case of metagenomic library screens this substrate might also act as inducer for expression of genes encoding phytases via endogenous promoters [23].

2. The number of fosmids carried by *E. coli* clones can be increased by adding L-arabinose (final concentration: 0.001%) or CopyControl™ Induction Solution (1000×). This might be advantageous during screening of large-insert metagenomic libraries as increased copy numbers of fosmids containing target genes might result in an increase of total phosphatase activity. Furthermore, higher DNA amounts can be extracted from clones carrying multiple copies of fosmids compared to those harboring a single fosmid.

3. To facilitate identification and selection of individual positive clones, we recommend growing a maximum number of approximately 10,000 colonies on screening medium plates (petri dishes 150×20 mm).

4. Due to endogenous phosphatase activity of host cells, all colonies grown on screening medium plates will change color after prolonged incubation times (more than 48 h). Positive clones show intense blue colony color, whereas false-positive colonies exhibit light blue or greenish color. Thus, it is possible that in some cases the presence of weakly expressed metagenome-derived phosphatases showing low catalytic activity is masked by the background reaction of the screening host. Nevertheless, we were able to identify a high number of clones carrying

recombinant phosphatase genes based on intense blue color developed by individual *E. coli* colonies.

5. It is highly recommended to use a proofreading polymerase to minimize mutations during amplification of putative phosphatase genes.

6. It is possible to spread some of the transformed cells directly on Sperber medium plates containing BCIP and ampicillin. Intense blue colonies growing on these plates indicate the presence of the targeted phosphatase gene.

7. The described conditions for heterologous expression were successfully tested for a number of phosphatase genes derived from function-based metagenomic library screening. Nevertheless, it might be necessary to vary different parameters such as temperature, IPTG concentration, and incubation time for improving heterologous expression of individual phosphatase genes.

8. The lysis buffer should be modified depending on intended further analysis. For instance, for affinity chromatography using a Ni-column 300 mM NaCl can be added.

References

1. McDowell LR (2003) Chapter 2 - Calcium and phosphorus. In: McDowell LR (ed) Minerals in animal and human nutrition, 2nd edn. Elsevier, Amsterdam, pp 33–100

2. Smil V (2000) Phosphorus in the environment: natural flows and human interferences. Annu Rev Energy Environ 25:53–88

3. Tarafdar JC, Marschner H (1994) Phosphatase activity in the rhizosphere and hyphosphere of VA mycorrhizal wheat supplied with inorganic and organic phosphorus. Soil Biol Biochem 26:387–395

4. Bagyaraj DJ, Krishnaraj PU, Khanuja SPS (2000) Mineral phosphate solubilization: agronomic implications, mechanism and molecular genetics. Proc Indian Nat Sci Acad B Rev Tracts Biol Sci 66:69–82

5. Cromwell GL (2009) ASAS Centennial Paper: landmark discoveries in swine nutrition in the past century. J Anim Sci 87:778–792

6. Lim BL, Yeung P, Cheng C, Hill JE (2007) Distribution and diversity of phytate-mineralizing bacteria. ISME J 1:321–330

7. Muginova SV, Zhavoronkova AM, Polyakov AE, Shekhovtsova TN (2007) Application of alkaline phosphatases from different sources in pharmaceutical and clinical analysis for the determination of their cofactors; Zinc and Magnesium ions. Anal Sci 23:357–363

8. Greiner R (2004) Purification and Properties of a Phytate-degrading Enzyme from Pantoea agglomerans. Protein J 23:567–576

9. Cho J, Lee C, Kang S, Lee J, Lee H, Bok J et al (2005) Molecular cloning of a phytase gene (*phy M*) from *Pseudomonas syringae* MOK1. Curr Microbiol 51:11–15

10. Cheng W, Chiu CS, Guu YK, Tsai ST, Liu CH (2013) Expression of recombinant phytase of *Bacillus subtilis* E20 in *Escherichia coli* HMS 174 and improving the growth performance of white shrimp, *Litopenaeus vannamei*, juveniles by using phytase-pretreated soybean meal-containing diet. Aquacult Nutr 19:117–127

11. Sarikhani M, Malboobi M, Aliasgharzad N, Greiner R, Yakhchali B (2010) Functional screening of phosphatase-encoding genes from bacterial sources. Iran J Biotech 8:275–279

12. Riccio ML, Rossolini GM, Lombardi G, Chiesurin A, Satta G (1997) Expression cloning of different bacterial phosphataseencoding genes by histochemical screening of genomic libraries onto an indicator medium containing phenolphthalein diphosphate and methyl green. J Appl Microbiol 82:177–185

13. Tan H, Mooij MJ, Barret M, Hegarty PM, Harington C, Dobson ADW, O'Gara F (2014) Identification of novel phytase genes from an

agricultural soil-derived metagenome. J Microbiol Biotechnol 24:113–118

14. Yao MZ, Zhang YH, Lu WL, Hu MQ, Wang W, Liang AH (2012) Phytases: crystal structures, protein engineering and potential biotechnological applications. J Appl Microbiol 112:1–14

15. Kennelly PJ (2001) Protein phosphatases – a phylogenetic perspective. Chem Rev 101:2291–2312

16. Huang H, Pandya C, Liu C, Al-Obaidi NF, Wang M, Zheng L et al (2015) Panoramic view of a superfamily of phosphatases through substrate profiling. Proc Natl Acad Sci U S A 112:E1974–E1983

17. Simon C, Daniel R (2010) Construction of small-insert and large-insert metagenomic libraries. Methods Mol Biol 668:39–50

18. Dower WJ, Miller JF, Ragsdale CW (1988) High efficiency transformation of E. coli by high voltage electroporation. Nucleic Acids Res 16:6127–6145

19. Altschul SF, Gish W, Miller W, Myers EW, Lipman DJ (1990) Basic local alignment search tool. J Mol Biol 215:403–410

20. Sayers EW, Barrett T, Benson DA, Bolton E, Bryant SH, Canese K et al (2012) Database resources of the National Center for Biotechnology Information. Nucleic Acids Res 40:D13–D25

21. Marchler-Bauer A, Zheng C, Chitsaz F, Derbyshire MK, Geer LY, Geer RC et al (2013) CDD: conserved domains and protein three-dimensional structure. Nucleic Acids Res 41:D348–D352

22. Heinonen JK, Lahti RJ (1981) A new and convenient colorimetric determination of inorganic orthophosphate and its application to the assay of inorganic pyrophosphatase. Anal Biochem 113:313–317

23. Vijayaraghavan P, Primiya RR, Prakash Vincent SG (2013) Thermostable alkaline phytase from Alcaligenes sp. in improving bioavailability of phosphorus in animal feed: in vitro analysis. ISRN Biotechnol 2013:6

Chapter 17

Activity-Based Screening of Metagenomic Libraries for Hydrogenase Enzymes

Nicole Adam and Mirjam Perner

Abstract

Here we outline how to identify hydrogenase enzymes from metagenomic libraries through an activity-based screening approach. A metagenomic fosmid library is constructed in *E. coli* and the fosmids are transferred into a hydrogenase deletion mutant of *Shewanella oneidensis* ($\Delta hyaB$) via triparental mating. If a fosmid exhibits hydrogen uptake activity, *S. oneidensis*' phenotype is restored and hydrogenase activity is indicated by a color change of the medium from yellow to colorless. This new method enables screening of 48 metagenomic fosmid clones in parallel.

Key words Metagenome, Function-based screen, Hydrogenase, Hydrogen uptake

---

1 Introduction

Hydrogen is the most abundant element on Earth. The vast majority of hydrogen is chemically bound in water, while some is bound in liquid or gaseous hydrocarbons and only less than 1 % exists in form of molecular hydrogen gas [1]. Molecular hydrogen is considered a highly promising chemical fuel, given its high energy output, relative to its molecular weight, and its combustion being free of environmental pollutants when burnt with oxygen [1, 2]. With the growing world's demand for energy, but limitations in fossil fuel availability and the problems associated with burning fossil fuels for the global climate, endeavors to develop alternative clean energy sources have increased. Hydrogen converting enzymes have attracted much attention in recent years due to their ability to produce H_2 from H_2O (biocatalyzed electrolysis) and because of their application in fuel cells to produce electrical energy (e.g., [3, 4]).

In prokaryotic and unicellular eukaryotic metabolisms hydrogen plays a key role. Its oxidation can be actively coupled to sulfur, nitrogen, and carbon cycling [5–8] and in fermentative processes it can be generated to recycle reducing equivalents [9]. These organisms have hydrogenase enzymes which can catalyze the

Wolfgang R. Streit and Rolf Daniel (eds.), *Metagenomics: Methods and Protocols*, Methods in Molecular Biology, vol. 1539, DOI 10.1007/978-1-4939-6691-2_17, © Springer Science+Business Media LLC 2017

reversible reduction of protons to molecular hydrogen following the equation $H_2 \leftrightarrow 2H^+ + 2e^-$ [10]. According to the active center of these metalloenzymes, hydrogenases can be categorized into three groups, namely [NiFe]-hydrogenases, [FeFe]-hydrogenases, and [Fe]-hydrogenases [10]. To date hydrogenases have been recovered mostly by sequence-based analyses from environmental samples [11, 12], by extraction from isolates [13] or by sequence-based identification and then subsequent cloning and heterologous expression of the hydrogenase gene fragments in a surrogate host [14]. The here described screen is the only currently published solely function-based approach to detect active recombinant hydrogenase enzymes from environmental metagenomic libraries independent of previous sequence identification.

2 Materials

2.1 Laboratory Equipment

1. General equipment for handling anaerobic cultures, e.g., gas attachments, syringes, needles, serum bottles (120 mL), butyl rubber stoppers, aluminum caps, crimping tool.

2. 96-well microtiter plates and 96-deep-well plates as well as a 48-pin replicator tool with flat pins (e.g., by Boekel scientific, Feasterville, PA, USA).

3. Centrifuge with rotor (adapter) for microtiter/deep-well plates.

2.2 Strains, Plasmids and Growth Media

1. *E. coli* strain EPI300™-T1R, phage T1-resistant (included in the CopyControl™ Fosmid Library Production Kit with pCC1FOS, Epicentre, Madison, WI, USA).

2. [NiFe]-hydrogenase deletion mutant *Shewanella oneidensis* Δ*hyaB*, available from M. Perner (University of Hamburg, Hamburg, Germany).

3. *S. oneidensis* Δ*hyaB*::pRS44_So_P5H2 (positive control for the screen: deletion mutant complemented with *S. oneidensis* hydrogenase operon), available from M. Perner.

4. Broad host range vector pRS44 [15], available from S. Valla (Norwegian University of Science and Technology, Trondheim, Norway).

5. Mobilization (helper) plasmid pRK 2013 for triparental mating (e.g., obtained as strain DSM No. 5599 in *E. coli* K-12 HBH101, DSMZ, Braunschweig, Germany).

6. Luria–Bertani (LB) medium: 10.0 g/L NaCl, 10.0 g/L tryptone, 5.0 g/L yeast extract, pH adjusted to 7.0. If necessary the medium is solidified with 1.5% (w/v) agar-agar and/or supplemented with 30 μg/mL kanamycin, 12.5 μg/mL chloramphenicol, 10 μg/mL gentamycin, 100 μg/mL IPTG and 50 μg/mL X-Gal. Prior to transduction, *E. coli* EPI300-T1R

cells are grown in LB supplemented with 10 mM MgSO$_4$ and 0.2% (w/v) maltose.

7. Freshwater enrichment (FW-) medium (modified according to ref. 16) (*see* **Notes 1–3**): 2.5 g NaHCO$_3$, 0.1 g KCl, 1.5 g NH$_4$Cl, 0.6 g NaH$_2$PO$_4$ × H$_2$O, 0.1 g CaCl$_2$×2H$_2$O, 3.0 g Fe(III)citrate, 0.02 g L-arginine-hydrochloride, 0.02 g L-glutamine, 0.02 g L-serine. The substances are dissolved in 900 mL H$_2$O (deionized) and the medium is boiled for 5 min. While cooling to room temperature the medium is flushed with oxygen-free N$_2$ gas (30–45 min) under vigorous stirring. The pH is adjusted to 7.0 with HCl and the medium is flushed with N$_2$ for another 15 min. 50 mL aliquots of the medium are distributed into 120 mL serum bottles (while flushing the bottles with N$_2$). The serum bottles are (crimp-)sealed with butyl rubber stoppers and aluminum caps. After autoclaving and cooling the medium, 1 mL of a mixture (50/50% (v/v)) of trace element solution and vitamin solution (sterilized by filtration) are added to each serum bottle. The headspace of the serum bottles is replaced by flushing the medium for 2 min with a gas mixture of H$_2$ and CO$_2$ (80:20% (v/v)).

8. Trace element solution [17]: 1.5 g nitrilotriacetic acid, 3.0 g MgSO$_4$×7H$_2$O, 0.5 g MnSO$_4$×2H$_2$O, 1.0 g NaCl, 0.1 g FeSO$_4$×7H$_2$O, 0.18 g CoSO$_4$×7H$_2$O, 0.1 g CaCl$_2$×2H$_2$O, 0.18 g ZnSO$_4$×7H$_2$O, 0.01 g CuSO$_4$×5H$_2$O, 0.02 g KAl(SO$_4$)$_2$×12H$_2$O, 0.01 g H$_3$BO$_3$, 0.01 g Na$_2$MoO$_4$×2H$_2$O, 0.03 g NiCl$_2$×6H$_2$O, 0.3 mg Na$_2$SeO$_3$×5H$_2$O. The nitrilotriacetic acid is dissolved in 900 mL of deionized water and the pH is adjusted to 6.5 with KOH. Afterwards the minerals are added to the solution, final pH of 7.0 is adjusted with KOH and deionized water is added to a final volume of 1 L.

9. Vitamin solution [17]: 2.0 mg biotin, 2.0 mg folic acid, 10.0 mg pyridoxine-HCl, 5.0 mg thiamine-HCl×2H$_2$O, 5.0 mg riboflavin, 5.0 mg nicotinic acid, 5.0 mg D-Ca-pantothenate, 0.1 mg vitamin B12, 5.0 mg aminobenzoic acid, 5.0 mg lipoic acid. The substances are dissolved in 1 L of deionized water.

10. 70% (v/v) glycerol stock solution, sterile.

11. DMSO (dimethylsulfoxide), sterilized by filtration (PTFE filter).

2.3 Kits and (Restriction) Enzymes

1. Copy control™ Fosmid Library Production Kit with pCC1FOS (Epicentre, Madison, WI, USA).

2. Plasmid isolation mini kit.

3. Gel/PCR DNA purification kit.

4. Restriction enzyme Eco72I (Thermo Scientific, Waltham, MA, USA).

5. Fast AP Thermosensitive Alkaline Phosphatase (Thermo Scientific, Waltham, MA, USA).

3   Methods

All steps for screening metagenomic libraries for hydrogen uptake activity are summarized in Fig. 1.

3.1   Construction of the Metagenomic Library with the Broad Host Range Vector pRS44

3.1.1   Preparation of the Broad Host Range Vector pRS44

1. Prior to ligation, the broad host range vector pRS44 has to be linearized and dephosphorylated: 1 μg of purified fosmid DNA (e.g., by means of a Plasmid isolation mini kit) is digested with 10 U Eco 72I with the corresponding buffer on a 20 μL scale and 1 μL of Fast AP Phosphatase is added.

2. The digestion/dephosphorylation is incubated for 2 h at 37 °C and inactivated at 80 °C for 20 min.

3. The success of the restriction digest is verified by running a standard 0.8 % TAE agarose gel (e.g., 100 V for 30 min).

4. The linearized and dephosphorylated vector is purified using a suitable Gel/PCR DNA purification kit.

5. The vector DNA should be eluted with nuclease-free, deionized water or Tris buffer (pH 8.0). The concentration of the purified vector DNA should at least be 100 ng/μL.

3.1.2   Preparation of Metagenomic DNA

1. The metagenomic DNA should be isolated according to the type of sample/habitat. The concentration should at least be 100 ng/μL and the size should be around 40 kbp.

2. The size of the isolated DNA can be checked by agarose gel electrophoresis (0.8 % TAE agarose gel, 80 V) in comparison to the 42 kbp Fosmid Control DNA provided with the CopyControl™ Fosmid Library Production Kit.

3. For the blunt-end ligation reaction into pRS44, an end-repair reaction has to be performed with the metagenomic DNA according to the manufacturer's protocol of the Copy control™ Fosmid Library Production Kit with pCC1FOS (Epicentre, Madison, WI, USA).

3.1.3   Ligation, Transduction, and Storing of the Metagenomic Library

1. The ligation reaction of the metagenomic DNA into the pRS44 vector and the packaging reaction of the vector construct can be done analogous to the protocol using the pCC1FOS vector. Prior to the "main transduction" the titer of the phage particles should be determined: 2.5, 5, and 10 μL of the packaging reaction are provided in microcentrifuge tubes and 100 μL of exponentially grown *E. coli* EPI300-T1R cells (grown in LB with MgSO₄ and maltose) are added to each tube.

2. The mixtures are incubated at 37 °C (shaking) for 30–60 min.

3. Subsequently the cells are plated onto LB plates containing kanamycin, chloramphenicol, and IPTG/X-Gal (for selection

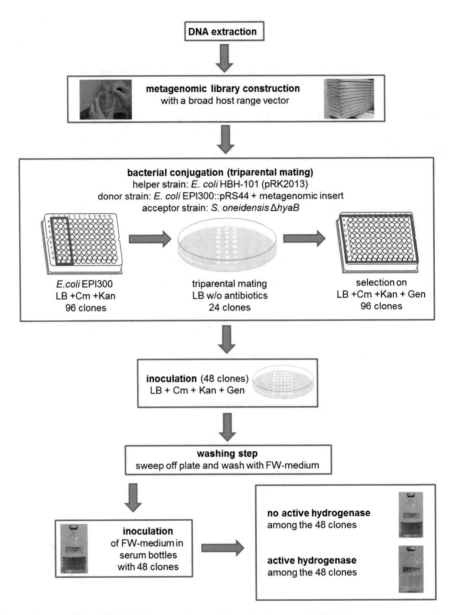

Fig. 1 Flow scheme of the [NiFe]-hydrogenase screening of metagenomic libraries

of clones containing the vector and blue–white screening). The numbers of white colonies (containing vectors with insert DNA) and blue colonies (containing empty vectors) are counted in order to determine the phage particle titer.

4. The final transduction is carried out with the volume of packaging reaction showing the best titer of transduced cells. The number of transduction reactions should be calculated in accordance to the desired number of clones of the metagenomic library.

5. Single white colonies are picked with a sterile toothpick and transferred into 96-well microtiter plates filled with 120 μL LB (+kanamycin and chloramphenicol) per well.

6. The microtiter plates are incubated at 37 °C overnight.

7. Afterward glycerol is added to a final concentration of 35 % (v/v) per well. The plates are stored at –70 °C.

3.2 Screening of Metagenomic Libraries for Hydrogen Uptake Activities

The screening method for hydrogen uptake active metagenomic clones is based on the complementation of the [NiFe]-hydrogenase deletion mutant of *Shewanella oneidensis* MR-1 (*S. oneidensis* Δ*hyaB*). *S. oneidensis* can couple the oxidation of molecular hydrogen to the reduction of Fe-compounds such as Fe(III)citrate [16, 18, 19]. The ability to reduce Fe(III)citrate (yellow) to Fe(II) citrate (colorless) under anaerobic conditions with hydrogen as the sole energy source is used for the detection of hydrogen uptake activity. A color change of the FW-medium from yellow to colorless during anaerobic chemolithotrophic growth shows the hydrogenase activity (Fig. 1, reaction scheme Fig. 2). In *S. oneidensis* Δ*hyaB* the structural gene of the [NiFe]-hydrogenase large subunit (*hyaB*) is deleted and accordingly no color change can be detected. The restoration of the wildtype phenotype by complementation of *S. oneidensis* Δ*hyaB* with the pRS44 vector harboring hydrogenase genes is possible and used for the screening for hydrogen uptake active enzymes. For the screening of metagenomic libraries, fosmids harboring metagenomic DNA are transferred into *S. oneidensis* Δ*hyaB* via triparental mating and pools of 48 conjugated clones are inoculated on FW-medium for the detection of hydrogen uptake activity.

3.2.1 Transfer of Metagenomic Fosmids into S. oneidensis Δ hyaB (See **Note 4**)

1. Precultures (5 mL) of *E. coli* K-12 HBH101 (with the helper plasmid pRK2013) are grown in LB containing kanamycin overnight shaking at 37 °C. *S. oneidensis* Δ*hyaB* (recipient strain) overnight cultures (5 mL) are grown in LB(+gentamycin) shaking at 28 °C. Microtiter plates with metagenomic *E. coli*

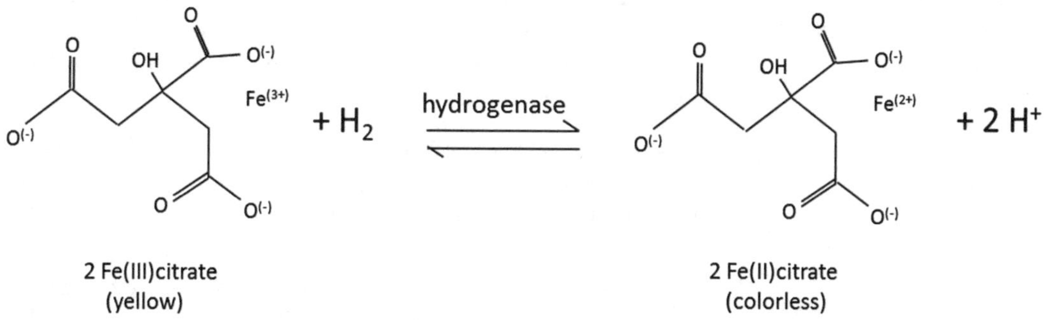

2 Fe(III)citrate (yellow) $+ H_2$ $\xrightarrow{\text{hydrogenase}}$ 2 Fe(II)citrate (colorless) $+ 2 H^+$

Fig. 2 Reaction mechanism of Fe(III)citrate with electrons generated by a hydrogen uptake hydrogenase

clones are inoculated on 96-deep-well plates, containing 1.2 mL LB + kanamycin and chloramphenicol per well, with a replicator tool and incubated shaking overnight at 28 °C.

2. Working cultures of the helper strain and the recipient strain with a volume of each 50 mL are inoculated with the respective overnight cultures and incubated until an OD_{600} of 0.6–0.8 (helper strain) and 4.0–4.5 (recipient strain) respectively is reached.

3. The donor strains (metagenomic *E. coli* clones) are harvested in the deep-well plates at $2250 \times g$ for 20 min at 4 °C and the supernatant is removed. The cell pellets are kept at 4 °C until further used.

4. The helper and recipient strains are harvested at $4500 \times g$ for 20 min at 4 °C and washed with 20 mL LB medium w/o antibiotics. Finally the cell pellets are resuspended in 20 mL of LB w/o antibiotics and pooled together.

5. 50 µL of the helper/recipient suspension per well are used to (column-wise) resuspend the metagenomic donor cells. Subsequently 5 µL of each the conjugation mixtures are pipetted onto LB plates (w/o antibiotics). We recommend to place three columns on one agar plate in order to avoid any mixing of conjugation reactions of individual metagenomic clones. The plates are allowed to dry under the clean bench and then incubated at 28 °C overnight.

6. Cell material of the conjugation reactions of each clone is transferred (e.g., via a multichannel pipette) into wells of a microtiter plate containing 175 µL LB medium + kanamycin, chloramphenicol, and gentamycin. These selection plates are incubated overnight at 28 °C.

7. A volume of 125 µL DMSO is added to each well of the selection plates (final concentration of 12.5 % (v/v)) and the *S. oneidensis* Δ*hyaB* clones now harboring metagenomic fosmids are stored at −70 °C.

*3.2.2 Detection of Hydrogen Uptake Active Clones (See **Note 2**)*

The hydrogen uptake activity of metagenomic *S. oneidensis* Δ*hyaB* clones is detected by a color change of the FW-medium during growth under anaerobic, chemolithotrophic conditions with hydrogen as the sole energy source.

1. *S. oneidensis* Δ*hyaB* harboring pRS44 fosmids with metagenomic inserts are inoculated on LB agar plates (+kanamycin, chloramphenicol, and gentamycin) by means of a 48-pin replicator. The plates are incubated at 28 °C overnight.

2. A negative control (the deletion mutant *S. oneidensis* Δ*hyaB* without any fosmid) is inoculated in 20 mL LB (+gentamycin) and grown overnight shaking at 28 °C.

3. The positive control (*S. oneidensis* Δ*hyaB*::pRS44_So_P5H2) is grown like the negative control but in LB-medium containing kanamycin, chloramphenicol, and gentamycin.

4. Pools of 48 colonies of the metagenomic *S. oneidensis* ΔhyaB clones are washed off the plates with 10 mL of FW-medium. Colonies are removed from the agar surface with a spatula and completely resuspended until they are harvested, in parallel with the negative and positive control, at $4500 \times g$ for 15 min at 4 °C.

5. The supernatants are removed and the cell pellets are washed each with 10 mL of FW-medium for two times. Finally the pellets are resuspended in 5 mL FW-medium and the OD_{600} of the suspensions is determined. If necessary, the suspensions are diluted to a final OD_{600} of 3.0 and four serum bottles per pool/control are inoculated with 400 µL (0.8%) of each of the respective suspensions. The cultures are incubated at 28 °C w/o shaking for a maximum of four weeks or until a color change of the medium occurs in all parallels. The color change of the positive control should occur within four days.

6. If a color change of all parallels occurs, the putative hydrogen uptake active single clone is identified by breaking down the clones in smaller pools in FW-medium, i.e., pools of 16, pools of four clones and then one clone. The putative positive single clones can then be further analyzed, e.g., with sequence analysis of the fosmids and measurements of the specific hydrogen uptake activities [20, 21] and hydrogen consumption rates [22].

4 Notes

1. The color of the FW-medium (prior to inoculation) may vary depending on the type of Fe(III)citrate used for the medium. Fe(III)citrate powder leads to a dark yellow/orange ("LB-like") color whereas the use of crystals results in a bright yellow medium.

2. It is essential to avoid any contamination of the FW-medium with organic compounds (apart from the three amino acids given in the recipe) as *S. oneidensis* is able to use a variety of organic compounds as electron donors and thus could circumvent the need for hydrogenase activity for chemolithotrophic growth. Contamination with organic compounds would therefore lead to false-positive results.

3. Contaminations of FW-medium with higher amounts of oxygen can be seen by a color change to green or black and the formation of precipitates resulting from Fe-oxidation. Cultures showing this color are not able to grow.

4. While pipetting the conjugation reactions onto agar plates avoid any mixing of the individual cultures as it would be very difficult to identify single hydrogen uptake active clones afterwards. We tested different ways for performing the conjugation (e.g., in deep-well and microtiter plates) but petri dishes were the most convenient option concerning the preparation of plates and also provided the best conjugational results.

Acknowledgments

We are indebted to Dr. Kai Thormann for providing us with the suicide vector pNTPS138-R6KT and the *Shewanella oneidensis* MR-1 strain. We also greatly appreciate that Prof. Svein Valla supplied the pRS44 broad-host range fosmid vector and the appendant pTA66 plasmid. We thank Nicolas Rychlik for constructing the *S. oneidensis* Δ*hyaB* mutant and for support with developing the screen. This work was supported by the research grant DFG PE1549-6/1 from the German Science Foundation.

References

1. Schlapbach L, Zuttel A (2001) Hydrogen-storage materials for mobile applications. Nature 414:353–358

2. Karyakin AA, Morozov SV, Karyakina EE, Zorin NA, Perelygin VV, Cosnier S (2005) Hydrogenase electrodes for fuel cells. Biochem Soc Trans 33:73–75

3. Armstrong FA, Belsey NA, Cracknell JA, Goldet G, Parkin A, Reisner E et al (2009) Dynamic electrochemical investigations of hydrogen oxidation and production by enzymes and implications for future technology. Chem Soc Rev 38:36–51

4. Wait AF, Parkin A, Morley GM, dos Santos L, Armstrong FA (2010) Characteristics of enzyme-based hydrogen fuel cells using an oxygen-tolerant hydrogenase as the anodic catalyst. J Phys Chem C 114:12003–12009

5. Tang KH, Tang YJ, Blankenship RE (2011) Carbon metabolic pathways in phototrophic bacteria and their broader evolutionary implications. Front Microbiol 2:165

6. Bothe H, Schmitz O, Yates MG, Newton WE (2010) Nitrogen fixation and hydrogen metabolism in cyanobacteria. Microbiol Mol Biol Rev 74:529–551

7. Dilling W, Cypionka H (1990) Aerobic respiration in sulfate-reducing bacteria. FEMS Microbiol Lett 71:123–127

8. Hügler M, Sievert SM (2011) Beyond the Calvin cycle: autotrophic carbon fixation in the ocean. Ann Rev Mar Sci 3:261–289

9. Hallenbeck PC (2009) Fermentative hydrogen production: principles, progress, and prognosis. Int J Hydrog Energy 34:7379–7389

10. Vignais PM, Billoud B (2007) Occurrence, classification, and biological function of hydrogenases: an overview. Chem Rev 107:4206–4272

11. Perner M, Gonnella G, Kurtz S, LaRoche J (2014) Handling temperature bursts reaching 464°C: different microbial strategies in the Sisters Peak hydrothermal chimney. Appl Environ Microbiol 80:4585–4598

12. Constant P, Chowdhury SP, Hesse L, Pratscher J, Conrad R (2011) Genome data mining and soil survey for the novel group 5 [NiFe]-hydrogenase to explore the diversity and ecological importance of presumptive high-affinity H(2)-oxidizing bacteria. Appl Environ Microbiol 77:6027–6035

13. Vargas W, Weyman P, Tong Y, Smith H, Xu Q (2011) A [NiFe]-hydrogenase from *Alteromonas macleodii* with unusual stability in the presence of oxygen and high temperature. Appl Environ Microbiol 77:1990–1998

14. Maroti G, Tong Y, Yooseph S, Baden-Tillson H, Smith HO, Kovacs KL et al (2009) Discovery of [NiFe] hydrogenase genes in

metagenomic DNA: cloning and heterologous expression in *Thiocapsa roseopersicina*. Appl Environ Microbiol 75:5821–5830

15. Aakvik T, Degnes KF, Dahlsrud R, Schmidt F, Dam R, Yu L et al (2009) A plasmid RK2-based broad-host-range cloning vector useful for transfer of metagenomic libraries to a variety of bacterial species. FEMS Microbiol Lett 296:149–158

16. Lovley DR, Phillips EJ, Lonergan DJ (1989) Hydrogen and formate oxidation coupled to dissimilatory reduction of iron or manganese by *Alteromonas putrefaciens*. Appl Environ Microbiol 55:700–706

17. Balch WE, Fox GE, Magrum LJ, Woese CR, Wolfe RS (1979) Methanogens: reevaluation of a unique biological group. Microbiol Rev 43:260–296

18. Myers CR, Myers JM (1993) Ferric reductase is associated with the membranes of anaerobically grown *Shewanella putrefaciens* Mr-1. FEMS Microbiol Lett 108:15–22

19. Meshulam-Simon G, Behrens S, Choo AD, Spormann AM (2007) Hydrogen metabolism in *Shewanella oneidensis* MR-1. Appl Environ Microbiol 73:1153–1165

20. Guiral M, Tron P, Belle V, Aubert C, Leger C, Guigliarelli B, Giudici-Orticoni MT (2006) Hyperthermostable and oxygen resistant hydrogenases from a hyperthermophilic bacterium *Aquifex aeolicus*: physicochemical properties. Int J Hydrog Energy 31:1424–1431

21. Ishii M, Takishita S, Iwasaki T, Peerapornpisal Y, Yoshino J, Kodama T, Igarashi Y (2000) Purification and characterization of membrane-bound hydrogenase from *Hydrogenobacter thermophilus* strain TK-6, an obligately autotrophic, thermophilic, hydrogen-oxidizing bacterium. Biosci Biotechnol Biochem 64:492–502

22. Hansen M, Perner M (2015) A novel hydrogen oxidizer amidst the sulfur-oxidizing *Thiomicrospira* lineage. ISME J 9:696–707

Chapter 18

Screening for *N*-AHSL-Based-Signaling Interfering Enzymes

Stéphane Uroz and Phil M. Oger

Abstract

Quorum sensing (QS)-based signaling is a widespread pathway used by bacteria for the regulation of functions involved in their relation to the environment or their host. QS relies upon the production, accumulation and perception of small diffusable molecules by the bacterial population, hence linking high gene expression with high cell population densities. Among the different QS signal molecules, an important class of signal molecules is the *N*-acyl homoserine lactone (*N*-AHSL). In pathogens such as *Erwinia* or *Pseudomonas*, *N*-AHSL based QS is crucial to overcome the host defenses and ensure a successful infection. Interfering with QS-regulation allows the algae *Delisea pulcra* to avoid surface colonization by bacteria. Thus, interfering the QS-regulation of pathogenic bacteria is a promising antibiotic-free antibacterial therapeutic strategy. To date, two *N*-AHSL lactonases and one amidohydrolase families of *N*-ASHL degradation enzymes have been characterized and have proven to be efficient in vitro to control *N*-AHSL-based QS-regulated functions in pathogens. In this chapter, we provide methods to screen individual clones or bacterial strains as well as pool of clones for genomic and metagenomic libraries, that can be used to identify strains or clones carrying *N*-ASHL degradation enzymes.

Key words *N*-acyl homoserine lactone, Quorum sensing, Quorum quenching, *N*-AHSL lactonase, *N*-AHSL acylase, *N*-AHSL amidohydrolase

1 Introduction

Gram negative bacteria couple gene expression to population density by a regulatory mechanism named quorum sensing (QS). QS relies upon the production and the perception of one or more signal molecules by the bacterial population [1, 2]. An important class of these signals is the N-acyl homoserine lactone (*N*-AHSL) class. QS regulates pathogenicity, or pathogenicity-related functions, in bacteria of medical or environmental importance such as the human pathogen *Pseudomonas aeruginosa*, or the plant pathogens *Erwinia carotovora* and *Agrobacterium tumefaciens* [3, 4]. If QS is an important component of the adaptation strategy of bacteria to their environment, one might suspect that competing bacteria/eukarya might have developed strategies to interfere with this communication system.

Wolfgang R. Streit and Rolf Daniel (eds.), *Metagenomics: Methods and Protocols*, Methods in Molecular Biology, vol. 1539, DOI 10.1007/978-1-4939-6691-2_18, © Springer Science+Business Media LLC 2017

Indeed QS interference was reported through the production of antagonists or the production of *N*-AHSL degradation enzymes (*N*-AHSLases) in various organisms from human, plant, and fungi to bacteria using cultivation-dependent [5–7] or cultivation-independent approaches [8, 9]. Whatever the physiological role of the *N*-AHSLases in their host, they have been used to interfere efficiently with the expression of QS regulated functions in bacteria [7]. Thus interfering with QS-regulation, a strategy coined the term quorum-quenching appears as one of the promising non-antibiotic-based therapeutic strategies for the future [8–10].

N-AHSLs exhibit a conserved structure, with a backbone composed of a lactone ring derived from the lactonization of homoserine, *N*-linked to an acyl chain via an amide bond (Fig. 1). Variation in *N*-acyl chain length and the oxidation status of *N*-AHSLs provides for specificity of the signal. Four chemical or enzymatic alterations of the structure are known to occur (Fig. 1), two of which, lactonolysis and amidohydrolysis, generate QS inactive molecules. Amidohydrolysis cleaves the *N*-AHSL molecule irreversibly into two QS inactive molecules, homoserine lactone (HSL) and the corresponding acyl chain. On the contrary, lactonolysis is a reversible reaction opening the lactone ring of the HSL moiety to yield *N*-acyl homoserine (*N*-AHS). It occurs

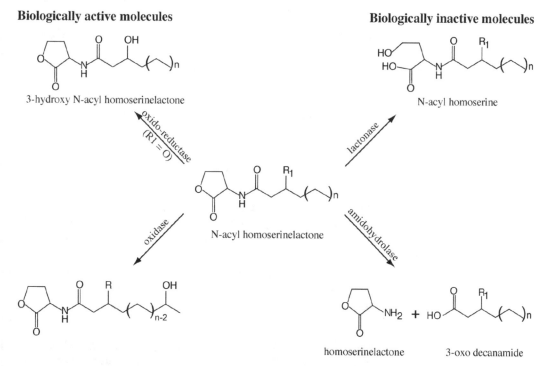

Biologically active molecules

3-hydroxy N-acyl homoserinelactone

Biologically inactive molecules

N-acyl homoserine

oxido-reductase (R1 = O)

lactonase

oxidase

N-acyl homoserinelactone

amidohydrolase

homoserinelactone   3-oxo decanamide

Fig. 1 *N*-AHSL chemical and enzymatic alterations. *Center.* Common structure of *N*-AHSLs (R1 = OH or 0; $0 \leq n \leq 6$). *Left.* Biologically active derivatives of *N*-AHSL following oxidase and oxido-reductase attacks. *Right.* Biologically inactive *N*-AHSL derivatives following lactonase or amidohydrolase degradation

spontaneously under basic pH, while low pH favors the recircular-
ization of the lactone [11]. Despite the large diversity of *N*-AHSL-
degrading organisms identified to date, only three families of
N-AHSL-inactivating enzymes have been described: the AiiA and
QsdA *N*-AHSL lactonase families [7, 12] and the AiiD [13]
N-AHSL amidohydrolase (or acylase) family. Since they irreversibly cleave the signal molecule, *N*-AHSL amidohydrolases have a
greater biotechnological potential than *N*-AHSL lactonases (*see*
Note 1). A short procedure, applicable from wild-type environmental isolates, genomic and metagenomic libraries to purified
proteins alike, allows to quickly screen for and characterize these
enzymes.

2   Materials

2.1   Strains and Growth Media for Cell Cultures

1. *N*-AHSL sensor systems (*see* **Note 2**): Sensor system for 3-oxo and 3-hydroxy *N*-AHSL (3O, and 3OH, *N*-AHSL respec-tively) *Agrobacterium tumefaciens* strain NTL4(pZLR4) [14]. This strain should be maintained and cultured on gentamycin 100 mg/L.

2. Sensor system for short chain *N*-AHSLs *Chromobacterium violaceum* strain CV026 [15]. This strain should be cultured on Luria Broth with 5 g NaCl per liter. It cannot be maintained for long periods on plates, and should be streaked regularly from frozen stocks.

3. Low salt Luria Broth (5 g NaCl/L, Gibco). When necessary this medium is buffered to pH = 6.5 with 100 mM phosphate buffer to avoid spontaneous degradation of *N*-AHSLs. To pre-pare 1 L of pH = 6.5-buffered LB dissolve 20 g of LB powder into 900 mL of water, then add 27.8 mL of 1 M K_2HPO_4 and 72.2 mL of 1 M KH_2PO_4. Sterilize by autoclaving.

4. AB minimal medium is prepared from stock solutions of 20× AB salts and 20× AB buffer and sterile water for liquid media and sterile water agar for solid media. 20× AB salts (per liter): 20 g NH_4Cl, 6 g $MgSO_4 \cdot 7H_2O$, 3 g KCl, 200 mg $CaCl_2$, 50 mg $FeSO_4 \cdot 7H_2O$; Sterilize by autoclaving. 20× AB Buffer (per liter): 60 g K_2HPO_4, 23 g NaH_2PO_4; Adjust the pH to 7 if necessary; Sterilize by autoclaving. 5 mM mannitol from a stock solution at 100 mM is added as a carbon source. When necessary gentamycin (100 mg/L) and X-gal (40 mg/L) are added to the medium.

5. Phosphate buffered saline solution (PBS 1×): 8 g NaCl, 0.2 g KCl, 1.44 g Na_2HPO_4, 0.24 g KH_2PO_4; Dissolve in 800 mL of distilled H_2O. Adjust the pH to 6.5 with HCl. Add H_2O to 1 L. Sterilize by autoclaving.

2.2 N-AHSL Degradation Assays

1. Transilluminator, 315 nm.
2. N-AHSL solutions in ethyl acetate (1 mM and 10 µM). Most N-AHSLs can be purchased from Sigma-Aldrich (Sigma-Aldrich, St. Louis, MO). The others can be purchased from Pr. Paul Williams (Nottingham University, UK).
3. Dansyl chloride (3.7 M in acetone stock solution).
4. HCl 5 and 0.2 M.
5. HPLC grade dichloromethane.
6. HPLC grade acetonitrile (Sigma-Aldrich, St. Louis, MO).
7. HPLC grade ethyl acetate (Sigma-Aldrich, St. Louis, MO).
8. Bradford kit for protein quantification (Sigma-Aldrich, St. Louis, MO).

2.3 Thin Layer Chromatography

1. Whatman 3MM filter paper (Whatman, Springfield Mill, UK).
2. Glass TLC Developing Tank for 20 cm×20 cm TLC plates (Whatman, Springfield Mill, UK).
3. Glass C18 coated TLC plates with 200 µm coating. We use Partisil® KC18 TLC plates, Silica gel 60 Å (Whatman, Springfield Mill, UK).
4. Methanol, analytical grade (Sigma-Aldrich, St. Louis, MO).
5. Overlay preparation: Sterilize by autoclaving 88 mL of soft water agar (7 g/L), then add to the medium 5 mL of each 20× AB salts and 20× AB buffer and 2 mL of 100 mM mannitol solution. Cool until it reaches ~50–55 °C, then add 150 µL of X-gal (40 mg/mL).
6. Custom made TLC overlaying container (*see* **Note 3**). This container is made out of 5 mm thick plexiglass. The base of the container is a 25 cm wide square, in which four 3 cm-wide holes placed approximately 5 cm from each corner along the diagonals have been drilled. These holes allow the user to access the plate from underneath and push to release it after the overlay has solidified. 2 cm wide bars are glued on top of the base form a 20.2 cm×20.2 cm 5 mm deep internal space which will accept the TLC plate. It is important to allow some extra spacing around the TLC to facilitate the extraction of the plate after solidification of the agar. The thickness of the overlay is 3 mm.

2.4 HPLC

1. Waters 625 HPLC system (Waters Corp., Millford, MA) coupled with a Waters 996 PDA photodiode array detector (operating with a Millennium 2010 Chromatography Manager) equipped with a Kromasil C8 5 µm column, 2.1×250 mm (Jones Chromatography, Mid Glamorgan, UK) or equivalent for the identification of amidohydrolysis degradation products.

2. Waters HPLC system equipped with a Waters separation module 2659 coupled to a Waters Micromass ZQ200 electrospray ionization-mass spectrometry detector and an Atlantis T3 Reverse-Phase column, 4.6 × 150 mm (Waters Corp., Millford, MA) for the detection of lactonolysis identification products.

3 Methods

Since the discovery of the QS regulation system, several very sensitive sensor strains have been designed for N-AHSL detection. These are based on the same principle: the gene responsible for the synthesis of the N-AHSL has been mutated, and can only respond to the exogenous N-AHSLs. Reporter genes can be either native, such as the production of the violacein pigment in the *Chromobacterium* sensor system [15], or engineered, such as to produce β-galactosidase in the *Agrobacterium* sensor system [14].

The screen for N-AHSL degradation enzymes proceeds in four steps if the screening is performed with bacterial strains or clones (individual tests), or five steps when using pools of clones from genomic and metagenomic libraries (mixed cloned tests). The four steps required for the identification of positive clones in individual tests include: First, a test to determine the capacity of bacterial strains or clones to inhibit one of the QS sensor systems (Subheading 3.1). This first step is not specific for N-AHSL degradation enzymes, but allows to screen the molecules/activities that may inhibit the detection of the N-AHSL by the sensor, including molecules that might interfere with its growth. Second, a test to determine the ability of each clone/strain to degrade N-AHSLs or inhibit their detection (Subheading 3.2). The third step allows to differentiate between lactonases and amidohydrolases (Subheading 3.3). The fourth step is a confirmation of this differentiation in which the degradation products of the N-AHSLs are characterized (Subheading 3.4). When screening genomic/metagenomic libraries, clones are tested in pools to increase the cost and time efficiency of the detection. The above procedure allows the detection of clone pools containing one or several positive clones, which are further identified by running each clone independently using the same procedure. Practically, we found that using pools of ca. 50 clones was the best compromise. It is thus better to have an estimate of the number of individual clones in the library to be tested. Assuming this, this approach allows a fast and cost-effective screen of high density libraries.

3.1 Preparation of Resting Cells (RC) and Cell Crude Extracts (CCE) for N-AHSL Degradation Assays [17]

3.1.1 Preparation of RC

1. Grow cells in LB until late exponential phase.

2. Pellet the cells by centrifugation. Resuspend the cells in PBS. Adjust the cell concentration to 10^9 cells/mL by measuring the OD at 600 nm.

3. Wash cells twice in 1/10th volume of PBS buffer (pH = 6.5).

4. Resuspend the cells in 1/10th volume of PBS buffer (pH = 6.5). Cell concentration of RC is 10^{10} cells/mL.

3.1.2 Preparation of CCE

1. Cycle the RC suspension five times in a cell disrupter (Constant Systems Cell Disrupter) under 15 kPa pressure.

2. Remove Cell debris by centrifugation (120 min, 4 °C, $10,000 \times g$).

3. Filter the supernatant through a 0.22 μm membrane.

4. Adjust the protein concentration to 0.5 mg/mL using the Bradford Protein Quantification method and store at 4 °C.

3.2 Microplate Fast Screening of N-AHSL Degradation Individual Clones [16] (Sub heading 3.2.1) or Mixed Pools of Clones (Subheading 3.2.2)

3.2.1 Screen of Pure Strains, Clones or Isolates

1. Grow the bacterial clones in 200 μL of LB supplemented with the appropriate antibiotics in microtiter plates for 24 h at 30 °C (or 37 °C for *E. coli*) (*see* **Note 4**).

2. Subculture the clones into 200 μL of fresh pH = 6.5-buffered LB medium without antibiotics but supplemented with 25 μM of the appropriate N-AHSL. Incubate for up to 2 days at 25 °C (*see* **Note 4**). Since N-AHSL may be spontaneously degraded in buffered LB medium over long incubation period, it is important to include a spontaneous degradation control. It consists of a non inoculated growth medium supplemented with the same amount of N-AHSL.

3. Transfer 5 μL aliquots of the bacterial suspensions to a 96-well microtiter plate containing 200 μL of solidified, pH = 6.5-buffered LB agar (16 g/L) medium. Kill the bacteria by UV irradiation by placing the microtiter plates upside-down on a transilluminator for 10 min.

4. Overlay the wells with 10 μL of an overnight culture of the reporter strain *Chromobacterium violaceum* CV026.

5. Monitor violacein (purple pigment) production after 24 h of incubation at 28 °C.

6. Wells in which no violacein production occurs are indicative of putative positive N-AHSL degrading clones/strains (Fig. 2). ATTENTION: The lack of violacein production may also reflect other activities due to molecules inhibiting the growth of the sensor, or inhibiting the recognition of the N-AHSLs by the sensor. Thus, the ability of the positive clones to effectively degrade the N-AHSLs needs to be confirmed by separating the degradation products by TLC (*see* Subheading 3.4).

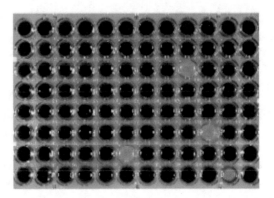

Fig. 2 *N*-AHSL degradation microplate assay of *E. coli* clones expressing a genomic bank of the *Rhodococcus erythropolis* strain W2 imaged after 24 h of incubation. Colorless wells indicate *N*-AHSL degradation [12]

3.2.2 Screen of Mixed Pools of Clones

1. Dilute the total library in the appropriate volume of pH = 6.5-buffered liquid LB supplemented with 12.5 mg/L of chloramphenicol, to reach ca. 50 cells per 150 μL.

2. Transfer 150 μL of this bacterial suspension in the wells of microtiter plates. Thus, each well will have a set of 50 cells. At this step it is important to know the number of independent clones present in your library, since it will determine the number of microtiter plates that you will have to set up to test all clones (*see* **Note 5**).

3. Grow the bacterial clones for 24 h at 37 °C.

4. From this step, the test of mixed pools is essentially the same as that described above for individual clones with an adaptation of volumes and incubation times.

5. Add 50 μL of pH = 6.5-buffered LB supplemented 100 μM the appropriate *N*-ASHL, to obtain a final concentration of 25 μM. Incubate for up to 2 days at 25 °C (*see* **Note 4**). Since *N*-AHSL may be spontaneously degraded in buffered LB medium over long incubation period or by the library host *E. coli*, it is important to include: (1) a spontaneous degradation control, which consists of a non inoculated growth medium supplemented with the same amount of *N*-AHSL; and (2) a well inoculated with *E. coli* with an empty vector.

6. Proceed as in **steps 3–6** of Subheading 3.1. *Important*: Remember to keep the microtiter plates containing the pools incubated in LB supplemented 25 μM *N*-ASHL at 4 °C to stop *E. coli* development until biosensor revelation, since it will be the source for the purification of the positive clones.

7. Wells in which no violacein production occurs are indicative of putative positive *N*-AHSL degrading pool. As it results from the activity of a mix of clones, the active clones need to be identified and isolated.

8. To avoid false positives, the activity of the positive pools are first confirmed. Localize the position of the positive pool(s) in the liquid LB growth medium in **step 4**, and perform an independent serial dilution (from 10^{-1} to 10^{-9}) in liquid LB supplemented 25 µM N-ASHL for each positive well.

9. Grow the serial dilutions for 24 h at 25 °C.

10. Repeat **steps 3–6** of Subheading 3.1.

11. Consider the dilution for which N-AHSL degradation is observed and plate the content of the related microtiter plate well on solid LB medium supplemented with chloramphenicol.

12. Recover independent clones by hand or using a colony picking system if available, and test each clone as described in Subheading 3.1 to identify N-AHSL degrading clones.

3.3 N-AHSL Lactonase and Acylase Activity Screen/N-AHSL Degradation Confirmation Test

Positive wells in the microplate assay group bacterial strains or clones capable of N-AHSL degradation as well as strains/clones with sensor interfering abilities. To detect the fraction of N-AHSL degraders, N-AHSLs and putative inhibitory molecules present in the growth medium are separated by thin layer chromatography, and detected using the QS sensor. Only clones with N-AHSL degradation abilities will fail to induce the QS sensor in both assays (For the detection of false-positive clones, proceed directly to Subheading 3.3.2, **step 10**).

The same approach is used to differentiate clones harboring lactonase and amidohydrolase activities. Lactonolysis of N-AHSLs yields N-acyl homoserine (Fig. 1). This reaction is reversible under low pH, and the N-AHSL molecule can thus be regenerated [12, 18]. On the contrary, the amidohydrolysis is irreversible. This divergence is exploited in a test to quickly differentiate lactonases from acylases in which one runs side by side on a TLC plate the products of a N-AHSL degradation reaction and a subsample acidified to induce lactonization (Fig. 3).

3.3.1 Preparation of the Samples [17]

1. To a clean 2 mL microcentrifuge tube add 50 µL of a 10 µM N-AHSL stock solution. Evaporate to dryness (*see* **Notes 6** and **7**).

2. Add 500 µL of RC to the tube. Vortex for 1 min to dissolve the N-AHSL (*see* **Note 8**).

3. Incubate for up to 6 h at 25 °C (*see* **Note 9**).

4. Centrifuge the tube at full speed to pellet the cells. Transfer the supernatant into two clean 2 mL microcentrifuge tubes (250 µL each).

5. In the first tube, add 1 volume of ethyl acetate to stop and extract the reaction. Vortex for 1 min. Allow the aqueous and ethyl acetate phases to separate for 10 min or centrifuge for 1 min. Transfer the upper phase to a clean tube and evaporate to dryness.

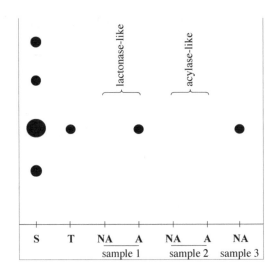

Separation by TLC
Detection with N-AHSL biosensor

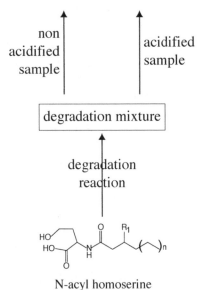

N-acyl homoserine

Fig. 3 *N*-AHSL Lactonase/acylase differentiation scheme. For each reaction, one sample is acidified (A) and the remnant is not (NA). Sample 1 and 2 present a sketch of results obtained for a lactonase and amidohydrolase respectively. S: *N*-AHSL set of synthetic standards. Sample 3 presents a sketch of results obtained for a false-positive clone in the microplate assay. T: Positive control, undigested *N*-AHSL

6. To the second tube add 5 M HCl to acidify the medium to pH = 2.

7. Incubate for 24 h at 4 °C.

8. Stop and extract the reaction as indicated in **step 5**.

9. Dissolve the residues in 100 µL of ethyl acetate (*see* **Note 10**).

1. These instructions assume the use of 20×20 cm glass TLC plates, an *Agrobacterium* based *N*-AHSL detection system and a custom made TLC overlaying container (*see* **Note 11**).

2. Transfer a single colony of the bacterial sensor strain into 5 mL of AB medium supplemented with 5 mM mannitol and genta-mycin (100 µg/mL). Incubate overnight at 30 °C under vigorous shaking.

3. The next morning, transfer the 5 mL preculture into 45 mL of the same medium. Incubate at 30 °C until late exponential phase, ca. 6 h.

4. Mark the spotting line on a clean TLC plate with a pencil. Care should be taken during the manipulations to avoid dropping organics accidentally onto the TLC plates. Samples should be spotted 2 cm from the bottom of the plate, 2 cm apart from each other. Mark a line 15 cm above from depot line as a guide to know when to stop the chromatography.

5. Spot 1 µL of each samples and standards. Standards should comprise at the least the original *N*-AHSL (*see* **Note 12**).

6. Wait until TLC is dry.

7. Fill the Glass TLC developing tank with 200 mL of running solution (methanol–water, 60:40, v:v).

8. Cover the inside of the glass TLC developing tank with running solution saturated Whatman 3MM paper. This step is important to get a linear running front in large TLC developing tanks.

9. Run the plate until it reaches the top line, approximately 2 h.

10. Take the plate out and dry in a fume hood for 10 min.

11. Mix the reporter strain culture (50 mL) with the cooled overlay medium (100 mL) by shaking gently to avoid the formation of bubbles.

12. Place the plate in the custom-made overlaying container, and gently pour the overlay on the plate. Remove the excess of medium and bubbles by running a plastic ruler over the container (*see* **Note 13**).

13. Wait until the soft agar has solidified.

14. Loosen the medium from the sides of the container with a flat spatula to take the plate out of the container.

15. Place the overlaid TLC plate in a plastic container with a paper towel at the bottom (*see* **Note 14**). The paper towel is used to help take the plate out of container after incubation.

16. Incubate the plate with lid closed overnight at 28 °C.

17. The plate should show blue dots according to the standard used. Plate are ready to be imaged, if the color is sufficiently

developed. The drying of the plate greatly improves the contrast, but may not be necessary if only presence or absence of a given spot is needed. It is however convenient for the storage of the revealed TLC. To dry the plates proceed as follows.

18. Remove the plate from the plastic container and place in the back of a fume hood to dry. Take the plate out of the hood when the plate is close to completely dried. Over-drying the plate results in the curling of the C18-layer and to crack. Let the plate sit at room temperature to completely dry slowly.

3.3.3 Interpretation of TLC Plates (See **Note 15**)

1. The presence of a lactonase activity will be evidenced by the presence of a blue spot in the acidified sample lane with a Rf identical to, e.g., migrating at the same distance as, the starting N-AHSL (Fig. 3, sample 1, lane A), concomitant with the absence of a spot in the non acidified sample (Fig. 3, sample 1 lane NA).

2. The absence of spots in both acidified and non-acidified lanes is evidence for a degradation activity not involving a lactonase, e.g., to date indication of an amidohydrolase activity (Fig. 3, Sample 2).

3. False-positive clones for the degradation of N-AHSLs will be evidenced after TLC separation by the presence of a spot with a Rf identical to the starting N-AHSL in the NA lane (Sample 3).

3.4 Identification of N-AHSL Lactonase Activities by HPLC-MS

1. N-AHSL degradation reactions are set as described above for the TLC plate assay, except that one should use 50 μL of a 1 mM N-AHSL solution, stop the complete reaction after the appropriate incubation time and dissolve the reaction in 50 μL of ethyl acetate (*see* **Note 8**).

2. Inject 10 μL of the reaction mixture into the HPLC system.

3. Elution: Water/formic acid 0.1 % (solvent A) and acetonitrile/formic acid 0.1 % (solvent B) under the following elution sequence: 100 % A 5 min; linear gradient 100 % A 0 % B to reach 80 % A and 20 % B 5 min; 80 % A and 20 % B 10 min. Between two samples, the column is rinsed by applying a linear gradient to reach 100 % B (2 min), and 100 % B (3 min). Column is then re-equilibrated with 100 % A for 7 min at a flow rate of 2 mL/min (*see* **Note 16**).

4. Under our experimental conditions, the C6-HS and C6-HSL harbors retention times of 15.81 and 21.00 min respectively (Fig. 4). Retention times and mass spectra for individual standard molecules in solution need to be obtained in the same conditions. Degradation of the N-AHSL is evidenced by the reduction of the surface of the N-AHSL characteristic peak and concomitant increase in the surface of the N-AHS peak.

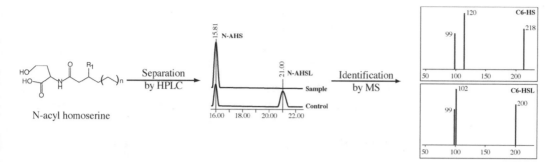

Fig. 4 Identification scheme for *N*-AHSL lactonase activities

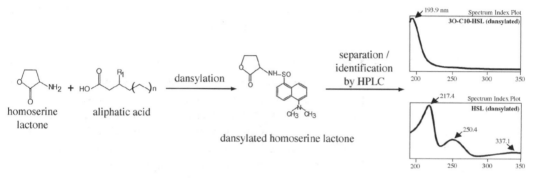

Fig. 5 Identification scheme for *N*-AHSL amidohydrolase activities

5. The identification of the degradation products is confirmed by mass spectrometry in comparison with those of the synthetic *N*-AHSL and *N*-AHS standards subjected to the same HPLC-MS/MS conditions. The specific fragments expected to appear in the mass spectra of *N*-AHSL and its corresponding *N*-AHS should differ in size by one water molecule, e.g., 18 units (see example in Fig. 4).

3.5 Detection of N-AHSL Acylase Activities by HPLC [17]

1. The scheme used to detect the degradation products of *N*-AHSL following amidohydrolysis involves the chemical trapping of the free amine of the newly formed HSL (Fig. 5). As a consequence, it is best to use crude or purified protein extracts at this step (*see* **Note 17**).

2. To a clean 2 mL microcentrifuge tube, add 50 μL of a 1 mM *N*-AHSL stock solution. Evaporate the ethyl acetate to dryness.

3. Add 500 μL of crude bacterial cell extract to the tube. Vortex for 1 min to dissolve the *N*-AHSL.

4. Incubate for up to 6 h at 25 °C (*see* **Note 9**).

5. Add 25 μL of dansyl chloride solution to a final concentration of 185 mM.

6. Perform a control reaction with synthetic HSL in the same reaction conditions.

7. Incubate for 1 h at room temperature with frequent shaking (*see* **Note 18**).

8. Extract the reaction with 1 volume of dichloromethane. Transfer the upper phase to a clean tube and evaporate to dryness.

9. Dissolve in 50 µL HCl 0.2 N to hydrolyze the excess of dansyl chloride.

10. Extract with 50 µL of acetone.

11. Inject 10 µL of the reaction mixture in the Waters 625 HPLC system equipped with the C8 column. Detection of the dansyl moieties is performed with the Waters 996 PDA photodiode array detector.

12. Elution of the sample is performed in isocratic conditions with acetonitrile/water (35% acetonitrile in water) over a 30 min period at a flow rate of 2 mL/min. In these experimental conditions, dansylated homoserine lactone harbors a retention time of 6.5 min. The confirmation of identification of the dansylated homoserine lactone is obtained by plotting the Spectrum Index Plot and comparing with the spectra obtained for the control reaction (Fig. 5).

4   Notes

1. Since the oxidoreduction of *N*-AHSLs generates alternate forms of the *N*-AHSL molecules, they have a lesser biotechnological potential. As a consequence of their retaining biological activity, the procedure described here will be inadequate to screen for these activities.

2. Several other sensors strains based on the same or different QS systems are available [20]. The procedure presented here could easily be adapted for these sensors.

3. If one does not have the use of a home made container, a single use container can be made out by taping all four sides of the TLC plate. Make sure the tape is properly sealed to avoid leaks. This is easily obtained if the tape also covers part of the reverse side of the TLC plate. This system does not allow the removal of bubble or the adjustment of the overlay thickness.

4. This screen can be used to screen virtually any type of microbial cell type/protein, from bacteria to fungi, from wild-type strains to clones overexpressing cloned *N*-AHSL degradation genes, from growing cells to purified proteins. Thus, it may be necessary to adjust the incubation time for each condition.

5. This step involves being able to know (1) the exact number of individual clones forming the library (titration) and (2) the number of colony forming unit of the library (cell density). For classical soil metagenomic libraries, titration of 10^5 clones is obtained. If the library considered is not subculti-vated, the number of clones is equivalent to the number of cfu. In this case, dilute the original library in a volume of LB to obtain 333 cfu per mL (equivalent to 50 cfu in 150 µL of culture medium). It is our experience that pools of 50 cfu give the best compromise between the cost and time reduction due to pooling and the reproducibility of the detection of N-AHSL degradation. If the library considered has been subcultivated, then the number of cfu will be higher than the actual tiration of the library. The number of microtiter plate wells to inoculate to test the library is calculated by dividing the titration by 50. Each well is inoculated as described above with 150 µL a 333 cells/mL dilution of the library. Thus, in both cases, the test of 10^5 clones will require ca. 300 mL of a suspension of 50 cfu/mL and ten 96-well microtiter plates. It is essential for the success of this approach that the number of cells inoculated in each well is around 50. If a higher number of clones is used, the degradation may fail due to the dilution of the positive clones. Furthermore, it may become difficult to recover individual clones from the pools.

6. The procedure to follow to assay for "false-positives" isolated in the microplate assay is essentially the same except that one just needs to run the original degradation reaction after extraction with 1 volume of ethyl acetate. Then proceed directly to **step 10**.

7. It is recommended to evaporate the N-AHSLs under a flux of nitrogen to avoid chemical alteration.

8. The same procedure can be followed with CCE or purified N-AHSL lactonases.

9. Incubation times and buffer conditions may have to be adapted to reflect these systems.

10. Sensor systems will differ from one sensor to the other. Reference concentrations for each N-AHSL can be found for the *Agrobacterium* and *Chromobacterium* sensor system in [19] and [15], respectively.

11. The TLC plate assay is easily adaptable to other sensor systems. To use it with the *Chromobacterium violaceum* sensor CV026 proceed as noted above with the following modifications. The sensor culture is a 5 mL culture of CV026 grown overnight at 30 °C. The overlay is composed of LB soft (7 g/L) agar (150 mL) to which the sensor culture is added.

12. The concentration of recircularized *N*-AHSL is difficult to estimate; since *N*-AHS might be further metabolized by some microorganisms. Thus it might be necessary to spot different volumes of the acidified sample. No more than 5 μL of sample should be spotted to limit the diffusion of the product in the TLC.

13. We have noticed that some batch of TLC plates have a tendency to form bubbles at the interface between the TLC layer and overlay. It is important to remove those bubbles because they prevent the contact between the overlay and TLC, thus the transfer of the *N*-AHSL into the overlay and subsequently the induction of the sensor. These bubbles may be removed with extreme care to avoid damaging the layer of the TLC using a small rounded spatula.

14. Square 245 mm culture dishes are most convenient. Dishes can be reused.

15. The TLC approach also has the potential to identify the oxido-reductase and oxidase activities since the Rf and shape of the spot of the QS-active derivatives are different from the starting *N*-AHSL. In this case, spots with specific Rf and shapes different from the *N*-AHSL would be seen in both A and NA lanes. However, clones harboring such activities do not pass the microplate screening step because they generate QS-active derivatives.

16. Elution conditions may need to be adapted for the best separation of different *N*-AHSLs.

17. The same procedure can be followed with purified proteins, but may require adaptation of buffer and incubation times.

18. The optimal temperature for the dansylation reaction is 37 °C. However, incubating at this temperature favors the opening of the lactone ring. Thus it is preferable to incubate at room temperature although the reaction is less efficient.

References

1. Winans SC, Bassler BL (2002) Mob psychology. J Bacteriol 184:873–883

2. Reading NC, Sperandio V (2006) Quorum sensing: the many languages of bacteria. FEMS Microbiol Lett 254:1–11

3. Hassett DJ, Ma JF, Elkins JG, McDermott TR, Ochsner UA, West SE et al (1999) Quorum sensing in *Pseudomonas aeruginosa* controls expression of catalase and superoxide dismutase genes and mediates biofilm susceptibility to hydrogen peroxide. Mol Microbiol 34:1082–1093

4. Beck von Bodman S, Farrand SK (1995) Capsular polysaccharide biosynthesis and pathogenicity in *Erwinia stewartii* require induction by an N-acylhomoserine lactone autoinducer. J Bacteriol 177:5000–5008

5. Rasmussen TB, Givskov M (2006) Quorum sensing inhibitors: a bargain of effects. Microbiology 152:895–904

6. Uroz S, Dessaux Y, Oger P (2009) Quorum sensing and quorum quenching: the yin and yang of bacterial communication. Chem biochem 10:205–216

7. Dong YH, Xu JL, Li XZ, Zhang LH (2000) AiiA, an enzyme that inactivates the acylhomoserine lactone quorum- sensing signal and attenuates the virulence of *Erwinia carotovora*. Proc Natl Acad Sci U S A 97:3526–3531

8. Tannières M, Beury-Cirou A, Vigouroux A, Mondy S, Pellissier F, Dessaux Y et al (2013) A metagenomic study highlights phylogenetic

proximity of quorum-quenching and xenobiotic-degrading amidases of the AS-family. PLoS One 8:e65473

9. Riaz K, Elmerich C, Moreira D, Raffoux A, Dessaux Y, Faure D (2008) A metagenomic analysis of soil bacteria extends the diversity of quorum-quenching lactonases. Environ Microbiol 10:560–570

10. Tang K, Zhang XH (2014) Quorum quenching agents: resources for antivirulence therapy. Mar Drugs 12:3245–3282

11. Yang F, Wang LH, Wang J, Dong YH, Hu JY, Zhang LH (2005) Quorum quenching enzyme activity is widely conserved in the sera of mammalian species. FEBS Lett 579:3713–3717

12. Uroz S, Oger P, Chapelle E, Adeline M-T, Faure D, Dessaux Y (2008) A *Rhodococcus* *qsdA*-encoded enzyme defines a novel class of large-spectrum quorum-quenching lactonases. Appl Environ Microbiol 74:1357–1366

13. Lin YH, Xu JL, Hu J, Wang LH, Ong SL, Leadbetter JR et al (2003) Acyl-homoserine lactone acylase from *Ralstonia* strain XJ12B represents a novel and potent class of quorum-quenching enzymes. Mol Microbiol 47:849–860

14. Luo ZQ, Su S, Farrand SK (2003) *In situ* activation of the quorum-sensing transcription factor TraR by cognate and noncognate acyl-homoserine lactone ligands: kinetics and consequences. J Bacteriol 185:5665–5672

15. McClean KH, Winson MK, Fish L, Taylor A, Chhabra SR, Camara M et al (1997) Quorum

sensing and *Chromobacterium violaceum*: exploitation of violacein production and inhibition for the detection of N-acylhomoserine lactones. Microbiology 143:3703–3711

16. Reimmann C, Ginet N, Michel L, Keel C, Michaux P, Krishnapillai V et al (2002) Genetically programmed autoinducer destruction reduces virulence gene expression and swarming motility in *Pseudomonas aeruginosa* PAO1. Microbiology 148:923–932

17. Uroz S, Chhabra SR, Càmara M, Wiliams P, Oger PM, Dessaux Y (2005) N-Acylhomoserine lactone quorum-sensing molecules are modified and degraded by *Rhodococcus erythropolis* W2 by both amidolytic and novel oxidoreductase activities. Microbiology 151:3313–3322

18. Yates EA, Philipp B, Buckley C, Atkinson S, Chhabra SR, Sockett RE et al (2002) N-acylhomoserine lactones undergo lactonolysis in a pH-, temperature-, and acyl chain length-dependent manner during growth of *Yersinia pseudotuberculosis* and *Pseudomonas aeruginosa*. Infect Immun 70:5635–5646

19. Shaw PD, Ping G, Daly SL, Cha C, Cronan JE Jr, Rinehart KL et al (1997) Detecting and characterizing N-acyl-homoserine lactone signal molecules by thin-layer chromatography. Proc Natl Acad Sci U S A 94:6036–6041

20. Winson MK, Swift S, Fish L, Throup JP, Jorgensen F, Chhabra SR et al (1998) Construction and analysis of *luxCDABE*-based plasmid sensors for investigating N-acyl homoserine lactone-mediated quorum sensing. FEMS Microbiol Lett 163:185–192

Chapter 19

Mining Microbial Signals for Enhanced Biodiscovery of Secondary Metabolites

F. Jerry Reen, Jose A. Gutiérrez-Barranquero, and Fergal O'Gara

Abstract

The advent of metagenomics based biodiscovery has provided researchers with previously unforeseen access to the rich tapestry of natural bioactivity that exists in the biosphere. Unhindered by the "culturable bottleneck" that has severely limited the translation of the genetic potential that undoubtedly exists in nature, metagenomics nonetheless requires ongoing technological developments to maximize its efficacy and applicability to the discovery of new chemical entities.

Here we describe methodologies for the detection and isolation of quorum sensing (QS) signal molecules from metagenomics libraries. QS signals have already shown considerable potential for the activation and "awakening" of biosynthetic gene clusters, bridging the existing divide between the natural product repertoire and the natural biosynthetic biodiversity hinted at by nature's blueprint. The QS pipeline from high-throughput robotics to functional screening and hit isolation is detailed, highlighting the multidisciplinary nature of progressive biodiscovery programs.

Key words Metagenomics, Quorum sensing signals, Secondary metabolites, High throughput, Biosensors, Natural product biodiscovery

1 Introduction

The metabolic pathways of microbial organisms have provided a rich source of bioactive compounds that have underpinned advances in such diverse areas as medicine, industry, cosmetics, food and agriculture, mariculture, textile and paper, and arts to name but a few [1, 2]. Addressing societal and commercial challenges, these bioactive molecules have proven hugely beneficial, and in the form of antibiotics, have supported a quantum leap in the quality of life of higher order organisms in general.

However, in recent years there has been a growing realization that the harvest of natural products has been limited at best, and that the natural ecosystem remains largely unexplored, based for the most part on the degree of genetic biodiversity encountered in metagenomics studies [3–5]. Indeed, the discovery of new natural chemical entities has undergone a steep decline in recent years, in

Wolfgang R. Streit and Rolf Daniel (eds.), *Metagenomics: Methods and Protocols*, Methods in Molecular Biology, vol. 1539,
DOI 10.1007/978-1-4939-6691-2_19, © Springer Science+Business Media LLC 2017

spite of an equally steep increase in biodiscovery programs [6, 7]. As a result, many of the compounds that are currently in use are still limited by such issues as chirality, sensitivity, selectivity, and the emergence of resistance in target systems. From a clinical perspective we are fast approaching a post-antibiotic era where the current stock of natural products can no longer protect us from even the most innocuous microbial challenge [8]. Even the so-called last frontier antibiotics, the polymyxins, have recently succumbed to transmissible resistance [9]. Therefore, there is an urgent and unmet need to develop sensitive and selective screening methodologies for the detection of the next generation of natural products from the previously inaccessible majority of the natural biodiversity we know to exist. Key to this would be the isolation of elicitors of silent or cryptic biosynthetic gene clusters (BGCs), potentially awakening a treasure trove of potential unseen activities for industrial and medical application [3, 10].

Quorum Sensing (QS) is a form of cell–cell communication used by microorganisms and is an important control point for secondary metabolism and biofilm formation in a broad spectrum of bacteria. QS signals have been shown to elicit activation of silent BGCs leading to the discovery of novel natural products [11]. Therefore, the isolation of QS-like molecules from metagenomic libraries has the potential provide unparalleled access to the silent microbial potential that exists. Of course, signal producing organisms exist within communities known as microbiomes, in which QS suppressing activities are also prevalent. Known as quorum quenching (QQ) compounds, these enzymes or small molecular mimics have demonstrated potential for the selective disruption of biofilm formation and virulence in a broad range of clinical pathogens. Biofilm formation is central to many serious and chronic refractory infections, with up to 80% of clinical infections existing as biofilms, resulting in exposure to lower concentrations of antimicrobials and substantially increased selective-pressure for antibiotic resistance. Therefore, there has been considerable interest in harnessing signals and their mimics that can bypass microbial resistance mechanisms such as biofilm formation and open communities to the activity of conventional drugs. Defining the signals that exist within these polymicrobial communities will provide the foundation knowledge upon which to interrogate beneficial QQ activities.

In this chapter, we describe the methodologies comprising a pipeline for the biodiscovery of QS compounds from metagenomics libraries. Two major classes of QS signal are described, the Acyl Homoserine Lactone (AHL) class which are widespread among microbial populations [12], and the more specialized Alkyl-Hydroxy-Quinolone class (AHQ) [13]. We provide a step-by-step guide from high-throughput screening to signal characterization, highlighting key bottlenecks in the process and the methodologies to overcome them.

2 Materials

Prepare the agar or broth medium using distilled water. The quorum sensing biosensor strains are stored long-term at −80 °C. AHLs are dissolved in DMSO or methanol, while AHQs are dissolved in methanol alone. 5-bromo-4-chloro-3-indolyl-β-D-galactopyranoside (X-gal) is dissolved in dimethylformamide (DMF). Antibiotics are dissolved in their corresponding solvents. All biological and chemical waste is disposed of properly, following the appropriate waste disposal regulations. The materials described below are sufficient to perform the tasks required to identify, extract, and validate QS signals from metagenomic libraries.

2.1 Culture Media Components

1. LB broth: 10.0 g/L of tryptone, 5.0 g/L of yeast extract, 5.0 g/L of sodium chloride. All components are added as dry powder and resuspended in distilled water prior to autoclaving at 121 °C for 15 min.

2. LB agar: 15 g/L of technical agar is added prior to placing in the autoclave.

3. To prepare LB soft agar, the concentration of agar used is 5 g/L.

2.2 Quorum Sensing Biosensor Strains

1. Short chain AHL detection: Biosensor reporter strain *Serratia marcescens* SP19 readily maintained at 30 °C on LB agar (*see* **Note 1**) [14].

2. Medium chain AHLs: Biosensor reporter strain *Chromobacterium violaceum* CV026 (*see* **Note 2**) [15]. Maintained as above.

3. Long chain AHLs: Biosensor strain *Agrobacterium tumefaciens* NTL4 (*see* **Note 3**) [16]. X-gal (40 μg/mL) and gentamicin (Gm, 30 μg/mL) are added to the media post-autoclave. Maintained as above.

4. AHQs: *Pseudomonas aeruginosa pqsA⁻* mutant carrying a *pqsA-lacZ* promoter fusion (*see* **Note 4**) [17]. This strain is maintained on LB supplemented with carbenicillin (Cb 200 μg/mL).

5. 90 mm petri dishes with 20 mL of LB agar for maintenance of biosensors (Gm used to maintain *A. tumefaciens* NTL4 and Cb used to maintain *P. aeruginosa pqsA⁻*).

2.3 High-Throughput Robotic Platform for Screening

1. QPix 400 series colony picking robot (Molecular Devices, UK). The QPix robot can be mounted with different picking heads (96 and 384).

2. 96- and 384-well plates compatible with the QPix system.

3. LB freezing medium: 36 mM K_2HPO_4 (anhydrous), 13.2 mM KH_2PO_4, 1.7 mM sodium citrate, 0.4 mM $MgSO_4$, 6.8 mM

ammonium sulfate, 4.4% (v/v) glycerol, LB broth (as above). Salts are added to 100 mL of LB as specified. Subsequently, 95.6 mL is added to another container to which 4.4 mL of glycerol is added. The resulting solution is mixed and filter-sterilized through a 0.2 μm membrane (Millipore).

2.4 Validation of QS Molecules

1. 0.2 μm membrane (Millipore).

2. 10 mL syringes.

3. A benchtop centrifuge capable of handling 50 mL tubes at 5000 rpm ($4,472 \times g$) or equivalent.

4. LB agar plates (20 mL).

5. Acidified ethyl acetate ACS grade (acidified with 10 mL/L glacial acetic acid).

6. Separation funnel.

7. Rotary evaporator.

8. Nitrogen gas.

9. Glass extraction vials (5 mL).

10. C18 reversed-phase TLC plates (Whatman, Clifton, NJ, USA).

11. 20× 20 silica gel T60 F_{254} thin layer chromatography plates (Analytical Chemistry).

12. Capillary tubes.

13. Glass TLC chamber.

14. UV Fluorescence imager.

15. Methanol (ACS grade).

16. Dichloromethane (ACS grade).

17. Biosensor strains.

18. AHL standards in DMSO or methanol and AHQ standards in acidified methanol.

2.5 High Performance Liquid Chromatography-Mass Spectrometry (HPLC-MS) Analysis and Characterization of AHL and AHQ Compounds

2.5.1 HPLC-MS Detection of AHLs

1. Agilent 1200 high performance liquid chromatography system (Agilent Technologies, Wilmington, DE, USA).

2. Agilent 6510 QTOF mass spectrometer (Agilent Technologies, Wilmington, DE, USA).

3. Agilent Zorbax Eclipse XDB C18 column (RP-HPLC), (2.1×100 mm, 5 μm) (Agilent Technologies, Wilmington, DE, USA).

4. Mobile phase: methanol and H_2O containing 0.2% (w/v) glacial acetic acid. All reagents and water are LC-MS grade.

5. MassHunter Workstation data acquisition software (Agilent Technologies, Wilmington, DE, USA).

2.5.2   HPLC-MS Detection of AHQs

1. Agilent Reverse phase C8 column 140×4.5 mm 1 mL/min flow rate.

2. Acidified methanol HPLC grade (acidified with 1 % glacial acetic acid by volume).

3. Acidified water HPLC grade (acidified with 1 % glacial acetic acid by volume).

4. MassHunter Workstation data acquisition software (Agilent Technologies, Wilmington, DE, USA).

2.6   Validation of QS Activity in Pathogen Systems

1. Permeabilization solution is prepared as 100 mM dibasic sodium phosphate (Na_2HPO_4), 20 mM KCl, 2 mM $MgSO_4$, 0.8 g/L CTAB (hexadecyltrimethylammonium bromide), 0.4 g/L sodium deoxycholate. β-mercaptoethanol (5.4 µL/mL, *see* **Note 5**) is added immediately prior to use. The solution is stored at 4 °C.

2. Substrate solution is prepared as 60 mM Na_2HPO_4 and 40 mM NaH_2PO_4, and stored at room temperature. *o*-nitrophenyl-β-D-galactoside (ONPG, 1 g/L, *see* **Note 6**) and β-mercaptoethanol (2.7 µL/mL) are added immediately prior to use.

3. Stop solution is prepared as 1 M sodium carbonate (Na_2CO_3), and stored at room temperature.

4. Plastic cuvettes (1 mm, Sarstedt).

5. Model strain, e.g., *Pseudomonas aeruginosa* carrying *lasR*- or *rhlR-lacZ* promoter fusion. Alternatively, *-lux* or *-gfp* based systems can be used.

3   Methods

3.1   Screening of Metagenomic Library for QS Active Clones

Classical screening strategies have not delivered the full potential of the natural environment. The advent of high-throughput robotic screening capacity and smarter more selective screening methodologies has underpinned a new wave of hit-discovery. Here we describe the screening methodology for isolation of AHL and AHQ like signal molecules from metagenomics libraries. The screening protocols described here, using multiple biosensors, are specifically designed to capture a broad spectrum of signals from the same library. For example, detection of short, medium, and long chain AHLs requires the use of three distinct biosensors, each with their own requirements and limits of detection. The protocols described below are broadly applicable to all the biosensors. Where differences exist, biosensor-specific requirements are included as appropriate. The necessary components needed to successfully complete the analysis are described in Subheadings 2.1–2.3.

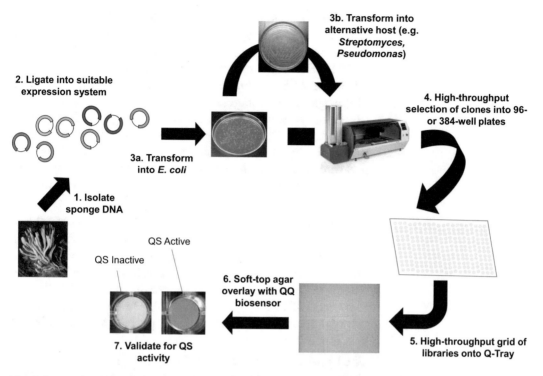

Fig. 1 Overview of the metagenomics mining process for QS activity. Isolation of good quality DNA precedes cloning into suitable expression systems and transformation into a compatible heterologous host. Robotics mediated high-throughput screening on Q-Tray plates facilitates the identification of QS active clones, depending on the biosensor strain used

1. The stock metagenomic library is removed from the −80 °C freezer and allowed to thaw at room temperature for 2–4 h, or until the frozen samples have reached a liquid state. Robot-compatible 96-well plates are filled with 135 μL of LB broth supplemented with the required antibiotic to maintain selection for the fosmid or plasmid (Fig. 1). The robot is used to transfer inoculum from the stock metagenomic library to the fresh plates which are then stacked and incubated static at 37 °C for 24 h. It is crucial that the plates are not allowed to dry out in this process as uniform transfer onto Q-tray plates becomes difficult.

2. Each QS biosensor strain is streaked on LB agar plates (supplemented with antibiotics as appropriate) from the −80 °C stocks and incubated at 30 °C for 24 h. Single colonies of the QS biosensors are used to inoculate 10 mL of LB broth (for *A tumefaciens* NTL4 supplemented with gentamicin at 30 μg/μL, for *pqsA-lacZ* supplemented with carbenicillin at 200 μg/μL), and these tubes are incubated shaking at 150 rpm for 24 h at 30 °C.

3. Q-tray plates are prepared by adding 250 mL of LB on a level surface (*see* **Note 7**) and allowed to dry for a period of 30 min

on a bench, followed by a further 30 min in a laminar flow system (*see* **Note 8**). The robotic platform replicates the metagenomic clones onto the Q-tray plates (X6023, capacity of 384–1536 colonies per plate), which are then incubated at 37 °C for 24 h, or until colonies have formed on the surface of the agar. At this stage, standard AHL or AHQ compounds (5 μL) can be spotted at the corner of the agar surface as positive controls. These positive controls are crucial in light of the sensitivity of the biosensor strains to factors such as temperature, media composition and growth interference from bioactive clones, thus avoiding large scale false negatives in the screening.

4. QS biosensor cultures are inoculated into 200 mL of LB soft agar at a final OD_{600nm} of 0.4. In the case of *A. tumefaciens* NTL4 the LB soft agar is also supplemented with X-gal at a final concentration of 40 μg/μL. Each biosensor is inoculated when the LB soft agar reaches approximately 50 °C. Both *S. marcescens* SP19 and *C. violaceum* CV026 are very sensitive to elevated temperatures and will not propagate if the LB soft agar is too hot.

5. The LB soft agar is overlaid on the Q-tray plates containing the already formed metagenomic library clones. The overlaid Q-tray plates are allowed to dry for 20–30 min in a laminar flow. The plates are then incubated at 30 °C and visually inspected periodically for the presence of positive clones after 24 and 48 h (*see* **Note 9**).

3.2 Extraction and Validation of QS Active Compounds

While the exact composition of solvents used in extraction methodologies for QS signals can vary considerably, they follow the general principal of using acidified organic solvents to separate compounds of interest from the aqueous phase. In general, ethyl acetate is the solvent of choice, with acidification achieved using formic or acetic acid at concentrations ranging from 0.01 to 1%. We routinely use 1% acetic acid acidification for both AHL and AHQ extractions but have also found formic acid to be efficient. Furthermore, buffering the LB with for example 50 mM 3-[*N*-morpholino] propanesulfonic acid (MOPS) at pH 6.5 can help prevent spontaneous lactonolysis of AHLs. The materials required for successful extraction and validation are listed in Subheading 2.4.

1. 500 mL sterile flasks with 100 mL LB broth supplemented with the required antibiotic, are inoculated with the positive clones at an OD_{600nm} of 0.05 and grown for 24 h at 37 °C.

2. Cultures are centrifuged at 10,000 rpm (15,180 × *g*) for 10 min at room temperature after which the supernatant is recovered and filter-sterilized using a vacuum filter system (pore size 0.22 μm) to achieve cell-free status.

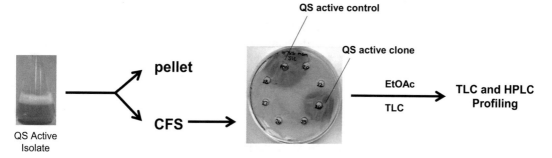

Fig. 2 Validation of QS activity. Individual clones are cultured overnight and fractioned into pellet and CFS following filtration through a 0.2 μm membrane filter. CFS is added to agar wells in a plate swabbed with QS biosensors. QS-active CFS is subsequently extracted and spotted on a TLC plate and visualized either by biosensor overlay or UV illumination

3. Wells are created in 20 mL LB agar plates swabbed with a biosensor strain (OD_{600nm} 0.1) using sterile P1000 tips. Aliquots (75 μL, *see* **Note 10**) of cell-free supernatants (CFS) are added to the wells and the plates are incubated upright for 24 h at 30 °C. Pigmentation is monitored visually. Commercial AHLs are used as positive controls (40 μL at 50 μM in DMSO), with media inoculated with 75 μL of DMSO providing the negative control (Fig. 2).

4. QS active CFS is mixed (1:1) with ethyl acetate acidified with 1% (w/v) of glacial acetic acid, and shaken for 10 min at 150 rpm at room temperature. After this step, a separating funnel is used to discard the aqueous phase (bottom phase) and then recover the organic phase (upper phase, *see* **Note 11**).

5. The organic phase is evaporated using a rotary evaporator, set at 40 °C, and residues are resuspended in 1 mL of DMSO.

6. Standard AHLs and AHQs in DMSO and methanol, respectively, are used as controls to identify the presence of specific QS molecules produced by the different positive clones.

7. Extracted AHL signal molecules are analyzed on C18 reversed-phase TLC plates. Aliquots of 5 μL are spotted using capillary tubes and the chromatograms developed with methanol:water (60:40, v:v) as mobile phase in a glass TLC chamber. After air-drying in a fume hood, the TLC plate is then placed in an empty sterile Q-tray plate and carefully overlaid with a thin film of LB agar (0.5% w/v) seeded with the appropriate AHL reporter strain. The agar should be cooled to approximately 50 °C and gently applied, as otherwise the surface of the TLC plate will be compromised. The lid is then placed on the Q-tray plate and following incubation at 30 °C for 24 h, AHLs are identified as pigmented spots on a white background.

8. AHQ extracted samples (5 μL) are applied to silica gel T60 F_{254} plates and run in a TLC glass chamber with dichloromethane–methanol (95:5) as the standard mobile phase. As above, samples are run to within 1 in. of the top of the TLC plate, the position of the solvent front marked in pencil, and the plate is subsequently visualized under UV illumination. Standard HHQ and PQS spots present with characteristic Rf values and appear dark and light purple, respectively.

9. Samples that are confirmed to be QS active are subsequently processed for analysis by HPLC.

3.3 HPLC Identification of QS Compounds

At this stage of the process, QS active extracts will have been confirmed and are ready for identification. This is generally achieved using HPLC-MS with standards available for AHL and AHQ discovery. As with the extraction protocols, several independent methodologies for the identification of QS molecules by HPLC have been described [18–20]. Materials are listed in Subheading 2.5.

3.3.1 HPLC Detection of AHLs

1. All the extracts from the positive clones are resuspended in 1 mL of methanol for AHL identification by HPLC. Aliquots (50 μL) of 10^{-1} and 10^{-2} dilutions from active extracts are loaded into HPLC glass vials. AHL standards are prepared as follows: using a 100 μM stock, dilute to 10, 100, and 500 nM in methanol and transfer 50 μL to HPLC glass vials [18].

2. AHLs are separated at 30 °C with a flow rate of 0.2 mL/min, using a gradient solvent system as mobile phase with increasing methanol concentration and with the effluent flowing directly into the mass spectrometer (mobile phase solvents: methanol and H_2O containing 0.2 % (v/v) glacial acetic acid). The gradient is increased linearly from 40 % (v/v) methanol–60 % (v/v) water–acetic acid to 80 % (v/v) methanol–20 % (v/v) water–acetic acid over 25 min.

3. AHLs are identified by comparison of the retention times and m/z values from extracts with those obtained for the standard AHLs.

3.3.2 HPLC Detection of AHQs

1. Transfer AHQ active extracts in acidified methanol (200 μL) into HPLC glass vials. Prepare AHQ standards as follows: using a 10 mM stock, dilute to 1, 10, 100, and 500 μM in acidified methanol (final volume 200 μL), and transfer to HPLC vials.

2. Standards (50 μL) are injected on the system, followed by a mobile phase wash, and finally injection of the test samples. A workflow of 60 % acidified methanol for 10 min, ramp up to 100 % in 5 min, hold at 100 % for 5 min, drop to 60 % in 1 min, and hold at 60 % for 3 min, has been previously reported [21].

3. The two primary AHQs, HHQ and PQS may be viewed by extracting the chromatogram at 325 nm.

4. Peak absorbance values are then plotted against AHQ standards to generate a standard curve. All samples points must be within the linear range of the curve.

3.4 Experimental Validation of AHL Compounds in a Model Pathogen System

The final stage of the QS signal validation and characterization involves the use of model pathogen strains such as *P. aeruginosa*, which encodes both AHL and AHQ based QS systems. The auto-inducing LasIR and RhlIR systems are activated by long and short chain AHLs, respectively. Therefore, extracted AHLs identified from the metagenomic library would be expected to enhance transcription of the respective AHL receptor genes *lasR* and *rhlR*. It is important to note that LasIR is activated early in the exponential growth phase while RhlIR is associated with entry to stationary phase. Therefore, it is crucial that kinetic experiments are employed to monitor changes in expression over time. Furthermore, *P. aeruginosa* is a Class II pathogen, therefore requiring certified clearance before use. Where this is not feasible, AHL encoding Class I model systems such as *Vibrio fischeri* can be used. All relevant materials required for this analysis are listed in Subheading 2.6.

1. *P. aeruginosa* carrying a *lasR-* or *rhlR-lacZ* promoter fusion (e.g., pMP220 or pMP190) is inoculated into LB media supplemented with the appropriate antibiotic and grown overnight at 37 °C at 150 rpm.

2. The culture is inoculated into 18 mL of fresh LB media (supplemented with antibiotic) at OD_{600nm} 0.05 in a 100 mL conical flask.

3. Extract or supernatant from the AHL positive clone is added to the inoculated conical flask (starting with 2 mL in 20 mL).

4. Each conical is placed on a 37 °C incubating shaker and growth is monitored into stationary phase. At 2 h periods, samples are removed for OD_{600nm} analysis (from 500 μL to 1 mL) from which 20 μL is added to a 1.5 mL microcentrifuge tube and stored in 80 μL of permeabilization solution at 4 °C for β-galactosidase analysis.

5. Once all samples have been collected, tubes are incubated at 30 °C on a heating block in a fume hood for 30 min. Meanwhile, ONPG and β-mercaptoethanol are added to substrate solution in a fresh container and incubated at 30 °C immediately prior to use.

6. Substrate solution (600 μL) is added to the incubated tubes in the heating block (Time 0) and the formation of a yellow color is monitored carefully over time. Upon the emergence of a yellow color, stop solution (700 μL) is added to the tubes and the time recorded.

7. Tubes are removed and spun by centrifugation at 13,000 rpm ($15,700 \times g$), after which 900 μL is transferred to a cuvette and the OD_{420nm} is measured.

8. Relative promoter activity is calculated as:

$$1000 \times \left[\frac{OD_{420nm}}{OD_{600nm} \times 0.02\,(\mathrm{ml}) \times T\,(\mathrm{min})} \right]$$

4   Notes

1. *S. marcescens* produces a QS-regulated red pigment, prodigiosin. *S. marcescens* SP19 (SP19) is an AHL-deficient triple mutant (*smaI*, *pigX*, and *pigZ*) that only produces prodigiosin in response to exogenous short chain AHLs.

2. *C. violaceum* produces a purple pigment, violacein, the production of which is also under the regulation of QS. *C. violaceum* CV026 is an AHL-deficient double mutant (putative repressor and *cviI*), thus only producing violacein when exogenous medium-chain AHLs are added.

3. *A. tumefaciens* NTL4 (AT NTL4) contains the pZLR4 plasmid with gentamicin resistance that carries a *traG::lacZ* reporter fusion. The addition of exogenous X-gal allows detection of long AHLs by monitoring activation of the *lacZ* gene, giving to the media the characteristic blue color.

4. The AHQ system in *P. aeruginosa* is auto-inducing and elicits activation of the *pqsA* promoter in a concentration dependent manner following co-induction of the PqsR transcriptional regulator by PQS and its biological precursor HHQ. A *pqsA*- mutant strain has lost the ability to produce both PQS and HHQ, and therefore, activation of the *pqsA* promoter in this strain can only occur in the presence of AHQ-type compounds.

5. β-mercaptoethanol is a hazardous liquid that is both corrosive and acutely toxic. It should be stored and handled appropriately in a properly ventilated fume-hood, and disposed of following the local safety guidelines.

6. ONPG is light sensitive and should be added to substrate solution immediately prior to use. Once added to the substrate solution it cannot be stored and reused. Therefore, the substrate solution should be stored as stock, with ONPG and β-mercaptoethanol added to aliquots as required on an experiment to experiment basis.

7. The volume of agar added to the Q-Tray is critical to the successful plating of the library. The contact distance between

the robot pins and the plate has to be calibrated to ensure the pins touch but do not penetrate the surface of the agar. Where this occurs, growth will be limited and phenotypes are not easily scorable if at all. Therefore, agar should be topped to the glass rim of the 250 mL bottle prior to pouring into a Q-Tray plate that has been levelled using a spirit-level or other measuring device.

8. LB media is suitable for the majority of heterologous hosts currently used to carry and express metagenomic libraries. As such, it is compatible with the use of LB soft top agar overlays. As advances are made in the development of heterologous hosts, other media requirements for growth of the library may lead to incompatibility issues with the biosensor overlays. In this case, efforts need to be made to find a common media composition to support the growth of both metagenomic clones and the biosensor.

9. A positive QS clone is that which display a colored ring around the colony. The ring color will depend on the AHLs production of the determined clone. Red color for the production of short chain AHLs, purple color for the production of medium chain AHLs, and blue color for the production of long chain AHLs.

10. The volume added must not exceed 80 % of the capacity of the well. Leakage over the wall of the well onto the surface of the agar will typically inhibit QS induction of the surrounding cells and thus interfere with the assay creating false negatives.

11. A teaspoon of anhydrous magnesium sulfate ($MgSO_4$) can be added to the recovered organic phase to remove excess water in the sample. The presence of water in the organic phase can generate problems downstream when the sample is undergoing evaporation, in addition to allowing possible carryover of unwanted material. Once the magnesium sulfate has been added, mix well, and allow to settle for 2 min. The organic phase is then recovered into a new receptacle avoiding the precipitate formed by the magnesium sulfate and water. Normally after this treatment the organic phase should be clarified.

Acknowledgments

The work described in this chapter was supported by grants awarded by the European Commission (FP7-PEOPLE-2013-ITN, 607786; FP7-KBBE-2012-6, CP-TP-312184; FP7-KBBE-2012-6, 311975; OCEAN 2011-2, 287589; Marie Curie 256596; EU-634486), Science Foundation Ireland (SSPC-2, 12/RC/2275; 13/TIDA/B2625; 12/TIDA/B2411; 12/TIDA/

B2405; 14/TIDA/2438), the Department of Agriculture and Food (FIRM/RSF/CoFoRD; FIRM 08/RDC/629; FIRM 1/F009/MabS; FIRM 13/F/516), the Irish Research Council for Science, Engineering and Technology (PD/2011/2414; GOIPG/2014/647), the Health Research Board/Irish Thoracic Society (MRCG-2014-6), the Marine Institute (Beaufort award C2CRA 2007/082), and Teagasc (Walsh Fellowship 2013).

References

1. Milshteyn A, Schneider JS, Brady SF (2014) Mining the metabiome: identifying novel natural products from microbial communities. Chem Biol 21:1211–1223

2. Reen FJ, Gutierrez-Barranquero JA, Dobson ADW, Adams C, O'Gara F (2015) Emerging concepts promising new horizons for marine biodiscovery and synthetic biology. Mar Drugs 13:2924–2954

3. Machado H, Sonnenschein EC, Melchiorsen J, Gram L (2015) Genome mining reveals unlocked bioactive potential of marine Gram-negative bacteria. BMC Genomics 16:158

4. Reen FJ, Romano S, Dobson ADW, O'Gara F (2015) The sound of silence: activating silent biosynthetic gene clusters in marine microorganisms. Mar Drugs 13:4754–4783

5. Rutledge PJ, Challis GL (2015) Discovery of microbial natural products by activation of silent biosynthetic gene clusters. Nat Rev Microbiol 13:509–523

6. Gaudêncio SP, Pereiraa F (2015) Dereplication: racing to speed up the natural products discovery process. Nat Prod Rep 32:779–810

7. Patridge E, Gareiss P, Kinch MS, Hoyer D (2015) An analysis of FDA-approved drugs: natural products and their derivatives. Drug Discov Today 21:204–207

8. Cooper MA, Shlaes D (2011) Fix the antibiotics pipeline. Nature 472:32

9. Liu YY, Wang Y, Walsh TR, Yi LX, Zhang R, Spencer J et al (2016) Emergence of plasmid-mediated colistin resistance mechanism MCR-1 in animals and human beings in China: a microbiological and molecular biological study. Lancet Infect Dis 16:61–168

10. Brakhage AA, Schuemann J, Bergmann S, Scherlach K, Schroeckh V, Hertweck C (2008) Activation of fungal silent gene clusters: a new avenue to drug discovery. Prog Drug Res 66:1–12

11. Williamson NR, Commander PM, Salmond GP (2010) Quorum sensing-controlled Evr regulates a conserved cryptic pigment biosynthetic cluster and a novel phenomycin-like locus in the plant pathogen, Pectobacterium carotovorum. Environ Microbiol 12:1811–1827

12. Bassler BL (2002) Small talk. Cell-to-cell communication in bacteria. Cell 109:421–424

13. Diggle SP, Matthijs S, Wright VJ, Fletcher MP, Chhabra SR, Lamont IL et al (2007) The Pseudomonas aeruginosa 4-quinolone signal molecules HHQ and PQS play multifunctional roles in quorum sensing and iron entrapment. Chem Biol 14:87–96

14. Poulter S, Carlton TM, Su X, Spring DR, Salmond GP (2010) Engineering of new prodigiosin-based biosensors of Serratia for facile detection of short-chain N-acyl homoserine lactone quorum-sensing molecules. Environ Microbiol Rep 2:322–328

15. McClean KH, Winson MK, Fish L, Taylor A, Chhabra SR, Camara M et al (1997) Quorum sensing and Chromobacterium violaceum: exploitation of violacein production and inhibition for the detection of N-acylhomoserine lactones. Microbiology 143:3703–3711

16. Farrand SK, Hwang I, Cook DM (1996) The tra region of the nopaline-type Ti plasmid is a chimera with elements related to the transfer systems of RSF1010, RP4, and F. J Bacteriol 178:4233–4247

17. McGrath S, Wade DS, Pesci EC (2004) Dueling quorum sensing systems in Pseudomonas aeruginosa control the production of the Pseudomonas quinolone signal (PQS). FEMS Microbiol Lett 230:27–34

18. Nievas F, Bogino P, Sorroche F, Giordano W (2012) Detection, characterization, and biological effect of quorum-sensing signaling molecules in peanut-nodulating Bradyrhizobia. Sensors 12:2851–2873

19. Rasch M, Andersen JB, Fog Nielsen K, Flodgaard LR, Christensen H, Givskov M et al (2005) Involvement of bacterial quorum-sensing signals in spoilage of bean sprouts. Appl Environ Microbiol 71:3321–3330

20. Lade H, Paul D, Kweon JH (2014) Isolation and molecular characterization of biofouling bacteria and profiling of quorum sensing signal molecules from membrane bioreactor activated sludge. Int J Mol Sci 15:2255–2273

21. Palmer GC, Schertzer JW, Mashburn-Warren L, Whiteley M (2011) Quantifying *Pseudomonas aeruginosa* quinolones and examining their interactions with lipids. Methods Mol Biol 692:207–217

ERRATUM TO

Cloning and Expression of Metagenomic DNA in *Streptomyces lividans* and Subsequent Fermentation for Optimized Production

Yuriy Rebets, Jan Kormanec, Andriy Luzhetskyy, Kristel Bernaerts, and Jozef Anne

Erratum to: Chapter 8 in Wolfgang R. Streit and Rolf Daniel (eds.), *Metagenomics: Methods and Protocols*, Methods in Molecular Biology, vol. 1539, DOI 10.1007/978-1-4939-6691-2_8, © Springer Science+Business Media LLC 2017

Erratum DOI 10.1007/978-1-4939-6691-2_20

In the original version of this chapter the name of the third author was misspelled. The name should read Andriy Luzhetskyy

The updated original online version for this chapter can be found at
DOI 10.1007/978-1-4939-6691-2_8

INDEX

Wolfgang R. Streit and Rolf Daniel (eds.), *Metagenomics: Methods and Protocols*, Methods in Molecular Biology, vol. 1539,
DOI 10.1007/978-1-4939-6691-2, © Springer Science+Business Media LLC 2017

Printed in the United States
By Bookmasters